A Practical Guide to the Therapy of Type II Diabetes

A Practical Guide to the Therapy of Type II Diabetes

Pathophysiology, Metabolic Syndrome, Differential Therapy, Late Complications

Edited by
M. Hanefeld

Contributions by
S. Fischer, M. Hanefeld, U. Julius, S. Meisel,
H. Rietzsch, H.-E. Schröder, J. Schulze, M. Weck

Walter de Gruyter
Berlin · New York 1995

Editor

Prof. Dr. med. habil. Markolf Hanefeld
Universitätsklinikum Carl Gustav Carus
der Technischen Universität Dresden
Fetscher Str. 74
01307 Dresden

Die Deutsche Bibliothek – Cataloging-in-Publication-Data

A practical guide to the therapy of type II diabetes : pathophysiology, metabolic syndrome, differential therapy, late complications / ed. by M. Hanefeld. Contributions by S. Fischer ... – Berlin ; New York : de Gruyter, 1995
Dt. Ausg. u. d. T.: Praxis der Therapie des Typ-II-Diabetes
ISBN 3-11-014592-8
NE: Hanefeld, Markolf [Übers.]; Fischer, Sabine

Medical science is constantly developing. Research and clinical experience expand our knowledge, especially with regard to treatment and medication. For dosages and applications mentioned in this work, the reader may rely on the authors, editors and publisher having taken great pains to ensure that these indications reflect the standard of knowledge at the time this work was completed.
Nevertheless, all users are requested to check the package leaflet of the medication, in order to determine for themselves whether the recommendations given for the dosages or the likely contraindications differ from those given in this book. This is especially true for medication which is seldom used or has recently been put on the market and for medication whose application has been restricted by the German Ministry of Health.

Typesetting: Arthur Collignon GmbH, Berlin. – Printing: Gerike GmbH, Berlin. –
Binding: Lüderitz & Bauer, Berlin – Cover design: Rudolf Hübler, Berlin. – Printed in Germany.

Preface

Type II diabetes, or in somewhat simpler terms – non-insulin-dependent diabetes (NIDDM) is a widespread disease, which strikes 4 to 10% of the middle-aged and elderly populations of countries with poor eating habits (overeating) and a lack of exercise. In contrast to coronary heart disease, the number of diabetics is not only increasing dramatically in the industrialized world, but also in many parts of the so-called third world. In Germany it is estimated that there will be over 4 million diabetics by the turn of the century – over 90% of whom will have NIDDM.

This implies that prevention, detection and treatment of NIDDM can only be obtained by the shared efforts of preventive medicine, practicing physicians and clinicians, and above all by a specially trained and motivated group of caregivers and dietary consultants. All of these efforts can only be successful if we work towards accomplishing them in a cooperative manner with our patients, the diabetic groups and other organizations in the public and private health care system.

Konrad Lorenz succinctly described this chain of recognition, transmission and regular execution, "Saying is not hearing, hearing is not understanding, understanding is not agreeing, agreeing is not action and action is a long way from continually maintained."

Our knowledge of the molecular and pathophysiological basis of type II diabetes, the chain of conditions which leads to its manifestation and defines its course has increased enormously in the last few years. The conception of the metabolic syndrome has contributed to a considerably improved understanding and expanded the perspective for an integrated diagnosis and treatment, the center of which is an intensified awareness of health. Treatment of NIDDM therefore does not always mean combating obesity, elevated blood pressure, dyslipoproteinemia and other associated disorders which are responsible for the fact that the excessive cardiovascular morbidity and mortality still lead to a type II diabetic with manifestations of the disease in middle age dying 5 to 10 years earlier than a non-diabetic.

This handbook strives to be a practical manual for avoiding complications and improving the quality of life. This consists of training, subtle diabetic control including associated risk factors and self-control.

One reason for this book was, however, to communicate the basis for a rational application of oral hypoglycemic agents and insulin in NIDDM. It is precisely this field which has witnessed a lively and sometimes controversial discussion in the last few years. This is a consequence of both new discoveries and new medications which make a differential therapy possible and necessary; a therapy whose aim is more than blood sugar cosmetics. As a result of its extraordinary importance for macro- and microangiopathy, the diabetes-adapted treatment of hypertension and dyslipoproteinemia is also dealt with. The same is true for the diabetic foot and nephropathy.

Markolf Hanefeld
Dresden, December 1994

Contents

1 Classification and epidemiology
M. Hanefeld
1.1 Introduction and classification 1
1.2 NIDDM sub-groups 2
1.3 Impaired glucose tolerance (IGT) 3
1.4 Epidemiology of NIDDM 3
1.5 Mortality and causes of death in NIDDM 4
1.6 Summary 5

2 Pathophysiology
M. Weck
2.1 Genetic and environmental factors 7
2.2 The triumvirate – B-Cells, musculature, liver – responsible for NIDDM 8
2.3 Cellular mechanisms of insulin resistance 14
2.4 The role of FFA in the pathogenesis of insulin resistance in NIDDM 16
2.5 Pathophysiological processes in the early stages of NIDDM 17
2.6 Glucose toxicity hypothesis 19
2.7 Summary 20

3 Course
Sabine Fischer 21

4 Uncomplicated type II diabetes: patient history and clinical findings
J. Schulze 25
4.1 Patient history 26
4.2 Clinical findings 28
4.3 Summary 29

5 The hormonal-metabolic syndrome in type II diabetes 31
5.1 Obesity
M. Weck 34
5.2 Dyslipoproteinemia
M. Hanefeld 42

5.3 Hypertension
J. Schulze 49

5.4 Hyperuricemia
H.-E. Schröder 56

5.5 Disturbances in the coagulation and the rheology
U. Julius 61

5.6 Disturbances in the liver and biliary system 68

6 Diagnostics

6.1 Clinical diagnostics
J. Schulze 71

6.2 Laboratory diagnostics and self-monitoring
M. Weck 74

7 Therapy 89

7.1 Health education and instruction
U. Julius 91

7.2 Weight reduction
M. Weck 98

7.3 Health promoting nutritional management
U. Julius 111

7.4 Physical exercise
M. Hanefeld 126

7.5 Oral hypoglycemics
M. Hanefeld, U. Julius 130

7.6 Insulin therapy
J. Schulze, H. Rietzsch 160

7.7 Differential therapy with antidiabetics
M. Hanefeld 169

8 Special therapeutic aspects

8.1 Treatment of hypertension
J. Schulze, Silke Meisel, M. Hanefeld 175

8.2 Treatment of dyslipproteinemia
M. Hanefeld 182

8.3 The treatment of hyperuricemia
H.-E. Schröder 189

8.4 Treatment of coagulation disorders and blood flow disorders
U. Julius 193

9 Late complications of diabetes
9.1 The diabetic foot
Sabine Fischer, H. Rietzsch 199
9.2 Diabetic polyneuropathy
H. Rietzsch 232
9.3 Retinopathy
J. Schulze 245
9.4 Nephropathy
J. Schulze 251

10 Medical-social aspects and legal determinations
Silke Meisel 257

Authors 262

1 Classification and epidemiology

M. Hanefeld

1.1 Introduction and classification

Diabetes mellitus is a chronic, genetically determined disease resulting from an absolute or relative lack of insulin, characterized by hyperglycemia and deep-rooted, complex disturbances in carbohydrate, lipid, protein and mineral metabolism. These disturbances can lead to diabetic coma in the short-term, infections in the middle-term and damage to the small and large vessels in the long-term. A. Bouchardat was first to note that there was no uniform clinical picture, but rather a syndrome and differentiated in his monography "De la glucosurie du diabète sucre: Son traitement hygiénique" – published in 1875 – between a "diabète maigre" and a "diabète gras" as the two basic forms of diabetes, which require different therapies. At the beginning of this century the terms "juvenile onset" and "maturity onset" were introduced, a differentiation which takes into account the fact that the two forms of diabetes not only differ significantly with respect to body weight, but with respect to age of manifestation as well. In 1936 Himsworth made the distinction between an "insulin resistant" and an "insulin sensitive" diabetes. A. Gudworth introduced the terms "type I" and "type II" diabetes for these two basic forms of diabetes in 1976. As a result of the difficulties in making this genetically determined classification in practice, the synonymous WHO classification from 1985 (tab. 1) [1] of "insulin-dependent diabetes mellitus" (IDDM) and "non-insulin-dependent diabetes mellitus" (NIDDM) are used.

The diagnosis of NIDDM does not, however, mean that these diabetics manage to get through their whole life without insulin. After 10–15 years of NIDDM 60–80% of the patients receive insulin. In cases of NIDDM requiring insulin the question is often raised as to whether it is not actually a matter of a slowly manifesting IDDM. According to our experiences in the Diabetes Intervention Study (DIS), C-peptide values of > 1.1 nmol/l can be detected after stimulation with glucagon in over 80% of the cases in patients who received insulin within the first 5 years after diagnosis of diabetes. Due to the fact that genetic markers still have not been found for type II (NIDDM) – in contrast to type I – the diagnosis of NIDDM must be made ex iuvantibus.

The genetic heterogeneity of NIDDM is likely, but is as yet unproven. Patients with manifestations before the age of 40 are at particular risk. Whether they represent a sub-group remains unproven [10].

Tab. 1: WHO classification of diabetes mellitus

A Clinical classes
Diabetes mellitus – Insulin-dependent diabetes mellitus (IDDM) – Non-insulin-dependent diabetes mellitus (NIDDM) (a) non-obese (b) obese – Malnutrition diabetes – Other types of diabetes associated with specific conditions and syndromes (pancreatitis, Cushings, etc.) – Gestational diabetes *Impaired glucose tolerance (IGT)* (a) non-obese (b) obese (associated with other conditions and syndromes)
B Statistical risk classes
Previous anomalies of the glucose tolerance Potential anomalies of the glucose tolerance

1.2 NIDDM sub-groups

NIDDM with obesity (*type IIb*) and *without obesity* (*type IIa*): Obesity often accompanies NIDDM. Depending upon the population the prevalence of obesity in NIDDM fluctuates between 30 and 50% [12, 13]. While the manifestations of type IIb are regularly characterized by hyperinsulinemia, insulin resistance and the cluster of the metabolic syndrome, a definite insulin deficit usually exists from the beginning with type IIa diabetes. The consequence is differing therapies. It should, however, be noted that comprehensive prospective studies including determination of the insulin resistance by CLAMP are still not available for type IIa.

Maturity Onset Diabetes of Young People (*MODY*): This special form of NIDDM, first described by Tattersal [11] in 1974, occurs in childhood and follows a dominant mode of inheritance. A NIDDM with presentation before the age of 25 years which does not exhibit any of the typical genetic or immunological markers for an IDDM and can be controlled for at least 5 years without insulin is defined as MODY. In the closed diabetes collective in the district of Erfurt Panzram and Adolph [7] found 61 cases (0.15%) which fulfilled the criteria for MODY amongst 40,927 diabetics. Based on the data available, there can be no doubt that MODY, with considerably less than 1% is a rare sub-form of NIDDM.

Gestational diabetes: We consider this to be a disturbance of the glucose tolerance which occurs for the first time during pregnancy and may disappear again thereafter. The majority of these cases will be later reclassified as NIDDM. Two concurring observations in Pima indians [8] and the DIS study indicate the special meaning of NIDDM during pregnancy: the frequency of NIDDM in the offspring of diabetic mothers is twice that of diabetic fathers; the reverse being the case with IDDM. This underlines the importance of optimal metabolic control of pregnant women as a fascinating possibility for diabetes prophylaxis of their children.

1.3 Impaired glucose tolerance (IGT)

The category IGT classifies a group of persons whose oral glucose tolerance test (see section 6.2) deviates from that of healthy adults. Only 10–30% of these persons develop diabetes within 5 to 10 years [12]. The peculiarity of these persons consists above all in the fact that they, along with the diabetes risk, exhibit an increased incidence of cardiovascular diseases, as shown in the Paris Prospective Study [2] and the Whitehall Study [4].

1.4 Epidemiology of NIDDM

At present there are over 3 million diabetics in Germany, about 95% of them NIDDM. With the increase of the portion of elderly and the higher life expectancy, an increase of up to 4 million should be expected by the year 2000. In a large-scale early diabetes detection campaign by Mehnert (1967) in Munich [5] only two of three diabetics were known. In the Diabetes Intervention Study, only 23% of the newly detected diabetics sought a physician as a result of diabetic symptoms [3a]. NIDDM is primarily a disease of the elderly. A glance at the geographical epidemiology shows that there are enormous differences in the various races (tab. 2) [13]. Along with the ethnic factors, there are environmental influences, and lifestyle obviously plays an important role. NIDDM was hardly known amongst the Polynesians or Pima indians before they succumbed to the western lifestyles of overeating and lack of physical activity. The effects of environmental influences and nutrition are demonstrated impressively in migration studies where NIDDM prevalence tripled in South African indians or Japanese who migrated to the U.S., compared to their contemporaries who remained in their native countries. The war and post war years demonstrated the influence of external factors with the decrease in diabetes during the war and the dramatic increase in the affluent society. Table 3 summarizes the factors which predispose to the development of NIDDM. When considering the role of obesity, one should not forget the large part that the lack of physical exercise plays in the diabetogenic potential of the overweight.

Tab. 2: Prevalence of NIDDM in various countries and ethnic groups (according to Zimmet [13])

Country	Age group (years)	Prevalence (%)
Papua New Guinea	20+	0.0
China	20+	1.3
Solomon Islands	18+	0.7
Indonesia	15+	1.7
Tanzania	20+	1.9
Australia	25+	3.4
Singapore (Chinese)	18+	4.0
Israel	30–65	4.1
Argentina	20–74	5.0
USA	20–74	6.6
Kiribati	20+	8.9
Malta	30–69	10.0
Fiji (Indians)	20+	13.5
Australia (Aborigines)	20+	15.6
USA (Mexican-Americans)	25–64	17.0
Nauru	20+	30.3
USA (Pima Indians)	20+	34.1

Tab. 3: Predisposing disease factors in NIDDM

Environment	Overeating
	Lack of exercise
	Malnutrition
	Alcoholism
Diseases	Insulin resistance syndrome (hypertension, obesity, hypertriglyceridemia)
	Chronic liver diseases
	Thyroid diseases
	Other endocrinopathies
Medications	Thiazide diuretics
	Steroid hormones
	Beta-blockers
	Nicotinic acid preparations

1.5 Mortality and causes of death in NIDDM

The life expectancy of the middle aged with NIDDM is still reduced by 5 to 10 years. This is for the most part attributable to an excessive mortality from cardiovascular diseases [6, 9], which is twice as high in diabetic men and 4 times as high in diabetic women than in non-diabetic persons. The multimorbidity of NIDDM in middle age at the point in time of the diagnosis of NIDDM is clearly shown in the unselected patients of the DIS study: 2.5% had already suffered an infarction at the time the diabetes was diagnosed, 1.3% a stroke, 0.3% exhibited gangrene and 8.8% cirrhosis of the liver and other diseases [3].

Cardiovascular diseases are the leading cause of death. According to a survey by Pyörälä and Laakso [9], 70 – 75% of the NIDDM cases worldwide die as a result of a macroangiopathy. The most important specific cause of death is coronary heart disease with about 30% (tab. 4), men and women being affected about

Tab. 4: Causes of death in diabetics in the Erfurt region, 1960 – 1970 (according to Panzram [6])

	Outpatient diagnosis n = 961		Clinical diagnosis n = 362		Autopsy n = 371	
Vascular disease		66.0		55.2		
				46.4		
– coronary heart disease	38.9		30.9		27.5	
– cerebrovascular disease	25.6		20.4		14.1	
– general sclerosis, incl. gangrene	1.5		3.9		4.8	
Kidney disease		0.9		4.7		6.2
Diabetic coma		1.4		4.7		
				6.2		
Infections		5.2		8.3		9.2
Tuberculosis		0.6		1.1		1.3
Neoplasia		8.8		8.6		14.3
Unnatural death		2.2		2.5		1.6
Other causes		9.4		13.8		14.6
Unknown		5.5		1.1		0.3

equally. Second is stroke with almost 15%, twice that of the non-diabetic population. Kidney disease occurs in about 5% of the cases as the cause of death, in the normal population about 2.9%. Overall, microangiopathies as a cause of death in NIDDM are of secondary importance. In the DIS study, cirrhosis of the liver was the second leading cause of death in patients between the ages of 35 and 60 years after a duration of 5 years of diabetes [3a].

From this we see that NIDDM is definitely not a mild form of diabetes, requiring no particular attention. On the contrary, multimorbidity, complexity and the possibility of effectively helping by means of a pathophysiologically oriented differential therapy, require vast experience and comprehensive knowledge.

1.6 Summary

Diabetes represents a heterogeneous clinical picture, the main representative of which is, in the WHO classification, non-insulin-dependent diabetes mellitus. Approximately 3% of the European population suffer from NIDDM. It affects about 95% of the diabetics. It is a genetic disease, whose genetic defect has still not been determined. NIDDM patients are multimorbid at diagnosis. The cluster of the risk factors of the metabolic syndromes can usually be detected in them. Macroangiopathy is the most important cause of death. It occurs more frequently in NIDDM, leading to a reduced life expectancy of 5 to 10 years.

References

[1] Diabetes mellitus. Report of the WHO Study Group. WHO Technical Report Series, No. 646. Geneva, Switzerland 1985.

[2] Eschwege, E., J. Richard, N. Thibult et al.: Coronary heart disease mortality in relation with diabetes, blood glucose and plasma insulin levels. The Paris Prospective Study, ten years later. Horm. Metab. Res. *15* (Suppl.) (1985) 41 – 46.

[3] Hanefeld, M., J. Schulze, S. Fischer et al.: The Diabetes Intervention Study (DIS). A cooperative multiintervention trial with newly manifested type II diabetics. In: R. W. James, D. Pometta (eds.): Dyslipoproteinaemias and diabetes. Monogr. on Atherosclerosis, 98 – 103. Karger, Basel 1985.

[3a] Hanefeld, M., S. Fischer, J. Schmechel et al.: Diabetes intervention study. Multiintervention study in newly diagnosed NIDDM. Diabetes Care *14* (1991) 732 – 737.

[4] Jarett, R. J.: Type 2 non-insulin-dependent diabetes mellitus and coronary heart disease – chicken, egg or neither. Diabetologia *26* (1984) 99 – 102.

[5] Mehnert, H.: Diabetes mellitus. In: H. Mehnert (Hrsg.): Stoffwechselkrankheiten. 115 – 258. Thieme Verlag, Stuttgart 1990.

[6] Panzram, G.: Mortality and survival in type 2 (non-insulin-dependent) diabetes mellitus. Diabetologis *30* (1987) 123 – 131.

[7] Panzram, G., W. Adolph: Results of clinical and genetic studies in 58 non-insulin dependent patients in childhood and youth. *21* (1981) 76 (Abstract).

[8] Pettitt, D. J., K. A. Aleck, H. R. Baird et al.: Congenital susceptability to NIDDM. Role of intrauterine environment. Diabetes *37* (1988) 622 – 628.

[9] Pyörälä, K., M. Laakso: Macrovascular disease in diabetes mellitus. In: J. Mann, K. Pyörälä, A. Teuscher (eds.): Diabetes in epidemiological perspective studies, 183 – 247. Churchill Livingstone, Edinburgh 1983.

[10] Rahilly, O., S. Spivey, R. S. Holman et al.: Type 2 Diabetes of early onset: a distinct clinical and genetic syndrome? Br. med. J. *294* (1987) 923 – 928.

[11] Tattersal, R. B.: Mild familial diabetes with dominant inheritance. Quart. J. Med. *43* (1974) 339 – 357.

[12] Zimmet, P., G. Dowse, C. Finch et al.: The epidemiology and natural history of NIDDM. Diabetes Metab. Rev. *6* (1990) 91 – 124.

[13] Zimmet, P. G. Dowse, R. La Porte et al.: Epidemiology. Its contribution to understanding of the etiology, pathogenesis, and prevention of diabetes mellitus. In: W. Creutzfeldt, P. Lefebvre (eds.): Diabetes mellitus: Pathophysiology and therapy, 5 – 26. Proc. of the Bayer AG Centenary Symposium, Edinburgh, U. K., May 25 – 28, 1988. Springer Verlag, Berlin, Heidelberg 1989.

2 Pathophysiology

M. Weck

2.1 Genetic and environmental factors

The genetics of NIDDM have received less attention in recent years than those of IDDM. Type I diabetes was long considered to be more strongly genetically influenced than type II diabetes. However, exactly the opposite is true. The following observations support this statement:

- a concordance of over 90% for NIDDM in monozygotic twins
- the intra-family aggregation of NIDDM
- pronounced differences between ethnic groups regarding diabetes prevalence
- in populations with the highest prevalence of NIDDM, an autosomal-dominant pattern of inheritance similar to MODY (maturity onset diabetes of the youth) can be assumed.

In comparison to IDDM, where well-defined HLA associations exist as markers of genetic susceptibility, such markers have not been found for NIDDM to date. However, suitable genetic markers for NIDDM are promised through the rapid development of molecular biology.

Insulin resistance is one of the earliest signs of the progression of diabetes. Structural and functional changes of the insulin receptor and of the so-called "post-receptor" area seem to be cellular causes of insulin resistance. For this reason, genetic research on NIDDM has been concentrated on the insulin receptor gene. Various mutations could bring different functional consequences with them.

The enormous significance of the environmental factors in the pathogenesis of NIDDM may well be documented by the saying: whoever gets old and fat enough will probably also become diabetic. Disturbed energy balance as a result of excessive calorie intake, decreased body activity, reduced energy use and the resulting increase in fat deposits, especially in the visceral-abdominal depot all count as essential sequence of the NIDDM pathogenesis. Increased food intake can thereby lead directly to the stimulation of insulin secretion. On the other hand, adipose cell hypertrophy has also been described as a partial cause of hyperinsulinemia and insulin resistance. The long-recognized metabolic syndrome has been referred to, in recent years, as syndrome X or insulin resistance syndrome. These terms are meant to more aptly indicate the central significance of insulin resistance, not only for disturbances in carbohydrate metabolism, but also for additional defects in lipid and protein metabolism (tab. 1).

Tab. 1: Diseases related to insulin resistance

Obesity
Hypertension
Hypertriglyceridemia
Glucose intolerance
HDL deficiency
Hyperuricemia?
Acanthosis nigricans

The importance of single genetic mutations or environmental factors may then determine which disease or symptoms of syndrome X (obesity, NIDDM, hypertriglyceridemia, hypertension) dominate. It should again be emphasized that as a possible central controlling element, insulin resistance can be genetically determined or acquired.

2.2 The triumvirate – B-cells, musculature, liver – responsible for NIDDM

The maintenance of normal glucose homeostasis depends on three simultaneous processes: insulin secretion, stimulation of glucose uptake in the peripheral tissues, the liver and intestine and the suppression of hepatic glucose production (tab. 2).

After glucose intake insulin secretion by the pancreas is stimulated and the resultant hyperinsulinemia with hyperglycemia stimulate glucose uptake by the peripheral (primarily the musculature) and visceral tissues (liver, intestine) thereby suppressing hepatic glucose production. This summary of the pathophysiological processes demonstrates that defects on the level of the B-cells, musculature or the liver can lead to glucose intolerance or the manifestations of diabetes. Or in other words, a more concrete and more frequently cited formulation: glucose intolerance can result from a defect in insulin secretion or resistance to the effect of the hormone on the target organs.

Tab. 2: Factors responsible for glucose homeostasis in humans

Insulin secretion
Glucose absorption
– peripheral tissues (musculature)
– glucose oxidation
– non-oxidative glucose utilization (glycogen synthesis, glycolysis)
– visceral tissues (liver, intestine)
Hepatic glucose production

These theoretical considerations have been supported clinically: in some NIDDM patients the primary defect began on the B-cell level and manifested itself as an impairment in insulin secretion. These patients are represented by the slim type II diabetics. In the larger group of NIDDM patients, the dominant defect is an impairment of the tissue sensitivity to insulin. These individuals are represented by the obese type II diabetics.

It must be noted that at the time of diabetes manifestation the patients are already in an advanced stage of the disease process and both defects – insulin resistance and (relative) secretion impairments – are shown to be present. In order to answer the famous question as to which of the two processes is the primum movens, "pre-diabetics" must be studied in follow-up investigations. To date, such a complete study design has not been accomplished.

2.2.1 Insulin secretion – the Starling Curve of the pancreas

It is generally known that hyperinsulinemia is present in obese NIDDM. However, this raised insulin level is too low in relation to hyperglycemia. The Starling Curve of insulin secretion [2] shows these processes (fig. 1). If one plots the fasting blood glucose as an index of the severity of diabetes against the average plasma insulin concentration during oGTT, the typical inverted U curve is produced. In an individual with a fasting blood glucose level of 4.4 mmol/l (80 mg/dl) one would expect an average plasma insulin concentration (oGTT) of about 50 μU/ml. If the fasting blood glucose level rises further, the B-cells recognize that the glucose homeostasis is disturbed and increase their insulin secretion in order to overcome the hyperglycemia. Accordingly, a patient with a fasting blood glucose level of about 6.6 mmol/l (120 mg/dl) (impaired glucose tolerance = IGT) or previous NIDDM secretes about twice as much insulin as the subject with

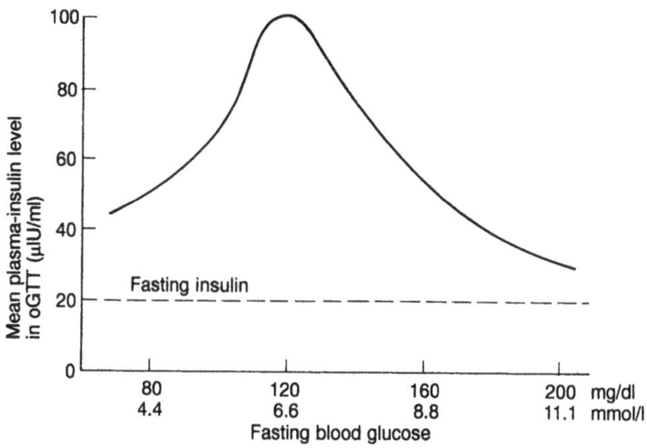

Fig. 1: Starling curve of insulin secretion (DeFronzo).

a fasting blood glucose of 4.4 mmol/l (80 mg/dl). If the blood glucose level exceeds the limit of 6.6 mmol/l (120 mg/dl), the B-cells can no longer maintain their accelerated insulin secretion and a further rise in blood glucose is linked with a progressive drop in the plasma insulin level. A diabetic with a fasting blood glucose of 8.3 – 8.8 mmol/l (150 – 159 mg/dl) secretes about as much insulin as a non-diabetic. With a further rise in the glucose concentration, the insulin response becomes increasing insulinopenic. By analogy to the Starling curve for the heart muscle, the term Starling curve of the pancreas was established. These data demonstrate that the absolute plasma insulin level is normal or raised in most diabetics with mild or moderate fasting hyperglycemia and therefore insulin resistance must play an important role in the development of glucose intolerance. It is, however, clear that isolated insulin level determination can lead to a misinterpretation of the stage of diabetes and thereby of the treatment strategy.

2.2.2 *Insulin sensitivity*

2.2.2.1 *Measuring insulin resistance*

By the end of the 1930s insulin resistance had already been documented by Himsworth and Kerr. The subjects received a standardized oral glucose dosage in combination with an i.v. bolus of regular insulin. The ability of this injected insulin to sufficiently reduce the glucose level was shown to be impaired in NIDDM patients as compared with healthy subjects.

Since the end of the 1970s, insulin resistance has been documented using the glucose clamp technique: the fasting insulin level is acutely raised by an i.v. insulin bolus and subsequently maintained at a level of approximately 100 μU/ml by continuous insulin infusion. Through the simultaneous infusion of glucose, the attempt is made to counteract the drop in blood glucose and to "clamp" the blood glucose at an euglycemic level, i. e. at about 5.5 mmol/l (100 mg/dl). Under these steady-state conditions, the amount of infused glucose corresponds to the glucose uptake of the tissues and is therefore a measure of insulin-mediated glucose metabolism or, in other words, the insulin sensitivity of the tissues or insulin resistance.

A patient who needs a large amount of glucose infused during such a clamp investigation to maintain euglycemia shows thereby only a slight insulin resistance, while the administration of only small glucose dosages shows pronounced insulin sensitivity (insulin resistance). Figure 2 shows the evaluation protocols of two euglycemic glucose clamp investigations for the patient groups described. The glucose clamp technique is reserved for very special inquiries and is only performed at a few centers.

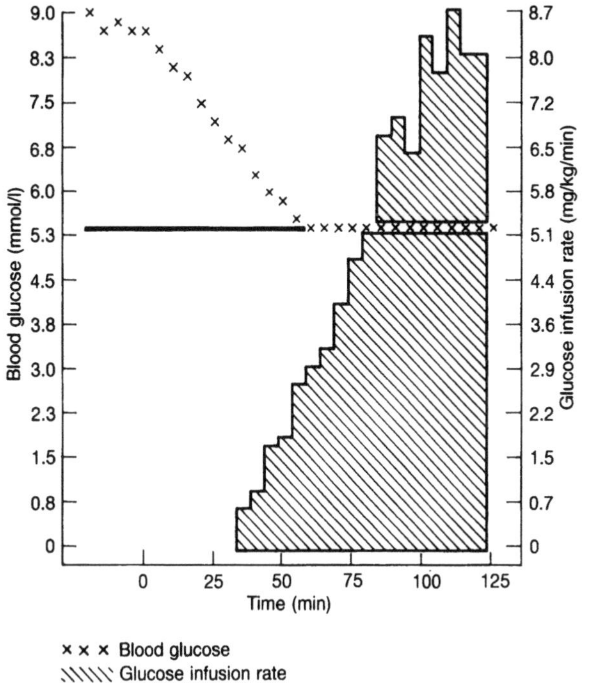

Fig. 2: Euglycemic glucose clamp technique: examples.

Fig. 2a: Patient with normal insulin sensitivity. G. M., 57 years old, male, height 177 cm, weight 78 kg, duration of diabetes 5 years, HbA_{1C} 8.8%, therapy: glibenclamide 7.5 mg/day.

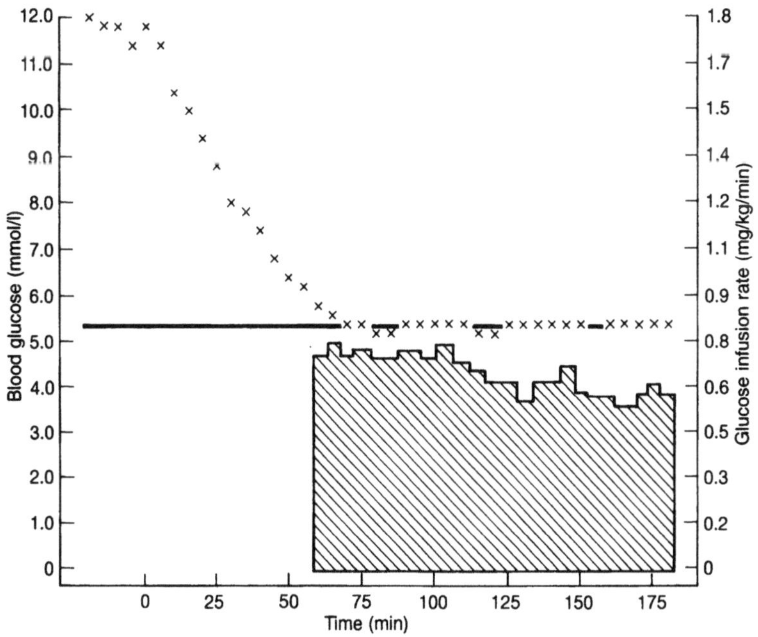

Fig. 2b: Patient with pronounced insulin resistance. H. W., 55 years old, female, height 166 cm, weight 77 kg, duration of diabetes 2 years, HbA_{1C} 10.9%, therapy: weight reduction.

2.2.2.2 *Sites of insulin resistance*

Insulin controls glucose homeostasis through three coordinated mechanisms, each of which can be the cause of insulin resistance:

- the suppression of hepatic glucose production
- the stimulation of glucose uptake by visceral tissue
- the stimulation of glucose uptake by peripheral tissue.

Hepatic glucose production (HGP)

In the basal condition, the liver produces the amount of glucose required in order to provide the brain with energy during the periods between meals. Against this, insulin is released directly after glucose intake in order to suppress HGP. If this does not occur, we have two sources of glucose – the liver and glucose absorbed through the digestive tract – and this results in pronounced hyperglycemia. In NIDDM, the increase in the fasting blood glucose is strongly correlated with the increase in HGP.

Two additional facts must be considered in order to understand this complicated interaction:

- the fasting insulin concentration in the plasma was approximately twice as high in NIDDM as in healthy subjects. Because insulin is the potent inhibitor of HGP, a pronounced insulin resistance of the liver must be present in order to explain the raised glucose output of the liver (the raised HGP).
- Hyperglycemia per se can also exert a suppressive effect on HGP. A “glucose resistance” must also be present in the liver.

From this data it can be concluded (and this has been experimentally supported) that

- With an increase in the stage of severity of NIDDM the disturbance of the inhibitory insulin effect on the HGP escalates and
- This defective suppression of HGP manifests itself even at low BG values in NIDDM with lower plasma insulin levels.

Excessive HGP mainly occurs in the night hours, when the patient sleeps and basal insulin levels have reached their minimum. Therefore, for patients who do not respond to diet or oral hypoglycemic agents, it seems theoretically practical to administer intermediary insulin during the sleeping hours in order to suppress nocturnal HGP and thereby morning hyperglycemia. The increased HGP is primarily caused by increased gluconeogenesis (to a lesser degree by glycogenolysis). A further therapeutic possibility would therefore be substances which primarily suppress hepatic gluconeogenesis.

Visceral glucose utilization

A further potential mechanism that could contribute to the impairment of insulin effect during the clamp investigation is a reduction in visceral glucose utilization. In any event it was proven in glucose clamp studies that only 7% of the glucose uptake of the entire body occurs in the visceral region. In practice this means that in NIDDM patients with mild to moderate hyperglycemia, neither the impairment of HGP suppression nor the reduction in visceral glucose utilization makes a significant contribution to the insulin resistance of the tissues and that finally the primary cause of insulin insensitivity is to be sought in the musculature.

Visceral glucose uptake, insulin sensitivity of these tissues and FFA are all closely related. It has been recently shown by Swedish [12] and American [6] authors that insulin binding to hepatocytes is strongly suppressed by FFA in physiological concentrations. Increased abdominal girth with its increased FFA mobilization into the portal circulation, is characterized by a decreased insulin uptake by the liver and successive hyperinsulinism. Because increased FFA also stimulates hepatic gluconeogenesis, these processes are of relevance in the development of hyperglycemia and insulin resistance. Detailed remarks on this problem are found in section 5.1.

Peripheral (muscle) glucose uptake

In healthy subjects, the glucose utilization of the musculature accounts for approximately 75–80% and adipose tissue 1% of the total glucose disposal. With the previously mentioned glucose clamp technique it has been clearly shown that the largest percentage of the impairment of the insulin-mediated glucose utilization in NIDDM is found in the musculature.

To summarize: tissue intolerance to insulin is an important pathogenetic factor of the glucose intolerance of NIDDM:

- The liver represents the primary location of insulin resistance in the basal (fasting) state. Increase in the HGP is the key factor for the increase of the fasting blood glucose level.
- After nutrient (glucose) uptake, i. e. in the insulin-stimulated state, the musculature is the primary site of insulin resistance. In diabetics with significant fasting hyperglycemia, an increase in the HGP is pathogenetic significant in the post-absorptive state as well.

From these conclusions result therapeutic points of intervention that should lead to an increase in glucose utilization and/or a reduction in insulin resistance:

- Supression of the basal HGP and
- Stimulation of glucose uptake in the musculature.

2.3 Cellular mechanisms of insulin resistance (tab. 3, fig. 3)

As a rough generalization, in the past it was assumed that – and this appears insightful – receptor defects and post-receptor defects contribute to insulin resistance. How is this to be understood in its particulars? Insulin exerts its biological effects on the target cells and thereby on glucose uptake and metabolism, especially in the musculature, via binding to special receptors. After the receptor binding, the glucose transport system is activated, so that an influx of glucose into the cells of the target tissue can actually take place. This inflowing glucose is then metabolized through the mediation of a cascade of enzymes, which are controlled by insulin. Most significant of these are glycogen synthetase (key enzyme of glycogen synthesis) and pyruvate dehydrogenase (key enzyme of glucose oxidation).

Tab. 3: Cellular mechanisms of insulin resistance: receptor and post-receptor defects

Receptor defects
Post-receptor defects
– reduced activity of the receptor kinase
– impairment of intracellular glucose transport and metabolism: glucose transport system, enzymes (glycogen synthetase, pyruvate dehydrogenase)

"Receptor defects"

In many previous studies, it has been shown that insulin binding to monocytes and adipocytes is reduced 20–30% in NIDDM. This reduced insulin binding has been attributed to a reduced number of insulin receptors. However, there are several instances in which this receptor hypothesis cannot be the essential factor in the development of insulin resistance:

- A decreased number of receptor sites was not found, in 30–50% of NIDDM patients.
- A correlation between reduced insulin binding and the severity of the insulin resistance could not be proven.
- Neither monocytes nor adipocytes are considered primary target cells for insulin.

"Post-receptor defects"

According to the commonly held opinion, the insulin receptor is composed of an alpha and a beta subunit. The alpha subunit displays the actual receptor attributes which are also extracellularly located. The beta subunit can then be attributed to the post-receptor region. This beta unit is a transmembrane protein with kinase activity [5]. The activation of this kinase by insulin stimulates glucose

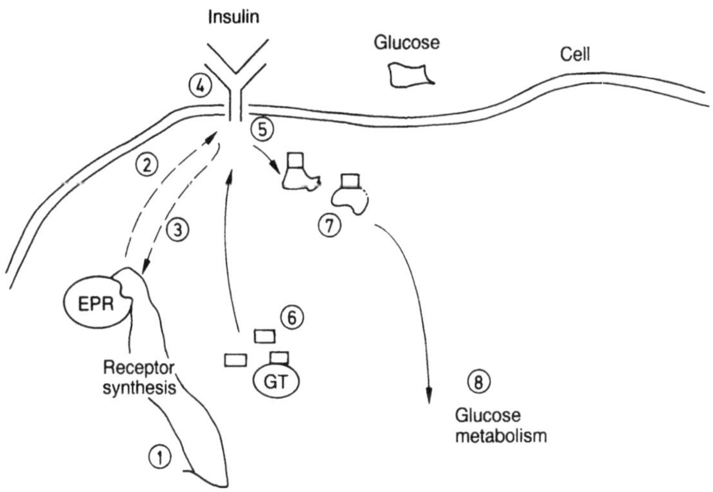

Fig. 3: Cellular and molecular causes of insulin resistance.
1 Disorder of the receptor synthesis in the endoplasmic reticulum (EPR)
2 Disorder of the transport of the receptors to the cell wall
3 Disturbed recycling of the receptors
4 Receptor alpha sub-unit: down-regulation of the insulin receptors
5 Receptor beta sub-unit: disorder of the kinase mechanism
6 Activation of the glucose transport system (GT) disturbed
7 Disorder of the postkinase signal transducer: glucose carrier defect
8 Disorder of the glucose metabolism: glycogen synthetase and pyruvate dehydrogenase

transport into the cell. Reduced activity of the receptor kinase appears to be the key mechanism of insulin resistance in NIDDM on a cellular level.

Recently, the mechanisms of intracellular glucose transport and glucose metabolism have become the subjects of intensive research projects. The glucose transport system has been given particular importance in these efforts. These glucose transporters are thought to be glycoproteins, the number of which appear to be genetically determined. The activity of this glucose transport system was found to be consistently reduced in NIDDM.

Distal to this glucose transport mechanism, the metabolism of glucose by the above mentioned enzymes takes place. The ability of insulin to stimulate the glycogen synthetase and the pyruvate dehydrogenase of adipocytes or muscle cells in patients with NIDDM is also reduced.

The following clinical-experimental findings suggest insulin resistance as the primum movens in NIDDM:

- In the course of the development of diabetes, the impairment of tissue sensitivity to insulin is the earliest metabolic abnormality.

- If patients of normal weight are overfed, a moderate to pronounced insulin resistance occurs.
- If overweight, insulinopenic diabetics are subjected to weight reduction, first the tissue sensitivity to insulin is improved and later insulin secretion recovers somewhat.
- In populations with higher NIDDM prevalence (Pima Indians) a general insulin resistance is present and appears to be genetically determined.

In summary, it appears that the receptor and post-receptor defects contribute to insulin resistance in NIDDM. Decreased insulin receptor binding is primarily a problem in patients with impaired glucose tolerance or very mild NIDDM, while with blood glucose values of > 7.7 mmol/l (140 mg/dl), post-receptor defects are primarily accountable for the insulin resistance of this patient group.

2.4 The role of FFA in the pathogenesis of insulin resistance in NIDDM (fig. 4)

FFA has three primary means of influencing insulin resistance:

- suppression of glucose oxidation
- reduced insulin suppressibility of lipolysis
- direct inhibition of insulin uptake.

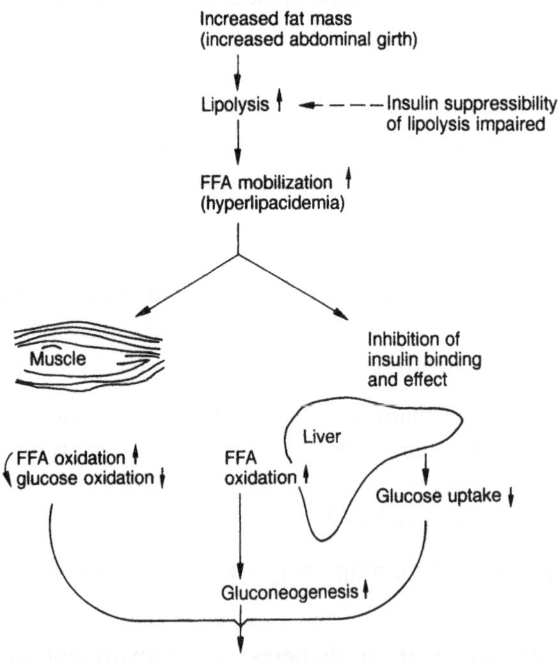

Fig. 4: Role of free fatty acids (FFA) in the pathogenesis of NIDDM.

More than two decades ago, Randle found that increased FFA oxidation inhibits glucose oxidation in the musculature, especially through the effect on different glycolytic enzymes. The classic investigations by Randle have been expanded and supplemented by new findings so that today we can be certain that increased FFA oxidation can affect all essential intracellular mechanisms of insulin resistance (reduced glucose transport, and decreased glycogen synthetase and pyruvate dehdrogenase activities). Not only are the basal FFA level and lipid oxidation increased, but an impairment of the normally present insulin suppressibility is also found.

Finally, as has already been mentioned several times, recent studies have demonstrated that FFA directly suppresses insulin binding and internalization in isolated hepatocytes.

In summary, it has been found that the elevated fat mass in obese subjects (diabetics and non-diabetics) is connected with increased lipolysis and sequential elevations in the FFA level in the blood (hyperlipacidemia). Lipid oxidation is stimulated by the increased cellular uptake of FFA. In the musculature, this leads to the suppression of insulin-mediated glucose utilization, while gluconeogenesis is stimulated in the liver. Together all these mechanisms create pronounced hyperglycemia and insulin resistance.

2.5 Pathophysiological processes in the early stages of NIDDM (fig. 5)

We have already shown that the manifestation of fasting hyperglycemia correlates with HGP. At this point, however, the diabetes process has been long underway and the question arises as to whether the increase in blood glucose in the early stages of NIDDM is caused by the increase in HGP or reduction of the glucose uptake of the tissue, i. e. insulin resistance. Comparing the HGP with the fasting blood glucose in healthy and NIDDM patients, it has been shown that with fasting blood glucose values under 7.7 mmol/l (140 mg/dl) the HGP of the diabetics and healthy subjects is comparable and only with blood glucose values > 7.7 mmol/l (140 mg/dl) does the increase in HGP occur. Excessive hepatic glucose production appears therefore not to be responsible for the fasting hyperglycemia of the early stages of diabetes.

The efficiency of glucose uptake in the early stages of NIDDM can be represented by the comparison of the fasting blood glucose level with the glucose clearance rate (measure of the glucose uptake of the tissues and thereby insulin resistance) gathered in clamp investigations. In diabetics with fasting blood glucose values in the range of 4.4 – 7.7 mmol/l (80 – 140 mg/dl) the glucose clearance rate falls

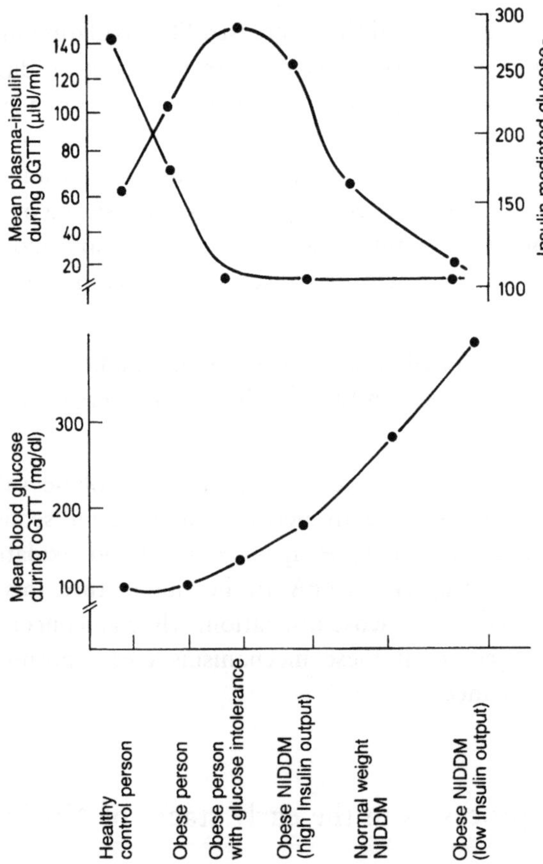

Fig. 5: Relationship between blood glucose, insulin and insulin sensitivity (according to DeFronzo).

proportionally to the increase in blood glucose, while with blood glucose values > 10 mmol/l (180 mg/dl) a plateau is reached. A decrease in the glucose uptake of the tissues or increase in insulin resistance is one of the earliest abnormalities in the NIDDM process.

The interaction between blood glucose, insulin secretion and tissue sensitivity to insulin are presented again in figure 6. A drastic drop in insulin sensitivity, i. e. an increase in insulin resistance, can already be demonstrated in obese non-diabetics. In spite of this, glucose tolerance remains constant because B-cell secretion increases. If the mildly glucose intolerant obese subject were to experience a further reduction in insulin sensitivity, then the further increase in insulin secretion would function to keep the blood glucose in bounds. The further progression to development of diabetes does not occur through an increase in insulin resistance, but rather, because the insulin secretion passes its peak and

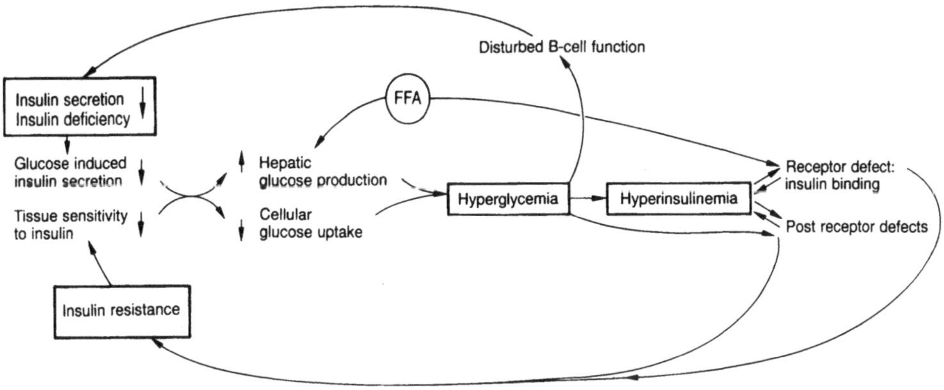

Fig. 6: Pathogenetic processes in NIDDM (according to DeFronzo).

declines thereafter. In obese NIDDM with lower insulin secretion, glucose tolerance is usually impaired. Insulin resistance is therefore an early characteristic of obesity and obese NIDDM. Accordingly, insulin resistance alone is not usually capable of causing a progression to NIDDM. In this case, an additional defect in insulin secretion must also be present.

2.6 Glucose toxicity hypothesis

In the last decade, the hypothesis that glucose possessed clear diabetogenic activity has been supported by experimental data. Chronic hyperglycemia could be important in the pathogenesis of NIDDM in several ways:

1. Down regulation of the glucose transport system in insulin target tissues: whereby a chronic hyperglycemia affects a drop in the glucose transporters of up to 50% and hypoglycemia leads to an increase in the number and activity of glucose transporters.

2. Desensitization of the B-cells to glycemic stimulus.

Chronic hyperglycemia could cause or aggravate both defects in insulin effect and insulin secretion (see fig. 6). For this hypothesis we are referring primarily to the results of therapy attempts in NIDDM, where a normalization of the blood glucose profile led to an improvement in insulin secretion independent of the treatment measures (weight reduction, physical conditioning, sulfonyl ureas, insulin). The hypothesis also had enormous practical consequences, because in a poorly-regulated diabetic with blood glucose values > 1.1 mmol/l (200 mg/dl), the indication for a drastic calorie reduction or short-term insulin therapy would be given in order to counteract the deleterious consequences of hyperglycemia on insulin secretion and resistance.

2.7 Summary

NIDDM is a heterogeneous syndrome which is triggered by two primary metabolic impairments:

- Defective insulin secretion by B-cells
- Defective action of insulin on the cellular level (insulin resistance).

Each of the mechanisms could count as a primary agent and alone is capable of inducing hyperglycemia. A number of findings point to insulin resistance as the primum movens in NIDDM.

Pronounced forms of NIDDM are always accompanied by impairments of both pathomechanisms, i. e. insulin secretion and insulin resistance, where each mechanism can act secondarily to the other and via several routes. For the individual patient it is rarely possible to locate the primary defect. It is a therapeutic imperative to interrupt the pathological chain which leads to NIDDM early on. As a rule this can occur through effective weight reduction and physical conditioning, as these can interrupt insulin resistance as well as give the damaged B-cells the possibility to recover and thereby increase insulin secretion. In advanced stages, the therapeutic administration of insulin should not be delayed.

References

[1] Björntorp, P.: The associations between obesity, adipose tissue distribution and disease. Acta Med. Scand. *723* (Suppl.) (1988) 121 – 134.

[2] DeFronzo, R. A.: The triumvirate: ß-cell, muscle, liver. A collusion responsible for NIDDM. Diabetes *37* (1988) 667 – 687.

[3] Editorial. Type 2 diabetes or NIDDM: Looking for a better name. Lancet I (1989) *589* – *591*.

[4] Ferrannini, E., S. M. Haffner, B. D. Mitchell et al.: Hyperinulinaemia: the key feature of a cardiovascular and metabolic syndrome. Diabetologia *34* (1991) 416 – 422.

[5] Häring, H. U.: Molecular biology of insulin action and resistance. In: E. Standl (Ed.): Perspectives of the hyperinsulinaemia/insulin resistance syndrome in NIDDM: From pathophysiology to clinical implications, 9 – 20. MMV Medizin Verlag, München 1990.

[6] Hennes, M. M., E. Shrago, A. Kissebah: Receptor and postreceptor effects of free fatty acids (FFA) on hepatocyte insulin dynamics. Int. J. Obesity *14* (1990) 831 – 41.

[7] Joost, H. G., T. M. Weber: The regulation of glucose transport in insulin-sensitive cells. Diabetologia *32* (1989) 831 – 838.

[8] Kissebah, A. H.: Mechanisms associating body fat distribution to glucose intolerance in diabetes mellitus. Window with a view. Acta Med. Scand. *723* (Suppl.) (1988) 79 – 89.

[9] Köbberling, J.: Genetik des Diabetes mellitus. Internist *28* (1987) 210 – 217.

[10] Reaven, G. M.: Role of insulin resistance in human disease. Banting lecture 1988. Diabetes *37* (1988) 1595 – 1607.

[11] Rizza, R. A., L. J. Mandarino, J. Genest et al.: Production of insulin resistance by hyperinsulinaemia in man. Diabetologia *28* (1985) 70 – 75.

[12] Svedberg, J., P. Björntorp, U. Smith et al.: Free fatty acid inhibition of insulin binding, degradation and action in isolated rat hepatocytes. Diabetes *39* (1990) 470 – 574.

[13] Unger, R. H., S. Grundy: Hyperglycaemia as an inducer as well as a consequence of impaired islet cell function and insulin resistance: implications for the management of diabetes. Diabetologia *28* (1985) 119 – 21.

3 Course

Sabine Fischer

Type II diabetes generally manifests itself in persons over 30 years old. Young patients with type II diabetes (MODY-type) are a true rarity. Type II diabetes is often an accidental diagnosis, with patients typically having no or limited clinical symptoms over a long period of time. It is to be assumed that the diabetic metabolic condition of many patients is present for a long period of time before the diabetes is discovered. The pre-diabetic phase is of special importance, since insulin resistance, hyperinsulinemia, and further risk factors already exist at this point. These are, however, often not known and therefore go untreated [1]. Blood vessel changes can also develop in this phase. The incidence of the disease increases with age. Acute infections or stress situations often cause manifestations of the disease to appear. The typical course of the disease is summarized in figure 1.

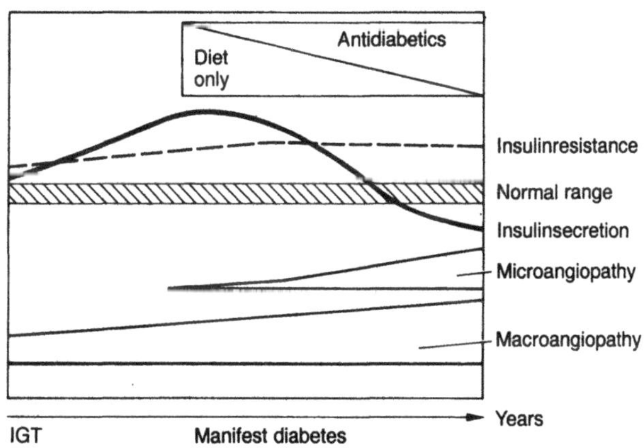

Fig. 1: Course of diabetes.

When the beta cells of the pancreas can no longer compensate for insulin resistance by increasing insulin secretion, the fasting blood sugar level increases and diabetes becomes manifest. Clinical symptoms can arise, are often limited, and can also be completely absent. The diabetes can often be regulated by diet over a certain period of time, however in addition to the patient's use of basal therapeutic principles, the degree of the insulin resistance must also be considered. Important for this are also genetic causes and the development of the obesity.

For a portion of patients with high blood glucose levels, oral hypoglycemic agents may be necessary at or shortly after the first clinical manifestation of diabetes. If the patient succeeds in reducing his/her body weight and maintains this reduced weight over an extended period of time, the insulin resistance is thus broken or at least decreased and the glucose control improves [2].

Since diabetes is a chronic progressive disease, the ability of the pancreas to produce sufficient insulin decreases over time and insulin resistance remains constant or even increases (i. e., the insulin sensitivity drops), and the blood sugar level increases as a result. Oral hypoglycemic agents are thus necessary to reduce the hyperglycemia. Glibenclamide stimulates insulin secretion by the pancreas; as a result, the B-cells are exhausted over a number of years. It is not presently known if this process can be stopped on a long-term basis by the other functioning principle of the acarbose medication. In the end, the endogenous insulin production does not suffice, despite the intake of oral anti-diabetics, to keep the blood sugar level within a respectable range. A true insulin deficiency arises and the introduction of insulin therapy becomes necessary. The regulation of diabetes with exogenous insulin intake is problematic due to the ongoing insulin resistance and the usually continued presence of obesity, so that a euglycemia is often not reached. Most important is whether the patient succeeds in effectively reducing his/her body weight and thus reducing the insulin resistance.

The course of the disease is influenced by many factors; in addition to the fateful progression of the disease and the eventual presence of secondary diseases and other risk factors, the behavior of the patient and his/her active influencing of the course of the disease has an important role, for example, through the change in habits, influencing other risk factors, weight reduction or self-monitoring. Good metabolic control is most important for the prevention of or the delay in the appearance of late complications, since a relationship exists between the quality of the metabolic control and the development of the micro- and macro-angiopathy. Good metabolic control increases the chance of preventing or delaying complications, but cannot, however, prevent them with absolute certainty due to the multiple influential factors. A decisive pathogenic factor for a good metabolic control is a normalization in weight.

Despite the major advances in the treatment of diabetes, the life expectancy of patients is still lower in comparison to the normal population; three quarters of all diabetics die of vascular diseases [4].

As can be seen in figure 1, the development of macrovascular complications already begins before the clinical manifestations of type II diabetes, in other words, in the stage of impaired glucose tolerance (IGT), while microvascular complications only begin to develop with the manifestation of diabetes mellitus, since they are heavily influenced by hyperglycemia. Microangiopathy develops after an average diabetes duration of 10 to 15 years [3].

Summary

In the majority of cases, type II diabetes manifests itself in patients over 30 years. At the time of manifestation, there are often no or limited clinical symptoms present. A percentage of the patients can primarily be regulated by diet, others immediately require metabolic compensation with oral hypoglycemic agents. Over a period of years, the hyperinsulinemia present in the first years decreases until an insulin deficiency develops as a result of the reduction in beta-cell function, which finally leads to a need for exogenous insulin application. The development of obesity, and the ability to influence it, is pathophysiologically important for the emergence and the course of the diabetes. The prognosis of diabetes is determined today by the micro- and macrovascular blood vessel complications, the appearance and course of which is decisively influenced by the quality of the metabolic regulation and the battle against the other risk factors. Macrovascular blood vessel complications have already begun to develop before the clinical manifestation of the diabetes, whereas the microvascular complications are dependent on hyperglycemia and therefore the duration of the diabetes.

References

[1] Hanefeld, M., H. Haller, J. Schulze et al.: Die Diabetesinterventionsstudie (DIS) – eine multizentrische Multiinterventionsstudie bei Typ-II-Diabetikern. 1. Mitteilung Dt. Gesundheitswesen *39* (1984) 1889–1894.

[2] Henry, R. R., B. Gumbiner: Benefits and limitations of very-low-calorie diet therapy in obese NIDDM. Very low Calory Diet Therapy in Obese NIDDM. Diabetes Care *14* (1991) 802–23.

[3] Mehnert, H. (Hrsg.): Stoffwechselkrankheiten. Georg Thieme Verlag, Stuttgart, New York 1990.

[4] Panzram, G., R. Zabel-Langhennig: Prognosis of diabetes mellitus in a geographically defined population. Diabetologia *20* (1981) 587–591.

4 Uncomplicated type II diabetes: patient history and clinical findings

J. Schulze

Type II diabetes is characterized by its appearance at adult age and its primary insulin independence. In contrast to its frequency and importance, type II diabetes is, as a result of its lack of obvious symptoms, often not diagnosed or diagnosed only long after its initial manifestation. Except for the few dramatic, hyperglycemic hyperosmolar imbalances or manifestations in the framework of fever-inducing concomitant illnesses, the uncomplicated type II does not exhibit classic diabetic symptoms for a long time.

The discovery of the disturbed glucose tolerance occurs either accidentally during routine screenings or check-ups in the course of general examinations or company physicals (fig. 1) or through the so-called selective screening of diseases which exhibit a close syntropy to type II diabetes such as obesity, hyperlipoproteinemia (HLP), hypertension or gout amongst others. Taking a detailed patient history may, retrospectively, uncover the first signs of diabetes-related symptoms and disease (tab. 1).

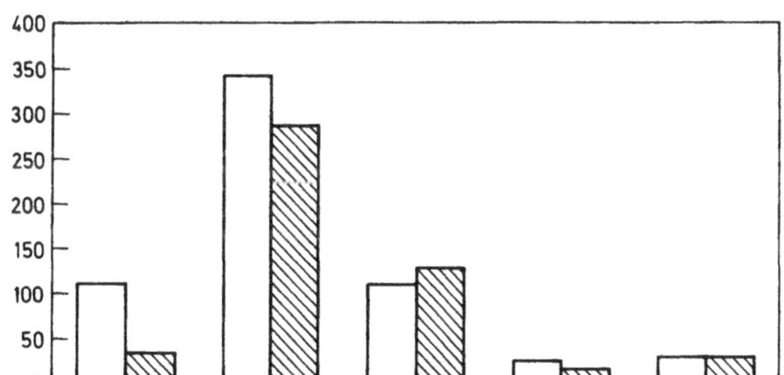

	Screening	Accidentally	Symptoms	Regular monitoring	Patient alone
Men	112	343	111	25	30
Women	34	288	129	16	29

Fig. 1: Modalities in diabetes detection (Diabetes Intervention Study, DIS).

Tab. 1: Medical history details and symptoms in diabetes mellitus

– Polydipsia, polyuria	– General susceptibility to infection (infections of the skin, urinary tract infections)
– Weight loss	– Pruritus
– Fatigue, decreased exercise tolerance	– Neurological symptoms (sensory disturbances)
– Increased appetite, polyphagia	– Decreased libido and impotence
– Nausea, vomiting	– Headaches, dizziness
– Abdominal pain	– Premature arteriosclerosis (claudication, angina pectoris)
– Muscle cramps	
– Transitory refraction anomalies	

4.1 Patient history

Family history

According to the representative data from the Diabetes Intervention Study (DIS) diabetes mellitus, obesity and hypertension occur with increased frequency in the maternal family history. Fathers, on the other hand, suffer myocardial infarctions at twice the rate of the mothers. These sex-specific differences indicate that genetic factors could be of importance for type II diabetes as well as for other illnesses and complications of the metabolic syndrome (tab. 2) [2].

Tab. 2: Family history of type II diabetics (DIS) regarding metabolic and cardiovascular diseases (in comparison: family history of randomly selected normal population group – Dresden study – [2])

	DIS (n = 1139)				Dresden study (n = 1216)		
	Mother %	Father %	Siblings %	Children %	Parents %	Siblings %	Children %
Obesity	46.4	24.8	35.3	15.8		not asked	
Diabetes mellitus	24.1	11.2	11.1	0.8	7.1	1.2	0.1
Hyperlipoproteinemia	0.7	0.7	1.1	0.1	0.4	–	–
Gout	1.6	1.1	0.7	0.1		not asked	
Myocardial infarction	4.5	9.2	2.3	0.2	6.2	0.8	–
Stroke	9.8	9.4	1.9	0	6.2	0.2	–
Hypertension	21.1	9.6	6.9	1.9	12.3	1.1	0.2

Patient history

Beyond determining diseases of the metabolic syndrome (see above) which are often causally associated with IGT or manifest diabetes mellitus, it is necessary to determine other diabetogenic and atherogenic noxia.

Here too, there is a considerably higher prevalence of associated risks at the time of diagnosis of type II diabetes compared to non-diabetics and partially in comparison to type I diabetics (tab. 3) [2].

Tab. 3: Patient self history of type II diabetics (DIS) regarding metabolic and cardiovascular diseases (in comparison: patient self histories from a randomly selected representative group of the general population – Dresden study – and from a group of insulin-dependent diabetics) [2]

	DIS (n = 1139) %	Dresden study (n = 1216) %	Insulin-dependent diabetics (n = 230) %
Hypertension	47.7	5.2	23
Hyperlipoproteinemia	7.8	0.5	3.5
Gout	5.3	not asked	not asked
Angina pectoris	17	2.8	19.6

Nowadays the acquired causes of diabetes mellitus are considered to be chronic liver and/or pancreatic disease, endocrine disorders, and administration of diabetogenic medication or hormones. Suspected diagnoses are also mentioned by specialists who are confronted with the typical findings of manifest micro- or macroangiopathy with as yet undetected diabetes mellitus:

Ophthalmologist:	microaneurysms, degenerative foci, cataracts, amongst others
Dermatologist:	pyodermas, boils, carbuncles, xanthomas, xanthelasmas
Neurologist:	polyneuritis, radicular or pseudoradicular syndromes
Gynecologist:	complications in pregnancy, vulvovaginitis, macrosomia
General medicine:	fatty liver, peripheral artery disease, coronary arteriosclerosis

The clinical picture is generally characterized by predisposing factors, concomitant illness (tab. 4) [1] and cardiovascular complications.

According to the results of the Diabetes Intervention Study (DIS) the rate of prevalence for hypertension was 53%, adiposis 49%, smokers 34%, hyperuricemia 22.5% and HLP 17.6% in newly diagnosed NIDDM.

In this representative type II segment of the age group 30–55 years there were already high rates of complications for cardiovascular and cerebrovascular events with the diagnosis, expressions of the actions of atherogenic risks.

Tab. 4: Predisposing factors of type II diabetes [1]

Obesity	
Diet	Overeating Deficiency of fibrous foods
Age	Increasing diabetes morbidity Decreasing glucose tolerance
Lifestyle	Stress Infections Operations Acute threatening conditions Decreased exercise
as well as	
Alcohol	Pancreatitis Obesity Liver cirrhosis
Iatrogenic diabetes	Corticosteroids Thiazide diuretics Oral contraceptives
Pregnancy	
Endocrine diseases	e. g. hyperthyroidism, acromegaly

4.2 Clinical findings

Of 1846 newly diagnosed diabetics, 2.5% had already had an infarction, 1.3% a stroke and 0.3% gangrene of the foot. By comparison, the prevalence of infarction in the same age group of non-diabetics was below 1% [3].

The reduced life expectancy of type II diabetics demands that the stage by stage progression of the metabolic vascular syndrome be unmasked as soon as possible.

From the clinical point of view there are, using the anamnestic, clinical and paraclinical findings for the most pathogenetically oriented characterization and treatment possible, two types of patients (see Chapter 1):

a) the overweight NIDDM with a short duration of diabetes (<5 years); insulin resistance, with compensatory hyperinsulinemia
b) the normal and underweight NIDDM with longer duration of diabetes (5 – 10 years); insulin resistance with worsening insulin deficiency and progressive weight loss.

The detection and classification of NIDDM according to these simple clinical definitions is an absolute prerequisite for differential therapeutic and diagnostic conclusions. Its distinction from a slowly manifesting type I diabetes is in some cases only possible by means of detailed investigations (tab. 5)

Tab. 5: Characteristics of NIDDM and IDDM

	NIDDM	IDDM
Age of onset	middle to old age	childhood and teens
Insulin dependency	most 2 – 3 years after diagnosis	mostly at onset
Genetic risk with a FDR[1)] with identical diabetes type	20.8 – 37.9%	3.5 – 4.5%
HLA association	–	DR 3 DR 4
Insulin and islet cell antibodies Antibodies to glutamate decarboxylase	– – –	+ + +
C-peptide after glucagon stimulation	> 1.1 nmol/l	0 – < 1.1 nmol/l
Microangiography	(+)	+
Cluster of the metabolic syndrome present at onset	+	–

[1)] first degree relative

4.3 Summary

Uncomplicated type II diabetes is the prototype of a frequently, clinically bland appearing complex metabolic disorder, which, as a result of the lack of apparent symptoms often remains undetected for years following its manifestation.

The early detection and classification of disturbed carbohydrate tolerance should serve to initiate examinations for associated risks of the metabolic syndrome (hypertension, obesity, smoking, hyperlipoproteinemia, hyperuricemia), because only in this manner can differential therapeutic and prognostic conclusions be drawn.

References

[1] Bruns, W., H. Mehnert, G. Use: Diabetestherapie heute, ein praktischer Leitfaden in Tabellen. Aktuelles Wissen Hoechst; Reihe Diabetes mellitus: 1. 5. Frankfurt 1991.

[2] Fischer, S., M. Hanefeld, J. Schulze et al.: Die Diabetesinterventionsstudie (DIS), eine multizentrische Multiinterventionsstudie bei Typ-II-Diabetikern. 2. Mitteilung. Z. Klin.Med. *42* (1987) 1613 – 1616.
[3] Hanefeld, M. H. Haller, J. Schulze et al.: Die Diabetesinterventionsstudie (DIS), eine multizentrische Multiinterventionsstudie bei Typ-II-Diabetikern. 1. Mitteilung. Dtsch. Gesundh.wes. *39* (1984) 1889 – 1894.

5 The hormonal-metabolic syndrome in type II diabetes

At the beginning of the 1970s our team, in the context of the Dresden Study, described the close association of obesity, diabetes mellitus (NIDDM), fatty liver, lipid metabolism disorders, hypertension and hyperuricemia which lead to arteriosclerotic manifestations and are defined as metabolic syndrome (fig. 1, tab. 1). As early as the 1960s the Frenchman Camus used the term "trisyndrome metabolique" (diabetes, hypertriglyceridemia, gout) and, referring to a similar constellation, the Munich group around H. Mehnert spoke of the "affluence syndrome".

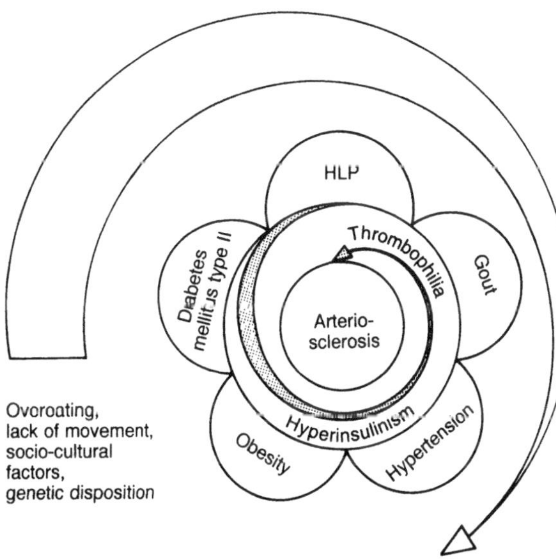

Fig. 1: The metabolic syndrome (Hanefeld and Leonhardt [3]).

More recently, the term Syndrome X has begun to appear in the literature to describe this cluster of metabolic disorders. This term was coined by Reaven and makes insulin resistance the central point. In the following, the current state of knowledge about the associations between the individual components of the hormonal-metabolic syndrome will be dealt with, taking NIDDM into special consideration. The paradigm (fig. 2) can serve as a summary of our current view of the syndrome.

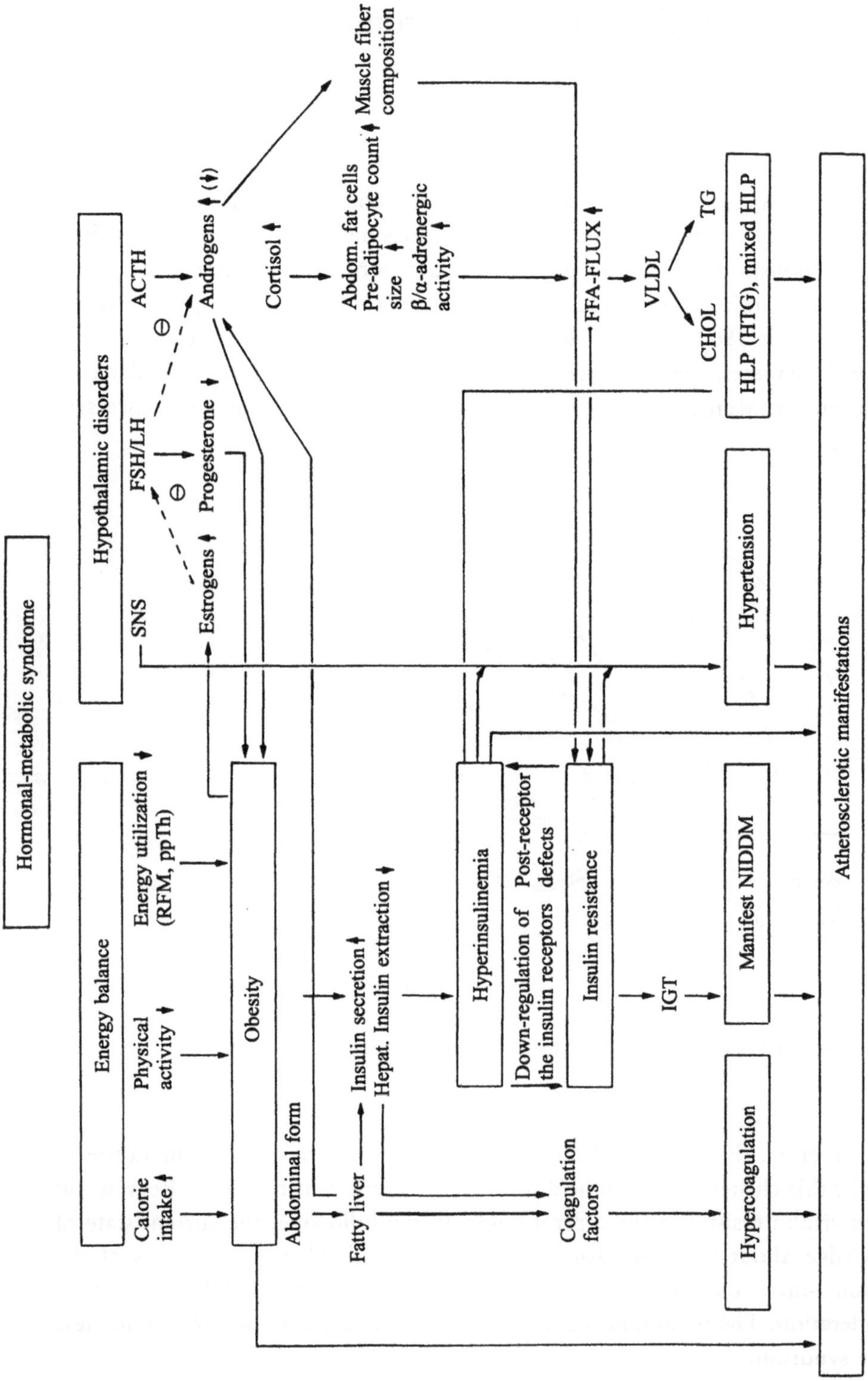

Fig. 2: The interactions of hormonal-metabolic disorders, hypertension and atherosclerosis.

Key: SNS ... Sympathetic nervous system
RFM ... Resting fasting metabolism
ppTh ... postprandial thermogenesis

Tab. 1: Prevalence of coronary risk factors (%) among DIS patients (n = 1139) upon inclusion in the study and among the general population (Dresden study, n = 1216)

Risk factor	DIS	Dresden study	Limits
HLP	17.6	7.6	Triglycerides ≥ 250 mg/dl and/or cholesterol ≥ 300 mg/dl
Hypertension	53.0	17.3	BP ≥ 160/95 mmHg and/or anti-hypertensives
HTG	11.3	3.4	
Hypercholesterolemia	3.5	3.7	
Mixed HLP	2.8	0.5	
Smoking	34.0	30.0	Tobacco consumption ≥ 1 g per day
Obesity	49.0	8.2	Ideal body weight index M > 1.2 F > 1.3
Hyperuricemia	11.5	3.8	Uric acid i. s. M > 7.0 mg/dl F > 6.0 mg/dl

HLP: Hyperlipidemia
HTG: Hypertriglyceridemia
DIS: Diabetes Intervention Study

5.1 Obesity

M. Weck

5.1.1 Genetic influences

Genetic influences affect the individual factors of the hormonal-metabolic syndrome directly and indirectly. Nowadays it is considered certain that the lower energy consumption which predisposes to obesity is frequently hereditary. Components of the energy consumption side of the energy balance are the resting metabolic rate, energy expenditures for physical activity and thermogenesis (ppTh). The latter is plainly visible as sweating after opulent meals and it is probably possible to show a genetic dependency for this component of the energy expenditure as well.

5.1.2 Obesity, adipose tissue distribution and NIDDM

Obesity is generally defined as increased masses of fat. However, only the abdominal and especially the intraabdominally located fat depot is closely connected with metabolic aberrations. The "waist-to-hip ratio" (WHR) is used as a measure of the distribution of body fat. A number of synonyms are used in the literature to describe the two forms of fat distribution in the obese. (tab. 2) The visceral adipose tissue mass can be quantified by means of CT. See section 7.2 for details about the measuring methods. The morphological and metabolical distinctions between abdominal and gluteal-femoral adipose tissue are shown in table 3.

The specific functional characteristics and the strategic localization of the visceral adipose tissue in the vena portae drainage region are related to its central position in the framework of the hormonal-metabolic syndrome. Clinical-epidemiological

Tab. 2: Synonyms for two forms of fat distribution in the obese

WHR > 1.0 (m) > 0.85 (f)	WHR < 1.0 (m) < 0.85 (f)
Abdominal	Gluteal-femoral
Android	Gynoid
Trunk-centered	Hip-centered
Central	Peripheral
Upper body	Lower body
Apple-shaped	Pear-shaped
Hypertrophic	Hyperplastic

Tab. 3: Morphological and metabolic differentiating characteristics between abdominal and gluteal-femoral fat tissue

	Abdominal-visceral		Gluteal-femoral
		fat tissue	
Insulin dynamics			
– Secretion		>	
– Hepatic extraction		<	
– Metabolic clearance		<	
Blood glucose regulation, insulin sensitivity			
– Blood glucose (oGTT)		>	
– Glucose utilization (M value)		<	
– Insulin resistance		>	
– Hepatic glucose production		<	
Fat tissue morphology and function			
– Fat cell volume		>	
– Lipolysis		>	
– Lipase activity		<	
Blood pressure			
– Hypertension		>	
Sexual hormones			
– Testosterone (m)		<	
– Testosterone (f)		>	
Coagulation data			
– PAI (plasminogen activator inhibitor)		>	
– Fibrinogen		>	

studies show that the abdominal fat accumulation is associated with a number of cardiovascular and secondary metabolic diseases. In general, men with abdominal obesity (the typical "beer belly") and women who lose their good figure and gain abdominal fat (fig. 3), exhibit an increased cardiovascular risk (tab. 4, 5).

The biochemical basis of these processes is shown in the following. Visceral-omental adipose tissue is particularly sensitive to lipolytic stimuli and demonstrates a reduced response to the antilipolytic insulin effect. Such a drastically increased FFA potential occurs in the portal circulation that several metabolic effects follow (fig. 4):

1) on hepatic insulin clearance
2) on carbohydrate metabolism
3) on hepatic lipoprotein synthesis

to 1) Effects of the portal FFA on the hepatic insulin clearance: obesity is associated with reduced hepatic insulin clearance. This can even be seen as a

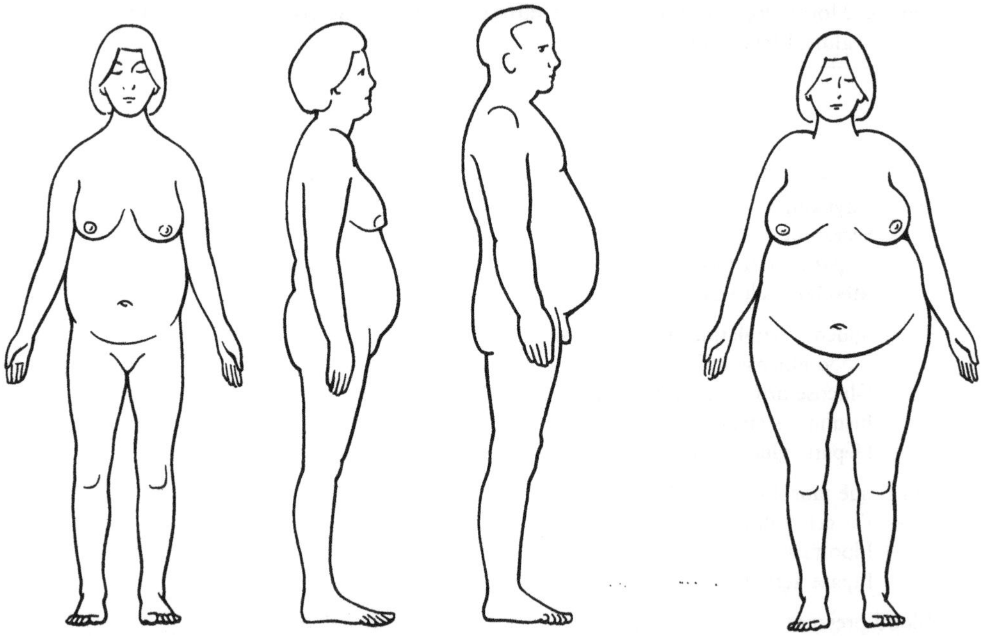

Fig. 3: Schematic representation of the types of fat distribution.

Tab. 4: Regression analysis (stepwise logistic regression) of 10 selected parameters in 286 men, who required a coronary angiography (Hauner et. al [6])

variable	p
LDL cholesterol	0.0001
Age	0.0005
WHR	0.013
Total cholesterol	0.154
BMI (body mass index)	0.197
Insulin	0.238
HDL cholesterol	0.243
Triglycerides	0.293
Systolic blood pressure	0.735
Diastolic blood pressure	0.973

characteristic of abdominal obesity. Independent of one another, a Swedish and an American group recently showed that in isolated liver cells, insulin binding in physiological concentration is severely limited by FFA. This FFA effect not only holds true for insulin binding, but for other processes of insulin internalization, breakdown and effect. Abdominal obesity is therefore associated with reduced insulin uptake in the liver. Consequently, there is portal and

Tab. 5: Correlations between cardio-vascular risk factors, end points and obesity (BMI) and their localization (WHR) (according to Björntorp) [1]

	BMI	WHR
Cardiovascular diseases	0	+
Apoplexy	0	+
Diabetes mellitus	+	+
Premature death	0	+
Hypertension	+	+
Cholesterol	0	+
Triglycerides	+	+
Insulin	+	+ +
Fibrinogen	0	+
Smoking	–	+

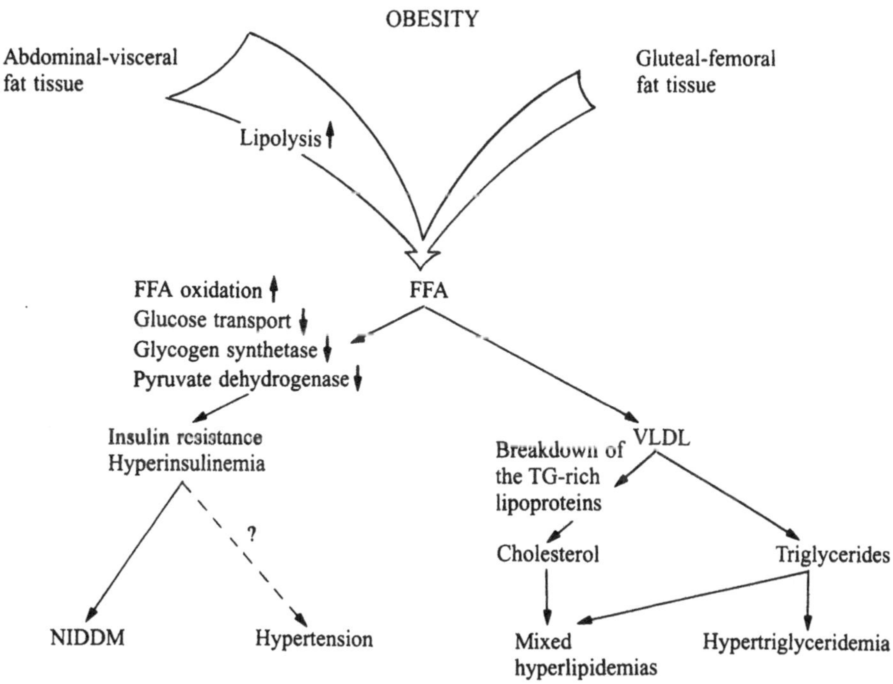

Fig. 4: Role of the adipose tissue system and FFA in the pathogenesis of NIDDM and the metabolic syndrome.

peripheral hyperinsulinism, which also can cause insulin resistance via the down regulation of insulin receptors. With the progressive disturbance in insulin and glucose homeostasis, the increased FFA flux and fatty acid oxidation can lead to increased strain on the pancreas and further to the development of hypoinsulinemia.

These disturbed insulin dynamics, in combination with the known stimulatory effect of the FFA on gluconeogenesis, promote relatively unopposed hepatic glucose production to the point of hyperglycemia. Portal hyperlipacidemia with subsequent hyperinsulinism and insulin resistance are central pathomechanisms of visceral obesity and NIDDM.

to 2) Effects of the FFA on carbohydrate metabolism: increased portal FFA increases blood glucose via stimulation of hepatic gluconeogenesis. Accordingly, lipolysis inhibitors (Acipimox, Olbemox®) effectively reduce blood glucose.

But not only the portal FFA concentrations are increased in abdominal obesity, the peripheral FFA is increased as well. The musculature may play an essential role in this defect, because it uses, for the most part, FFA as the oxidative substrate in healthy persons. Reduced muscular FFA consumption would lead to increased plasma FFA and increased lipid oxidation with subsequently increased glucose production and therefore represents a mechanism which associates defects in the musculature and liver with NIDDM.

to 3) Effects of the portal FFA on hepatic lipoprotein synthesis: portal hyperlipacidemia leads to increased production of VLDL and TG, whereby the availability of FFA determines the VLDL synthesis rate. Consequently, there is an increase in the concentration of LDL and ApoB-100, established risk factors of arteriosclerotic manifestations.

5.1.3 Hormonal regulation of the adipose tissue distribution

In recent years neuroendocrine regulatory processes have again been taken into consideration for the pathogenesis of obesity. On the one hand, certain types of stress, high alcohol consumption and nicotine abuse are associated with hormonal imbalances and a preponderance of adipose tissue in the abdomen, on the other hand, the size of the fat deposits are dependent on the number of fat cells and the lipid content.

Lipoprotein lipase (LPL) is the key enzyme for fat deposition and lipolysis. Lipid release is determined by the lipolytic system, which is primarily activated by the sympathetic nervous system and principally inhibited by insulin. These enzymatic processes are conducted by hormones, and above all, by steroid hormones as well as adrenocortical and sex hormones. In the end, the effects of these hormones depent on the density and affinity of receptors on the target organs, i. e. the adipose tissue.

5.1.3.1 Corticosteroids

It is known from patients with Cushing's Disease that cortisol increases LPL activity. This disease exhibits a drastically increased activity of this enzyme in abdominal adipose tissue. If this data is followed, cortisol would, by means of its high density of receptors in visceral adipose tissues, promote LPL activity and as a result fat accumulation in this region. Of course the net deposit of fat is just as dependent on the lipolytic system, whereby it is assumed that corticosteroids increase lipolysis through a permissive effect on the catecholamine-stimulated release of glycerol. The lipolysis of the abdominal fat depot was significantly lower in Cushing patients than in healthy women and beyond that did not differ from the femoral depot. Finally the corticoids play an important role in the development of hyperplastic obesity. Preadipocytes can be converted into mature fat cells by physiological glucocorticoid concentrations in the presence of insulin.

5.1.3.2 Testosterone

Testosterone appears to have regionally differing effects on adipose tissue metabolism. An inhibition of the LPL and stimulation of lipolysis in the abdominal depot has been described, whereby both mechanisms would lead to deposition of fat. Obese men exhibit low serum testosterone levels and these are inversely correlated with the degree of obesity; they normalize following weight reduction. It has recently been proven that the blood level of free and total testosterone, as well as SHBG (sex hormone binding globulin) are correlated negatively with the WHR, the size of the visceral fat depot and increased blood glucose, insulin and C-peptide values in men [13].

In contrast to men increased levels of total and free testosterone and low SHBG are characteristic for abdominally obese women and are not observed in gluteal-femoral obesity. Low SHBG was an independent risk factor for the development of NIDDM in women in the Göteborg study. Recent studies have demonstrated a positive correlation between free testosterone and the insulin resistance of obese women, measured by means of glucose clamp technique. The effect of the increased androgen level is above all on the muscles. Muscle mass and muscle fiber composition of these women exhibit male characteristics, i. e. an increase in type II muscle fibers, which have a lower insulin sensitivity than type I fibers [9].

5.1.3.3 Progesterone

Progesterone causes an increase in LPL activity in the gluteal-femoral region.

5.1.3.4 Estrogens

Definite evidence of an abnormal secretion of estrogens has not been found in obesity. Only in excessive obesity (BMI $>$ 40) have increased estrone and estradiol values been reported. However, adrenal androgens are converted to estrone by adipose tissue and this conversion is of course increased as a consequence of increased fat mass.

Glucocorticoids and sex hormones have very different effects on the regulation of adipose tissue metabolism in both of the main regions. Disturbances in the balance of the two hormone groups also cause aberrations in the adipose tissue metabolism. Cortisol appears to cause the accumulation of fat in the intraabdominal region, while the sex hormones work against this. Progesterone leads to an accumulation of fat in the periphery.

These biochemical findings are mirrored by well-known clinical features. The Cushing Syndrome, with its massive fat deposits in the abdominal region, is associated with glucocorticoid-related, drastically increased LPL activities in this region. The menopause (normal cortisol, decreasing testosterone) is counted amongst these hormonal imbalances which are accompanied by changes in the regional fat deposition.

The abdominal, especially the visceral adipose tissue, act on the one hand as a target organ, and on the other hand as potentiator for the aberration of the endocrine-metabolic syndrome described above and its subsequent disturbances, cardiovascular diseases and NIDDM.

5.1.4 Summary

The individual components of the hormonal-metabolic syndrome represent risk factors for atherosclerosis and its subsequent diseases. Increased abdominal girth with increased FFA-influx into the portal circulation, hyperinsulinism and insulin resistance are central pathogenetic mechanisms of the metabolic syndrome described. It is not the obesity as such, but the central accumulation of fat, measurable by means of the WHR (waist-to-hip ratio), which is associated with increased cardiovascular risk.

References

[1] Björntorp, P.: Obesity and diabetes. In: K.G.M.M Alberti, L. P. Kral (eds.): The diabetes annual/5, 373–395. Elsevier, Amsterdam 1990.

[2] Haffner, S. M., D. Fong, H. P. Hazuda et al.: Hyperinsulinaemia, upper body adiposity and cardiovascular risk factors in non-diabetics. Metabolism *37* (1988) 338–345.

[3] Hanefeld, M., W. Leonhardt: Das metabolische Syndrom. Dt. Gesundh.-Wesen *36* (1981) 545–551.

[4] Hanefeld, M.: Untersuchungen zur Fettleberproblematik unter besonderer Berücksichtigung metabolischer Gesichtspunkte. Habilitation, Medizinische Akademie, Dresden 1973.

[5] Hauner, H.: Fettgewebsverteilung und Adipositasrisiko. Dtsch. med. Wschr. *112* (1987) 731–735.

[6] Hauner, H., K. Stangl, C. Schmatz et al.: Body fat distribution in men with angiographically confirmed coronary artery disease. Atherosclerosis *85* (1990) 203–210.

[7] Jequier, E., Y. Schutz: New evidence for a thermogenic defect in human obesity. Int. J. Obesity *9* (1985) (Suppl. 2) 1–7.

[8] Kissebah, A. H., A. N. Peiris, D. J. Evans: Mechanism associating body fat distribution to glucose intolerance and diabetes mellitus. Window with a view. Acta Med. Scand. *723* (1988) (Suppl.) 79 – 89.

[9] Krotkiewski, M., P. Björntorp: Muscle tissue in obesitiy with different distribution of adipose tissue. Effects of physical training. Int. J. Obesity *10* (1986) 311 – 341.

[10] Peiris, A. N., R. A. Mueller, M. F. Struve et al.: Relationships of androgenic activity to splanchnic insulin metabolism and peripheral glucose utilization in premenopausal women. J. Clin. Endocrinol. Metab. *64* (1987) 162 – 169.

[11] Ravussin, E., S. Lilioja, W. C. Knowler et al.: Reduced rate of energy expenditure as a risk factor for body weight gain. N. Engl. J. Med. *318* (1988) 467 – 472.

[12] Reaven, G. M., B. B. Hoffmann: A role for insulin in the aetiology and course of hypertension. Lancet II (1987) 435 – 436.

[13] Seidell, J. C., P. Björntorp, L. Sjöström et al.: Visceral fat accumulation in men is positively associated with insulin, glucose and C-peptide levels, but negatively with testosterone levels. Metabolism *39* (1990) 897 – 901.

[14] Svedberg, J., P. Björntorp, U. Smith et al.: Free-fatty acid inhibition of insulin binding, degradation and action in isolated rat hepatocytes. Diabetes *39* (1990) 570 – 574.

[15] Weck, M.: Abdominale Fettsucht im Rahmen des metabolischen Syndroms. Gewichtiger kardiovaskulärer Risikofaktor. Therapiewoche *42* (1992) 1560 – 1566.

5.2 Dyslipoproteinemia

M. Hanefeld

NIDDM, lipid metabolism disturbances and atherosclerosis are closely tied to one another. E.P. Joslin's statement from 1927 still holds true, "I think the main reason for the premature development of arteriosclerosis in diabetics, which hinders attaining old age, is an excess of fat in the body, adiposis, too much fat in food, too much fat in the blood. Diabetics die with an excess of fat, previously of coma, now of arteriosclerosis."

5.2.1 *Epidemiology*

Dyslipoproteinemia in type II diabetes occurs for the most part in two forms, as hypertriglyceridemia and as a lack of HDL [1,4]. There is no direct relationship to familial hypercholesterolemia. In 40 – 80% of patients, one finds triglyceride and/or cholesterol elevations which are above the threshold values of the European Atherosclerosis Society (tab. 1) [3]. The prevalence of pronounced hyperlipoproteinemia (HLP) (triglyceride concentrations $\geq$ 2.9 mmol/l, cholesterol $\geq$ 7.8 mmol/l) with well-adjusted diet-controlled NIDDM was, with 17.6%, three times that of the normal population [4]. Among the patients in the Diabetes Intervention Study, 12% had an HDL cholesterol value < 0.9 mmol/l 5 years after determination of the diabetes, despite intensive therapy. There is an obvious syntropy between NIDDM and primary hypertriglyceridemia. Between 30 and 70% of the patients with familial hypertriglyceridemia, familial combined hyperlipidemia and familial dysbetalipoproteinemia (type III) exhibit impaired glucose tolerance or mild NIDDM [5]. Even after optimizing the diabetes therapy in the near-normoglycemic range, about 10% of the patients still exhibit a hypertriglyceridemia, or an abnormal composition of the lipoproteins exists. Therefore, even after optimal diabetic adjustment, it is not always possible to separate primary and secondary dyslipoproteinemia. As clearly demonstrated in prospective studies, hypertriglyceridemia with IGT is a risk factor for the subsequent manifestation of diabetes as well as for hypertension and atherosclerosis [14].

With respect to the importance of lipids and lipoproteins as risk factors for atherosclerosis in NIDDM, the results of prospective studies published in the recent past have clearly shown that beside the "classic" indicators LDL-cholesterol and HDL-cholesterol, triglycerides are a serious independent risk factor [7]. In the Paris Prospective Study [4a] the combination of high triglycerides and high cholesterol values proved to be an explosive risk constellation for cardiac death.

Tab. 1: Frequency of hyperlipidemias at the time of diagnosis of type II diabetes: the Diabetes Intervention Study [3]. Categories of the European Atherosclerosis Society.

n	mg/dl	mmol/l	Men (n 606)	Women (n 479)	Significance
A	Cholesterol (TC)				
	200 – 250	5.2 – 6.5			
	+ Triglycerides (TG)		30.2%	30.5%	n. s.
	< 200	< 2.3			
B	TC 250 – 300	6.5 – 7.8			
	+ TG < 200	< 2.3	12.4%	13.4%	n. s.
C	TC < 200	< 5.2		3.5%	
	+ TG 200 – 500	2.3 – 5.6	3.5%		n. s.
D	TC 200 – 300	5.2 – 7.8			
	+ TG 200 – 500	2.3 – 5.6	13.5%	16.5%	n .s.
E	TC > 300	> 7.8	1.3%	0.42%	
	and/or TG	> 5.6			n. s.
	> 500				
	Total		60.9%	64.3%	n. s.

The same is true for the combination hypertriglyceridemia-hyperinsulinemia [4]. An analogy can be found in the Helsinki Heart Study where the highest rate of infarction occurred in the sub-group with a total cholesterol/HDL-cholesterol ratio > 5 and triglycerides above 2.0 mmol/l [10]. The rate of infarction in the group with poorly controlled triglycerides (> 2.3 mmol/l) was 3.3 times higher than that of well-adjusted patients (< 1.7 mmol/l) in the Diabetes Intervention Study [7]. To what degree ApoB-elevations and $ApoA_1$ insufficiencies are relevant as independent risk factors requires further clarification.

There can no longer be any doubt in the importance of a raised Lp(a) as an independent risk factor for NIDDM. Table 2 offers a summary of the lipoprotein anomalies for which a role as risk factor has been proven in epidemiological studies.

The special importance of lipid anomalies in NIDDM is obvious from the comparison of the relative risk of increased cholesterol in diabetics and non-diabetics in the MRFIT [12], the largest prospective study of coronary heart disease performed to date. According to this study, after adjusting to the same risk level, the individual cholesterol concentrations in diabetics were subject to a three-fold higher rate of infarction as in non-diabetics. Santen [11] pointed out in 1972 that diabetics require a significantly lower triglyceride level to remain free of the clinical manifestations of atherosclerosis than do non-diabetics.

Tab. 2: Anomalies in the lipoprotein profile with effect on the risk of atherosclerosis in NIDDM.

Total cholesterol	=↑	Apo A1	↓
LDL cholesterol	=↑	Apo B	↑
HDL cholesterol	↓	Apo A/B	↑
Triglycerides	↑ ↑	HDL C/A1	↓
VLDL			
– Core			
– Triglycerides	↑		
– Cholesterolester	↓		
– Surface			
– Free cholesterol	↑		
– Phospholipids	↓		
– Anomalies of the apo-lipid proteins (CIII/CII ↑)			
– Percentage of small dense VLDL ↑			
LDL			
TG	↑		
Small dense LDL subfractions ↑			
HDL			
TG	↑		
HDL 2	↓		
Lp(a)	=↑		

5.2.2 Pathophysiology of lipid metabolism in NIDDM

The diabetes-induced changes affect, above all, the metabolism of triglyceride-rich lipoproteins (fig. 1) and the HDL. The regulation and disturbances of the VLDL-metabolism in NIDDM are very complex [8, 6]. The VLDL-synthesis is dependent to a large extent on the level of insulin secretion and insulin resistance, glucose control and obesity. The typical android obesity leads to increased influx of free fatty acids to the liver and promotes, along with hyperglycemia, the synthesis of triglycerides. As long as sufficient insulin is secreted, the increased hepatic VLDL-synthesis is the most important determinant of triglyceride concentration. Despite hyperinsulinemia, however, the fractional removal rate is also reduced [13]. The explanation for this is to be found in the insulin resistance of the musculature and liver, which lead to a relative lipoprotein lipase deficit. The consequence of this is an increase in VLDL and chylomicron remnants. The VLDL over-production decreases with a lack of insulin secretion and it dominates the removal defect, i. e. the anomalies in kinetics approach those of type I diabetes with absolute insulin deficit (fig. 2).

The fact that the composition of the VLDL changes is of importance in atherogenesis. The VLDL become richer in triglycerides and cholesterol, whereby their breakdown shifts in the direction of macrophages and myointimal muscle cells of the vessel wall (fig. 3) [2].

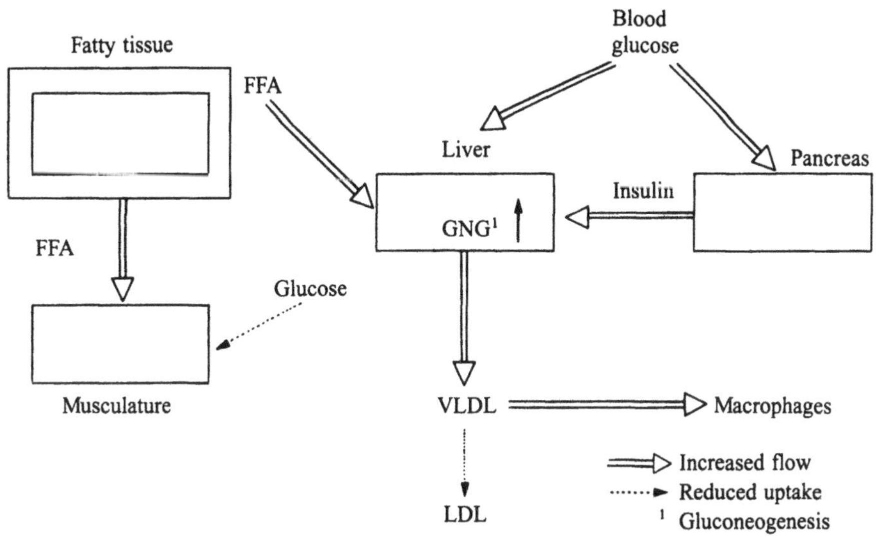

Fig. 1: Pathophysiology of lipoprotein metabolism in NIDDM with hyperinsulinism.

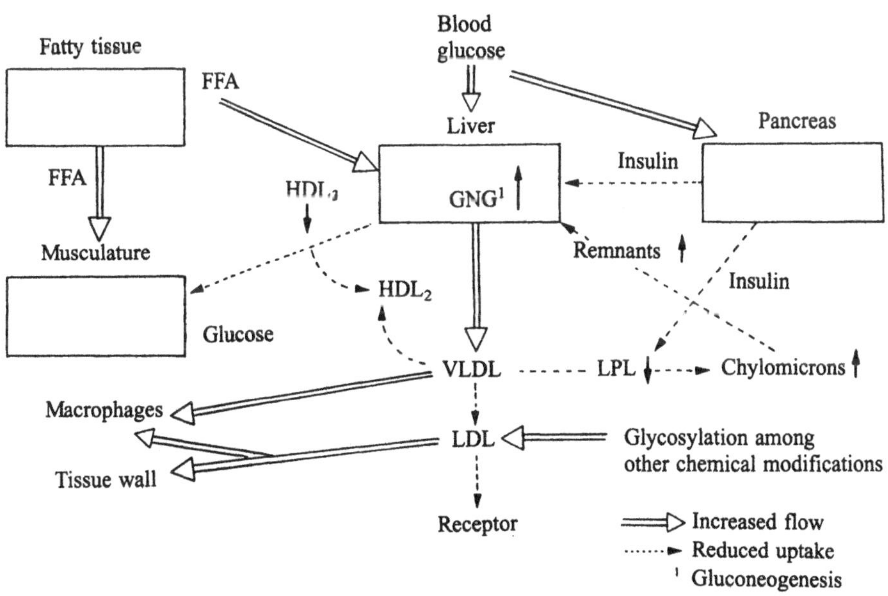

Fig. 2: Pathophysiology of lipoprotein metabolism with insulin deficiency.

The LDL-metabolism is only slightly changed when a certain level of insulin secretion is still present. Dependent on the glycemic state, non-enzymatic binding of glucose to apoprotein B occurs. The glycosylation reaches 5 – 10% maximum and leads to delayed LDL-breakdown, which, however, does not cause any

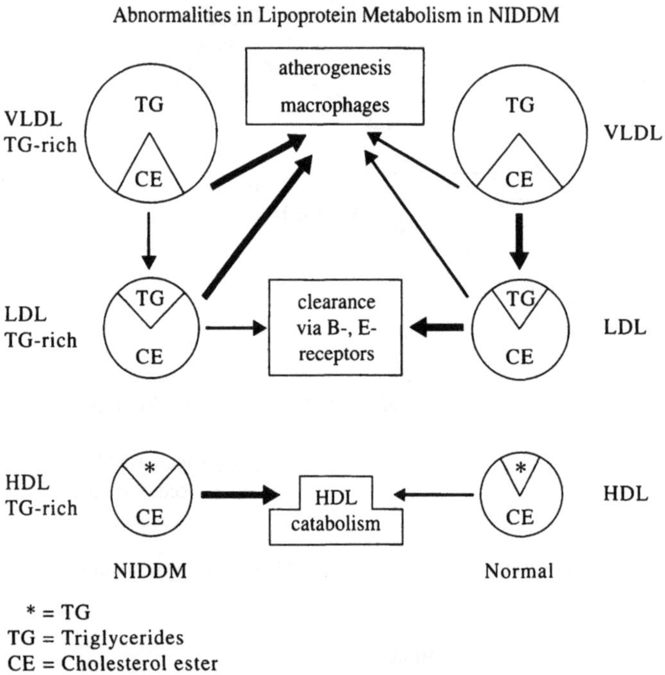

Fig. 3: Disorders of the VLDL, LDL and HDL metabolism in NIDDM with hypertriglyceridemia (modified from Eisenberg [15]).

significant increase in the LDL-cholesterol as a result of the increased shunting into the scavenger pathway. The importance of other chemical modifications is not very well known. The low HDL levels are to some extent explained by an accelerated breakdown as a result of glycosylation [9]. To summarize the available knowledge about dyslipoproteinemia in NIDDM, the consequences for the interaction of vessel wall and lipoproteins of the blood can be characterized as negative synergism. The excessive synthesis of abnormally composed and chemically modified VLDL leads to increase in and the deterioration of remnants and smaller, denser LDL, which enter macrophages and smooth muscles cells of the vessel wall, for the most part via the scavenger pathway. There, deposits of crystalline cholesterol are built up because the reverse transport capacity has been reduced by the HDL deficiency and the anomalies of the HDL molecules. In addition, the glycosylation of intercellular substances (collagen) acts like a net for LDL-cholesterol. Recently, a further dimension of the negative effects of the hypertriglyceridemia has been established: the inhibition of fibrinolytic activity.

These are all plausible biochemical explanations for the increased atherogenic potential of disturbances of the lipoprotein metabolism in NIDDM compared to non-diabetics.

5.2.3 *Summary*

Dyslipoproteinemias can be found in 60 – 80% of persons with NIDDM. Anomalies in the area of triglyceride-rich lipoproteins and HDL-deficiencies are the most common. Increases in LDL-cholesterol and triglycerides and HDL-deficiencies have a higher atherogenic potential for diabetics than for non-diabetics. Along with genetic defects, insulin resistance, hyperinsulinemia, obesity and lack of movement are the most important pathogenetic factors of the hypertriglyceridemia in the beginning of diabetes. Later the insulin deficiency plays an increasingly important role. The atherogenic effect of the dyslipoproteinemia is potentiated if disturbances in the VLDL-LDL transfer are combined with HDL deficits and their simultaneous occurrence with other risk factors, in particular hyperinsulinemia. Chemical modifications of the lipoproteins, with poor metabolic control, above all glycosylation, further accelerate the atherogenesis.

References

[1] Assmann, G., H. H. Schulte: The prospective cardiovascular Münster (PROCAM) study: prevalence of hyperlipidemia in persons with hypertension and/or diabetes mellitus and the relationship to coronary heart disease. Am. Heart J. *116* (1988) 1713 – 1724.

[2] Eisenberg, S.: Very low density lipoprotein metabolism. Proc. Biochem. Pharmacol. *15* (1979) 139 – 165.

[3] Fischer, S. et al.: Hyperlipidämien bei Typ-2-Diabetes. Submitted.

[4] Fontbonne, A., M. A. Charles, N. Thibult: Hyperinsulin aemia as a predictor of coronary heart disease mortality in a healthy population: the Paris Prospective Study, 15-year follow-up. Diabetologia *34* (1991) 356 – 361.

[4a] Fontbonne, A., E. Eschwege, F. Cambien et al.: Hypertriglyceridemia as risk factor for coronary heart disease mortality in subjects with impaired glucose tolerance or diabetes: results from the five year follow-up of the Paris Prospective Study. Diabetologia *32* (1989) 300 – 304.

[5] Haller, H., M. Hanefeld: Primäre HLP mit diabetischer Stoffwechselstörung. In: H. Haller, M. Hanefeld, W. Jaroß (Hrsg.): Lipidstoffwechselstörungen. Diagnostik, Klinik, Therapie, 252 – 254. G. Fischer Verlag, Jena 1983.

[6] Hanefeld, M.: Diabetes, obesity and dyslipoproteinemia. Implications for atherosclerosis. Clin. Invest. Arteriosclerosis *3* (1991) 171 – 177.

[7] Hanefeld, M., H. Schmechel, U. Julius et al.: Five-year incidence of coronary heart disease related to major risk factors and metabolic control in newly diagnosted non-insulin-dependent diabetes. The Diabetes Intervention Study (DIS). Nutr. Metab. Cardiovasc. Dis. *1* (1991) 135 – 140.

[8] Howard, B. V.: Lipoprotein metabolism in diabetes mellitus. J. Lip. Res. *28* (1987) 613 – 628.

[9] Kesaniemi, A.: Pathophysiology of low density lipoprotein and high density lipoprotein glycosylation. In: R. W. James, D. Pometta (eds.): Dyslipoproteinaemias and diabetes. Monogr. Atheroscler. No 13. Proceedings of the European Atherosclerosis Group Meeting, Montreux, March, 15 – 16, 1985, 63 – 73. Karger, Basel 1985.

[10] Manninen, V., O. Elo, H. Frick et al.: Lipid alterations and the decline in the incidence of coronary heart disease in the Helsinki Heart Study. JAMA *260* (1988) 641 – 651.

[11] Santen, R. J., P. W. Willis, S. S. Fajans: Atherosclerosis in diabetes mellitus. Correlations with serum lipid levels, adiposity and serum insulin level. Arch. Intern. Med. *130* (1972) 833 – 843.

[12] Stamler, J.: Epidemiology, established major risk factors and the primary prevention of coronary heart disease. In: W.W. Parmley, P.A. Chatterjee (eds.): Cardiology, 1 – 41. Lippincott, Philadelphia, PA. 1987.

[13] Taskinen, M. R., W. F. Beltz, I. Harper et al.: The effects of non-insulin-dependent diabetes mellitus on VLDL triglycerides and VLDL apoB metabolism: studies before and after sulfonylurea therapy. Diabetes *35* (1986) 1268 – 1277.

[14] Wilson, W. F., W. B. Kannel, K. M. Anderson: Lipids, glucose intolerance and vascular disease: the Framingham study. In: R. W. James, D. Pometta (eds.): Dyslipoproteinaemias and diabetes. Monogr. Atheroscler. No 13. Proceedings of the European Atherosclerosis Group Meeting, Montreux, March, 15 – 16, 1985, 1 – 11. Karger, Basel 1985.

5.3 Hypertension

J. Schulze

5.3.1 *Introduction*

Arterial hypertension is a frequent and serious risk and progression factor in diabetes mellitus, which considerably reinforces the atherogenic potential for the development of macro- and microangiopathy that is already present. The increased cardiovascular morbidity and mortality of diabetics in comparison to non-diabetics must first of all be viewed in connection with three-fold prevalence of hypertension [1, 5]. Recent discoveries in epidemiology, pathophysiology and prognosis of hypertension in diabetes mellitus indicate this dangerous synergism, which must be met with new therapeutic concepts [20].

5.3.2 *Epidemiology*

Interactions between diabetes and hypertension have been known and investigated again and again since the beginning of the century. It has been proven in a number of studies that disturbed carbohydrate tolerance and diabetes occur more frequently with hypertension than under normotension [2]. Viewed from the other perspective arterial hypertension has been detected in over 50% of persons with NIDDM [6, 8, 15].

Anamnestic data of essential hypertension with concomitant diabetes show that in 63% the hypertension preceded the disturbed glucose tolerance [2]. As early as 1922 Maranon [9] raised the suspicion that arterial hypertension might represent a pre-diabetic condition.

Results from the Framingham Study show the morbidity rates from cardiac and vascular complications in hypertensive diabetics are 5-fold higher than those of normotensive non-diabetics. This rate increases if left-ventricular hypertrophy is present (fig. 1) [18]. In the PROCAM study, middle aged men with both diabetes and hypertension were found to have double the risk of infarction [1]. Hypertension was the most important independent risk factor in the Diabetes Intervention Study [6]! The incidence of myocardial infarction was 18/1000 patients/year with blood pressure values < 140/90 mmHg, 57/1000 with 140 – 159/90 – 94 mmHg and BP > 160/95 mmHg 92/1000 patients/year in the first 5 years after diagnosis of NIDDM [7]. The disappointing results of an effective antihypertensive drug treatment on the CAD mortality in several intervention studies – the so-called "CAD paradox" – was attributed to the lack of or insufficient control of other risk factors and to some extent the unfavorable side effects of the

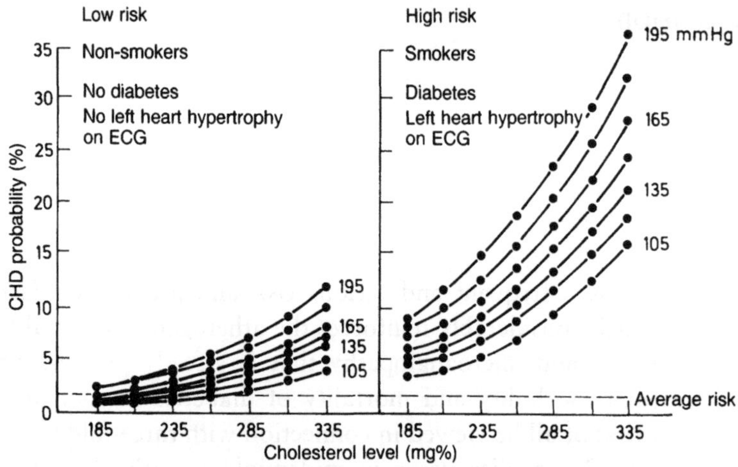

Fig. 1: Coronary risk, as dependent on high blood pressure and other risk factors, Framingham Study, initially 40 year old men, 16-year follow-up [18].

antihypertensives on carbohydrate and lipid metabolism. It was found that while beta-blockers and thiazide diuretics, which were primarily used in the study, not only effectively control the high blood pressure and therefore reduce the incidence of stroke by 30–80%, they also cause negative metabolic influences which had unfavorable cardiac effects [16, 17]. Another important component of vascular risk appears to be hyperinsulinemia. A number of large-scale epidemiological studies [4,7,8] have shown that hyperinsulinemia in diabetics is a serious coronary risk factor which is also closely correlated with hypertension and hyperlipoproteinemia.

5.3.3 Importance of insulin resistance for the pathogenesis of hypertension

In the last few years, diabetes research groups have been able to show that insulin resistance or hyperinsulinemia with disturbed glucose tolerance function as a link between essential hypertension, android obesity, HLP and accelerated atherogenesis [10, 19]. A well-founded hypothesis that essential hypertension per se is connected with a reduced insulin sensitivity can be derived from a number of studies.

The presently known mechanisms, which could lead to an increased blood pressure through a compensatory hyperinsulinemia, are

1. increased tubular sodium retention
2. increased sympathetic tone
3. change in transmembrane ion transport.

to 1) The antidiuretic effect of insulin on sodium may lead to a hypervolemic hypertension via an increase in the extracellular space. (note: also "insulin edema"!)

to 2) Elevated insulin concentrations increase the activity of the sympathetic nervous system (hypothalamic insulin effect?) and lead via elevated norepinephrine concentrations to vasoconstriction and an increase in heart rate and blood pressure.

to 3) The insulin-dependent transmembrane ion transport for cations and anions also contributes to vasoconstriction via elevated intracellular sodium concentrations and altered salt concentrations in the vascular endothelia (fig. 2), [10, 11].

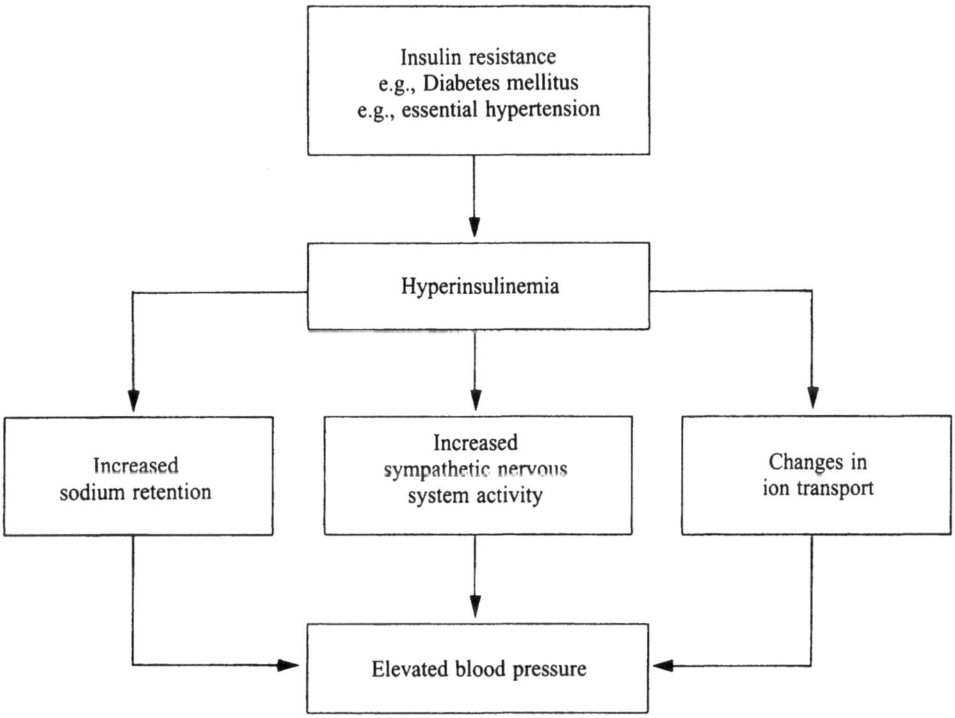

Fig. 2: Insulin resistance and hypertension [11].

According to the illustration of the etiopathogenesis of hypertension in insulin resistance with compensatory hyperinsulinemia, it could be either a combination of volume and resistance mechanisms corresponding to a systolic-diastolic or an isolated occurrence of systolic or diastolic hypertension. The current picture of hypertension in disturbed glucose tolerance results from the dysregulations and compensations of the pressoric and depressoric systems whereby the insulin resistance as the pathophysiologic primary event influences the etiology as well as the course and prognosis of the blood pressure.

5.3.4 *New demands on diagnostics*

The measurement of blood pressure is still performed for the most part conventionally, i. e. by occasional measurements in the physician's practice while seated. The diagnosis of hypertension should only be made when at least three values $\geq$ 160/95 mmHg are measured at two different appointments, whereby the precision of the readings must be within 2 mmHg. With respect to an autonomic neuropathy, in diabetics an additional measurement of the blood pressure while standing must be performed to complete the diagnosis. The patient's own blood pressure monitoring allows, in contrast to office monitoring, for a day-to-day profile of the blood pressure. The values of the patient's own measurements are lower than those from the practice, however these differences are greater in hypertensives than by normotensives.

Along with measurement of the occasional blood pressure and self-monitoring by the patients, 24-hr blood pressure profiles with automatic measurement devices have proven themselves well-suited for individualized blood pressure therapy [14]. Only devices which have been tested by the Physical-Technical Federal Agency have been licensed, e.g. Space-Labs, Medilog ABF (Oxford), Accutracker II/104 (Reynolds/Suntech), whereas the devices which measure only oscillometrically (Space-Labs 90207) are preferred. These allow for measurements in diabetics with frequent disturbances in the daily rhythm, waking hypertension and autonomic neuropathy, recognizable by the loss of the nocturnal drop in blood pressure. Figures 3a-c show three typical profiles of blood pressure in NIDDM.

As a cardiovascular risk profile with higher prevalence of the metabolic syndrome is already to be seen in the diagnosis of IGT or manifest type II diabetes, [6], all the examinations which contribute to the characterization of the insulin-resistance-syndrome are recommended for the precise planning of therapy. The parameters of the so-called "Euro-Norm" from the NIDDM Policy Group [3] represent a diagnostic process which satisfies these demands for the characterization of the metabolic situation. The determination of smoking habits and the measurement of the waist/hip ratio (WHR, men > 1; women > 0.85 correspond to the pathological findings of android obesity) would be a reasonable and necessary supplement to these control guidelines.

To assess the overall situation, it is necessary to perform a detailed history (cardiovascular diseases in the family, renal and metabolic diseases) and determine important clinical and other paraclinical findings (creatinine, electrolytes, urine findings, renal sonography, including duplex, ECG, thorax x-ray, echocardiography, funduscopy) (see Chapter 6). The exclusion of secondary hypertension should be conducted by hormone analyses with suspicion of hyperthyroidism, pheochromocytoma, Cushing Syndrome, Conn's Syndrome or acromegaly.

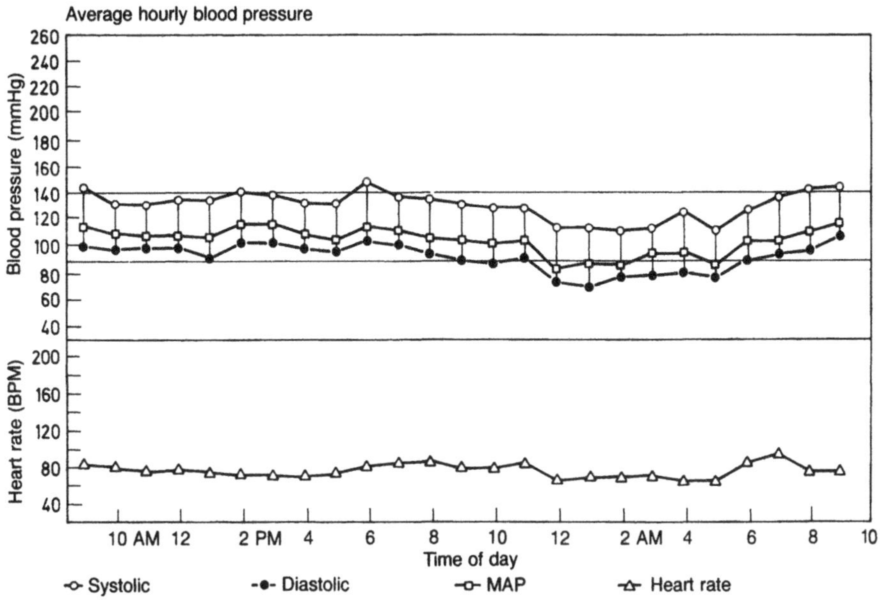

Fig. 3a: Diabetic with physiological blood pressure regulation.

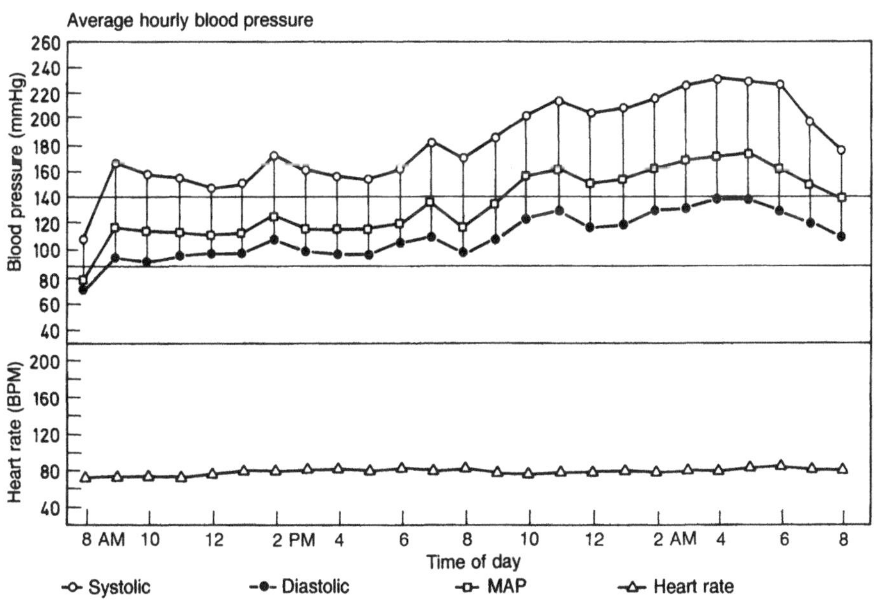

Fig. 3b: Hypertensive diabetic with nocturnal blood pressure imbalances with neuro- and nephropathies.

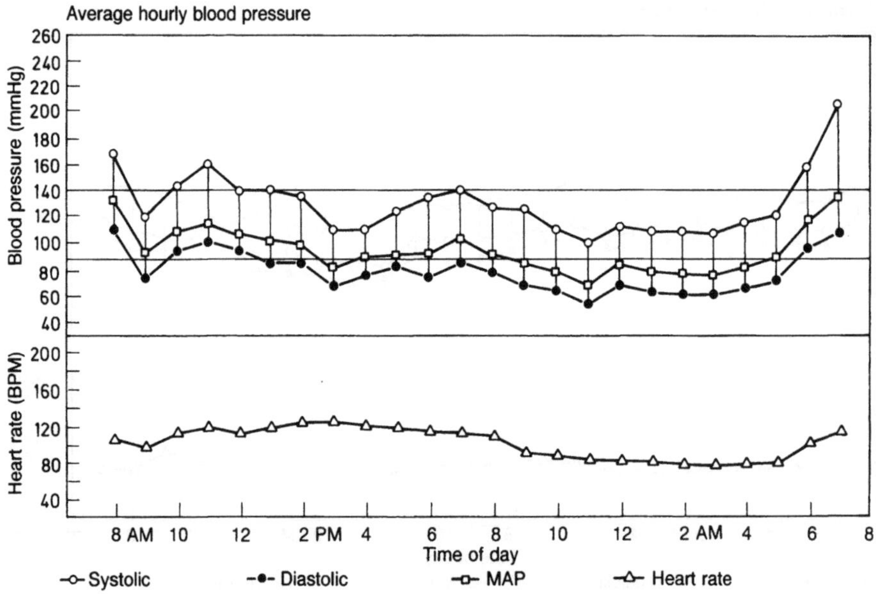

Fig. 3c: Diabetic with irregular hypertension and "waking" hypertension

The *earliest possible determination* of all the pertinent risk factors and concomitant diseases for the prognosis allows for a hypertensive treatment which is more than just lowering blood pressure.

5.3.5 *Summary*

With respect to the prognosis of the macro- and microangiopathy, there is a dangerous synergism with type II diabetes *and* hypertension. According to data from the Framingham Study, there are 5-fold the number of cardiovascular complications in hypertensive diabetics as in normotensive non-diabetics. Further studies (DIS and PROCAM, for example) demonstrate that, in the presence of multiple risks there is a potentiating influence on the coronary-heart morbidity. A genetically determined insulin resistance with various stages of disturbed insulin secretion could be established as the connecting feature between essential hypertension and type II diabetes in the last few years. Along with blood pressure profiles and a subtle check of the renal function, the diagnostic parameters of the NIDDM Policy Group could be recommended.

References

[1] Assmann, G., H. Schulte: PROCAM-Studie. Panscientia Verlag, Hedingen, Zürich 1986.

[2] Baumann, R., C. Graff: Die Vergesellschaftung des Frühstadiums der essentiellen Hypertonie mit latenten und asymptomatischen diabetischen Kohlenhydrat-Stoffwechseldefekten. Dtsch. Gesundh. wes. *34* (1968) 2390–2398.

[3] European NIDDM Policy Group: A Desktop Guide for the Management of NIDDM. IDF Bulletin *35* (1990) 9.

[4] Fontbonne, A., E. Eschwege, F. Cambien et al.: Hypertriglyceridemia as a risk factor of coronary heart disease mortality in subjects with impaired glucose tolerance or diabetes. Results from the 11-year follow-up of the Paris Prospective Study. Diabetologia *32* (1989) 300–304.

[5] Hanefeld, M., S. Fischer, H. Schmechel et al.: Diabetes Intervention Study – Multi-Intervention Trial in Newly Diagnosed NIDDM. Diabetes care *14* (1991) 308–317.

[6] Hanefeld, M., H. Haller, J. Schulze et al.: Die Diabetesinterventionsstudie (DIS) – Eine multizentrische Multiinterventionsstudie bei Typ-II-Diabetikern. I. Mitteilung Dtsch. Gesundh. wes. *39* (1984) 1889–1894.

[7] Hanefeld, M., H. Schmechel, U. Julius et al.: Five-year incidence of coronary heart disease related to major risk factors and metabolic control in newly diagnosed non-insulin-dependent diabetes – The Diabetes Intervention Study (DIS). Nutr. Metab. Cardiovasc. Dis. *1* (1991) 135–140.

[8] Janka, H. U.: Herz- und Kreislaufkrankheiten bei Diabetikern. Urban und Schwarzenberg, München – Wien – Baltimore 1986.

[9] Maranon, G.: Über Hypertonie und Zuckerkrankheit. Zentralbl. Inn. Med. *43* (1922) 169–176.

[10] Reaven, G. M.: Role of insulin resistance in human disease. Diabetes *37* (1988) 1595–1607.

[11] Simonson, D. C.: Etiology and prevalence of hypertension in diabetic patients. Diabetes Care *11* (1988) 821–827.

[12] Standl, E., H. U. Janka, H. Mehnert: Verbesserung der Lebenserwartung von Diabetikern durch Präventionsmaßnahmen. Nierenhochdruckkrankheiten *14* (1985) 310.

[13] Langhlin, K. D., P. J. Sherrard, L. Fisher: Comparison of clinic and home blood pressure levels in essential hypertension an variables associated with clinic-home differences. J. Chron. Dis. *33* (1975) 197–206.

[14] Schrader, J., G. Scholl: 24-Stunden-Blutdruckmessung, Einsatz in Diagnostik und Therapie. Akuelles Wissen Hoechst, 20–21.

[15] Uusitupa, M.: Coronary heart disease and left ventricular performance in newly diagnosed noninsulin-dependent diabetics. Publications of the university of Kuopio, (Ac. Diss.) 1983.

[16] Lithell, H., C. Berne: Diabetogenic drugs. In: C. E. Mogensen, E. Standl (eds.): Pharmacology of diabetes, 57–74. De Gruyter, Berlin, New York 1991.

[17] Middeke, M., P. Weisweiler, P. Schwandt et al.: Serum lipoproteins during antihypertensive therapy with beta blockers and diuretics: A controlled longterm comparative trial. Clin. Cardiol. *10* (1987) 94–98.

[18] Kannel, W. B.: Status of risk factors and their consideration in anti-hypertensive therapy. Am. J. cardio. *59* (1987) 80 A – 90 A.

[19] Rett, K., M. Wicklmayr, G. Dietze: Das verkannte Stoffwechselsyndrom essentielle Hypertonie – Chronologie einer interdisziplinären Meinungsänderung. Med. Klin. *86* (1991) 86–91.

[20] Schulze, J.: Typ-II-Diabetes und Hypertonie, ein gefährlicher Synergismus. Therapiewoche *42* (1992) 1542–1548.

5.4 Hyperuricemia

H.-E. Schröder

5.4.1 *Epidemiology and genetic background*

The combination of a type II diabetes with hyperuricemia is not a rare event. The Diabetes Intervention Study proved this again in recent times [1]. In contrast to a control group in which hyperuricemia, according to the selected threshold values occurred in only 3.8% of the cases, the frequency of hyperuricemia in the diabetes group was 22.5%.

In contrast, patients with primary hyperuricemia more frequently demonstrate a disturbance in carbohydrate metabolism than does the normal population [4, 7]. The prevalence of the purine metabolism disorder appears to increase with time. We found a disturbance of the glucose metabolism in 20% of the patients with hyperuricemia and 33% of the patients with gouty arthritis (duration of disease 5 – 10 years longer) [5].

It is therefore imperative that in patients with type II diabetes or with purine metabolic disorders the assumption be made that multiple disorders in latent or clinical manifestation are present [4,7]. In patients with primary hyperuricemia we have, on the basis of long-term observations, been able to determine that the individual metabolic derangements frequently appear in stages. The purine metabolic disorder occurs in puberty or in early adulthood. The second derangement is the dyslipoproteinemia or hyperlipoproteinemia, while the disorders of glucose tolerance do not occur until middle-age or older.

Which disorders occur first certainly depends upon the combination of genetic abnormalities and factors which favor the disease. The hormonal-metabolic syndrome is often a matter of polygenetic disorders with slight deviations in the protein functions which first become phenotypically apparent as a result of the factors which favor disease [6]. The genetic defect with the strongest deviation is therefore the leading symptom. The various accumulations of metabolic disorders in the specific groups investigated can at present best be explained on this basis.

5.4.2 *Pathophysiology*

Primary and secondary causes can be separated pathogenetically. In the primary forms, the regulatory cycle between uric acid formation and uric acid excretion is disturbed by congenital defects and, in the secondary forms, by overriding

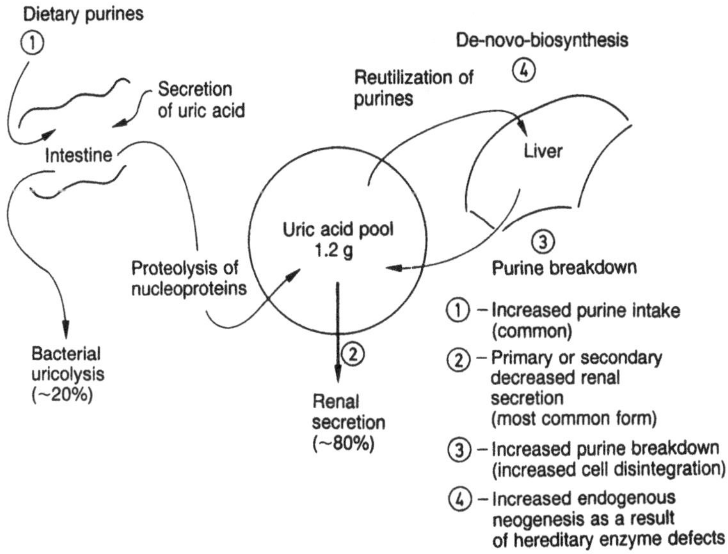

Fig. 1: Scheme of the normal uric acid metabolism and the most important disturbing factors.

diseases, or drug influences. If a primary hyperuricemia is accompanied by a secondary form, the serum uric acid values are usually very high. The uric acid excretion is 80% renal, the remainder is excreted via the intestine (fig. 1).

Hyperuricemia can be traced back to two basic forms, excessive uric acid production and renal excretion dysfunction. About 20% of primary hyperuricemias are the result of an exogenously and/or endogenously induced excess uric acid production. About 80% are due to a congenital renal excretion defect. In the renal form of hyperuricemia, a carrier for the active transport of the uric acid into the tubular lumen is either partially or completely blocked [3].

Secondary forms of hyperuricemia are also attributable to renal uric acid blockage, when the uric acid formation is greater than the maximum renal elimination or the renal uric acid excretion is directly lowered [2]. The most important causes for secondary hyperuricemia are summarized in tab. 1. In contrast to the primary forms of hyperuricemia, the uric acid concentration normalizes itself in secondary forms if the causes are eliminated.

5.4.3 Clinical picture

Hyperuricemia is first of all a biochemical disorder. Depending on the level of the serum uric acid concentration and the duration of the disorder, gout-specific organ manifestations may develop. They occur in the region of the skeletal system, most frequently in the form of acute gout attacks (fig. 2). The serious tophus forms with a destructive bone or joint gout are observed only rarely

Tab. 1: Important causes of secondary hyperuricemia

Increased formation of uric acid	Increased renal uric acid secretion
– Myeloproliferative diseases – Malignant lymphoma – Leukemia – Radiation sickness	– Chronic kidney diseases with reduction in kidney function – Isolated tubular defects – Ketoacidosis – Hyperlactacidemia – Respiratory insufficiency – Poisoning

Secondary hyperuricemia as a result of medications

Increased formation of uric acid	Increased renal uric acid secretion

– Cytostatic agents
– Fructose
– Sorbitol
– Xylite
(Cytostatic agents, Fructose, Sorbitol: Higher doses)
	– Diuretics
	  – Thiazide
	  – Loop diuretics
	– Anti-tuberculosis drugs
	  – Pyrazinamide
	  – Ethambutol
	– Cyclosporine
	– Low doses of
	  – Salicylic acids
	  – Probenicid
	  – Phenylbutazone
	– H_2 receptor blockers
	  – Cimetidine
	  – Ranitidine

nowadays thanks to improved diagnostics and therapies (fig. 3). The renal disorders are more important, because they are frequently overlooked. They express themselves in the form of proteinuria (often only intermittently detectable), urolithiasis or an impairment in renal function. A result of this disorder might be the development of hypertension. Comparable renal changes occur in diabetes (see section 5.3), so that in patients with type II diabetes and hyperuricemia, the renal function parameters must be particularly carefully monitored.

5.4.4 *Summary*

Hyperuricemia occurs more frequently in type II diabetics than in the normal population. There are, however, probably not any common genetic aberrations. Among the organ manifestations, the role of the kidneys is important in type II diabetes, because they can clearly increase the risk of hypertension.

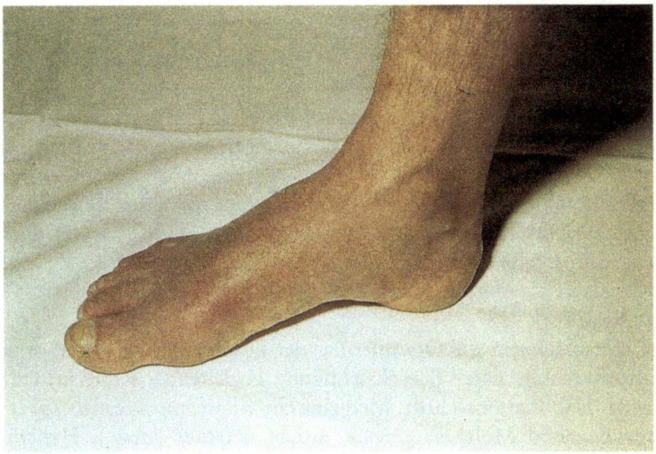

Fig. 2: Acute gout attack.

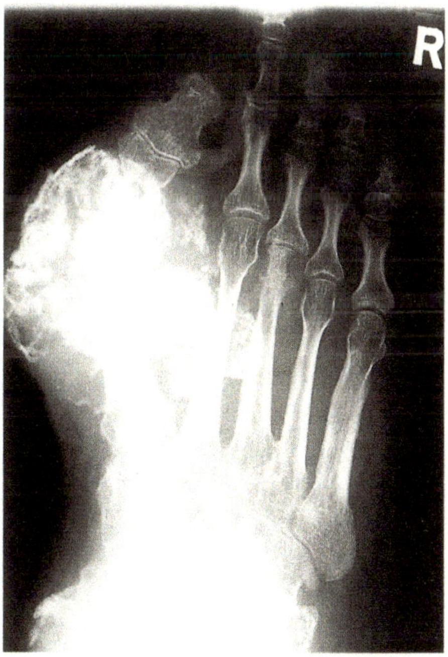

Fig. 3: Bone destruction with plaque-shaped calcifications of the metacarpals 2 and 5.

References

[1] Fischer, S., M. Hanefeld, J. Schulze et al.: Die Diabetesinterventionsstudie bei Typ-II-Diabetikern. II. Mitteilung. Z. klin. Med. *42* (1987) 127 – 137.

[2] Gröbner, W.: Sekundäre Hyperurikämie. In: N. Zöllner (Hrsg.): Hyperurikämie, Gicht und andere Störungen des Purinstoffwechsels, 234 – 252. Springer, Berlin, Heidelberg, New York 1990.

[3] Lang, F., R. Greger, H. Oberleithner et al.: Renal handling of urate in healthy man in hyperuricaemia and renal insufficiency: circadian fluctuation, effect of water diuresis and of uricosurie agents. Eur. J. Clin. Invest. *10* (1980) 285 – 292.

[4] Mertz, D. P.: Primäre Gicht als Allgemeinkrankheit. In: D. P. Mertz (Hrsg.): Gicht, 151 – 178. Thieme, Stuttgart, New York 1987.

[5] Schröder, H.-E.: Untersuchungen zur Optimierung der Diagnostik und Therapie von Störungen des Purinstoffwechsels unter Berücksichtigung begleitender Krankheiten und der Nierenfunktion. Med. Habilitationsschrift, Medizinische Akademie Dresden 1982.

[6] Schuster, H.: Vererbung und Molekulargenetik. In: N. Zöllner (Hrsg.): Hyperurikämie, Gicht und andere Störungen des Purinhaushalts, 81 – 115. Springer, Berlin, Heidelberg, New York 1990.

[7] Thiele, P.: Assoziierte Krankheiten bei Störungen des Purinstoffwechsels. In: P. Thiele, G. Heidelmann, H.-E. Schröder (Hrsg.): Hyperurikämie und Gicht, 67 – 74. Fischer, Jena 1986.

5.5 Disturbances in the coagulation and the rheology

U. Julius

5.5.1 *Disturbances in the coagulation*

Disorders in hemostasis and in blood-flow properties are important for the manifestation of micro- and macroangiopathy [2, 6]. This is especially true for type II diabetics, who are generally elderly and also present with other symptoms which also have an influence on these systems.

5.5.1.1 *Partial systems of hemostasis*

Hemostasis embodies a very complex regulated system which normally impairs the formation of thrombus in flowing blood, but can, under certain conditions, quickly cause blood coagulation.

Course of the thrombus formation in
artery:
endothelial lesion → thrombocyte adhesion and aggregation →
secondary fibrin thrombus
vein:
slower blood flow → primary fibrin thrombus
(which includes the erythrocytes)

An increased blood viscosity (e.g. in polyglobulianism) also aids the formation of thrombi in the arteries and in the veins (tab. 1).

Coagulative and fibrinolytic functions result from the interaction between the partial systems mentioned. The in vitro measureable fibrinolytic capacity is essentially determined by the relationship of tissue plasminogen activator (tPA) and plasminogen activator inhibitor (PAI). For details refer to the appropriate literature.

5.5.1.2 *Coagulation components as risk factors*

In a prospective study [3] the relationship between episodes of ischemic heart disease (IHD) and activated factor VII and the fibrinogen level proved themselves to be stronger than those of cholesterol within 5 years after the beginning of the study. Interestingly, a high-fat diet can influence factor VII activity. In other prospective studies, an interaction between fibrinogen and blood pressure with respect to coronary artery disease and apoplexy could be established. The plasma fibrinogen level represents an important and independent risk factor for myo-

Tab. 1: Subsystems contributing to hemostasis

Subsystem	Function	Essential components
– Coagulation	Formation of fibrin thrombus	Classical coagulation factors
– Inhibitors of coagulation	Suppression of coagulation	Anti-thrombin III, Protein C, Protein S, α_2 macroglobulin
– Fibrinolysis	Dissolution of a fibrin thrombus	Tissue plasminogen activator, plasminogen
– Inhibitors of fibrinolysis	Suppression of fibrinolysis	α_2 antiplasmin, α_2 macroglobulin, plasminogen activator inhibitor
– Thrombocytes	Release of mediators, aggregation, formation of thrombocyte thrombus	Factor 4, β-thromoglobulin, prostanoids
– Endothelial cellls	Release of mediators, interactions with blood cells, integrity of the vessel wall	Factor VIII-ass. antigen, prostanoids

cardial infarction. The effect of the fibrinogen level compares with the risk factors blood pressure and hypercholesterolemia.

In prospective observations, higher values for spontaneous thrombocyte aggregation, factor VIII-associated antigen and fibrinogen had a significant predictive value for new vascular occlusions and vascular death in diabetic men [7]. Elevations in factor VII-associated antigen are particularly associated with peripheral vascular diseases in diabetic women. The risk profile for cerebrovascular diseases for diabetic men includes, along with age and high blood presure, increased platelet aggregation [7].

An increased plasma fibrinogen level is closely connected with microangiopathy in diabetics [2].

Elevated fibrinogen level has been associated with many "risk factors" for deep vein thrombosis: age, adiposis, varicosities, tumors, coronary insufficiency, myocardial infarction, stroke, pregnancy, oral contraceptives, nephrotic syndrome, trauma, and operations. However, despite hyperfibrinogenemia, neither smokers nor diabetics have an increased risk of deep vein thrombosis.

5.5.1.3 Hemostasis in diabetes mellitus

It is possible that a number of type II diabetics have disturbances in all these partial systems [5, 7]. At present it is not possible to draw a conclusive picture of the pathogenetic connections or the interrelations between the partial systems.

This is also due to methodological reasons, because many of the studies only investigate partial aspects or individual components and do not consider all the possible influencing factors [5]. Beyond that, there is the fact that concentrations of a component to be measured do not necessarily reflect its activity in vivo.

It is generally accepted that the following constellation is frequently present in type II diabetics [4, 7]:

- activation of the coagulation system
- impairment of fibrinolytic capacity
- increased tendency of thrombocytes to aggregation.

Overall then there is the finding "thrombophilia" (hypercoagulability) [1].

The following factors can, in individual cases, modify the severity of the aberrations mentioned:

- age
- sex
- acute concomitant illness (e.g. bacterial infection)
- level of the hyperglycemia
- degree of the insulin deficit or hyperinsulinism
- fatty acid metabolic disorders
- concomitant (primary or secondary) hyperlipoproteinemia
- increase in lipoprotein(a)
- increased abdominal girth
- hypertension
- degree of physical activity or inactivity
- presence of atherosclerotic vascular lesions
- pharmaceutics (diuretics, anticoagulants, antirheumatics)
- genetic defects (e.g. protein C or S deficiency)
- chronic liver or renal diseases
- neoplasia, immunological diseases
- post-operative and post-traumatic conditions
- stress

This list contains the essential components of the metabolic syndrome.

5.5.1.4 Diagnostic recommendations for the practice

Not all determinable parameters permit direct therapeutic intervention. An imminent threat of thrombosis cannot be predicted with certainty by any test. A venous blockage of longer duration can have considerable influence on the data collected.

The following parameters should be measured for control of thrombophilia:

1. Quick, partial thromboplastin time
2. Thrombocyte aggregation (standardization still difficult)

3. Fibrinogen level
4. Factor VIII-associated antigen

These parameters are especially important in the presence of a vascular disease. However, they also serve for the estimation of risk in the framework of a complex investigation of a patient with metabolic syndrome.

5.5.1.5 *Summary*

The assessment of risk for macro- and microangiopathy in the type II diabetic must definitely include coagulation parameters (fibrinogen, factor VIII-associated antigen), which are relatively easy to determine. Many investigations are being conducted in this area, so it can be expected that more subtle coagulation/fibrinolytic analyses (e.g. plasminogen-activator-inhibitor activity) will soon find their way into clinical practice. The interpretation of these parameters must be performed under consideration of a number of possible influences.

References

[1] Barthels, M., H. Poliwoda: Gerinnungsanalysen. Thieme-Verlag, Stuttgart, New York 1987.
[2] Jones, S. L., C. F. Close, M. B. Mattocket et al.: Plasma lipid and coagulation factor concentrations in insulin dependent diabetics with microalbuminuria. Brit. Med. J. *298* (1989) 487–490.
[3] Meade, T. W., S. Mellows, M. Brozovic et al.: Haemostatic function and ischaemic heart disease: principal results of the Northwick Park Heart Study. Lancet *II* (1986) 533–537.
[4] Mehnert, H.: Stoffwechselkrankheiten. Thieme-Verlag, Stuttgart, New York 1990.
[5] Ostermann, H., J. van de Loo: Factors of the Hemostatic System in Diabetic Patients. Haemostasis *16* (1986) 386–416.
[6] Pyörälä, K.: Diabetes und Herzerkrankungen. In: C. E. Mogensen, E. Standl (Hrsg.): Spätkomplikationen des Diabetes mellitus, 167–186. De Gruyter, Berlin, New York 1990.
[7] Standl, E., H. Stiegler, H. U. Janka et al.: Erkrankungen zerebraler und peripherer Gefäße unter besonderer Berücksichtigung des diabetischen Fußes. In: C. E. Mogensen, E. Standl (Hrsg.): Spätkomplikationen des Diabetes mellitus, 187–220. De Gruyter, Berlin, New York 1990.
[8] Van Wersch, J. W. J., J. Rompelberg-Lahaye, F. A. Th. Lüstermans: Plasma concentration of coagulation and fibrinolysis factors and platelet function in hypertension. Eur. J. Clin. Chem. Clin. Biochem. *29* (1991) 375–379.
[9] Wysocki, M., M. Krotkiewski, M. Braide et al.: Hemorheological disturbances, metabolic parameters and blood pressure in different types of obesity. Atherosclerosis *88* (1991) 21–28.

5.5.2 *Disturbances in the rheology*

5.5.2.1 *Blood flow properties*

Blood is not a homogeneous fluid, its composition as well as vascular and circulatory parameters (e.g. vessel diameter, internal physical properties, flow rate) modify its flow behavior. Blood rheology is influenced by several determinants (fig. 1):

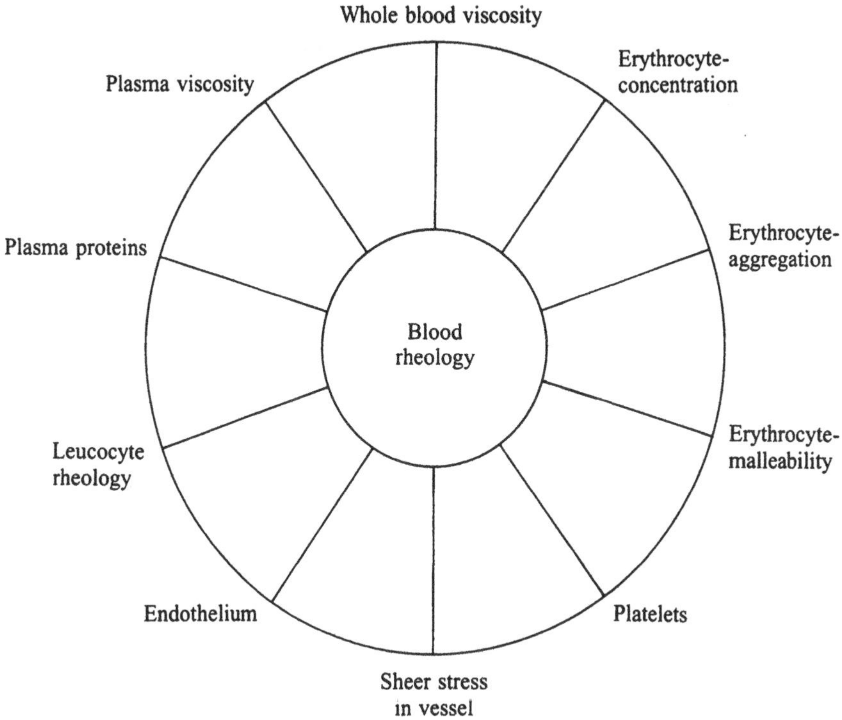

Fig. 1: The interrelations of hemorheological determinants ([1]).

The decisive parameter which goes into plasma viscosity is the fibrinogen concentration, other macromolecules, e.g. lipoproteins, also play a role to varying degrees. Adhesion and aggregation are essential functions of the platelets. The flow in larger vessels is influenced by the total viscosity of the blood, the microcirculation on the other hand mainly by the plasma viscosity and the erythrocyte properties. The interactions between blood components, plasma flow and vascular properties are detectable at the capillary-microscopic level.

A hyperinsulinism with android obesity can apparently negatively influence the malleability of the erythrocytes [6].

5.5.2.2 *Rheological particularities with diabetes mellitus*

Diabetics have rheological particularities which above all can be attributed to an increased plasma viscosity (elevated fibrinogen) and an increased erythrocyte aggregation (also as a possible result of elevated fibrinogen [5]) [2, 3, 4]. The severity of the hyperglycemia is of importance for the blood flow properties; the highest blood viscosity is measured in diabetic coma (also as a result of the dehydration).

Microcirculatory disorders are coupled with blood flow abnormalities. The distension of the capillaries in diabetic late-syndrome leads to stasis, which, among other things allows for interaction between blood cells and endothelial cells. Such interactions have also been observed in microaneurysms. Changes of rheological parameters were measured in the presence of a macroangiopathy or a myocardial infarction, the classification of which as primary or secondary is not possible in the individual case [1,4]. It is conceivable that in these cases previously impaired circulatory reserves will be further limited by a worsening of the blood's flow properties.

Comparable to the coagulation disorders, a number of additional factors lead to changes in the blood rheology. Among other factors, smoking may contribute to the increase in the erythrocyte count, without influencing the plasma volume. Long-term physical exercise has very definite positive effects on blood flow properties.

5.5.2.3 *Diagnostic recommendations for the practice*

Two parameters of basic prognostic importance can be measured everywhere:

1. Hematocrit
2. Fibrinogen concentration

Elevated hematocrit or hemoglobin concentrations proved themselves to be indicators of increased stroke risk in the Framingham Study. The prognostic importance of the fibrinogen concentration was already mentioned in the discussion of the coagulation system.

There are relatively simple procedures for the determination of the plasma viscosity. Other, very interesting parameters from the pathophysiological perspective have not been sufficiently standardized and are still reserved for special laboratories.

5.5.2.4 *Summary*

Two primary factors (hematocrit and fibrinogen), which decide the rheological properties of the blood, can be determined by means of simple procedures. Blood flow properties are important for the therapy of individual patients in that, in cases where ischemia (change of the vessel wall) is present, tissue necrosis may be directly connected with a worsening of the rheological situation.

References

[1] Dormandy, J. A.: Cardiovascular diseases. In: S. Chien, J. Dormandy, E. Ernst et al. (eds.): Clinical Hemorheology, 165 – 194. Martinus Nijhoff Publishers, Dordrecht, Boston, Lancaster 1987.

[2] Janka, H. U.: Epidemiologie und klinische Bedeutung diabetischer Spätkomplikationen bei Typ-II-(nicht-insulinabhängigem) Diabetes mellitus. In: C. E. Mogensen, E. Standl (Hrsg.): Spätkomplikationen des Diabetes mellitus, 33 – 45. De Gruyter, Berlin, New York 1990.

[3] Koenig, W.: Hämorheologische Parameter und kardiovaskuläres Risiko. Münch. med. Wschr. *130* (1988) 867 – 870.

[4] Leschke, M., B. E. Strauer: Die Bedeutung rheologischer Mechanismen in der Atherogenese. Arzneimittel-Forschung *40* (1990) 356 – 362.

[5] Lowe, G. D. O.: Thrombosis and hemorheology. In: S. Chien, J. Dormandy, E. Ernst et al. (eds.): Clinical Hemorheology, 195 – 226. Martinus Nijhoff Publishers, Dordrecht, Boston, Lancaster 1987.

[6] Wysocki, M., W. Krotkiewski, M. Braide et al.: Hemorheological disturbances, metabolic parameters and blood pressure in different types of obesity. Atherosclerosis *88* (1991) 21 – 28.

5.6 Disturbances in the liver and biliary system

M. Hanefeld

5.6.1 Liver diseases

The most prominent and frequent change of the liver in the course of the metabolic syndrome in NIDDM is the fatty liver (tab. 1) [4]. Knick [5] pointed out the close association of steatosis hepatica and disturbances in carbohydrate tolerance in the late 1960's. At the same time as Beringer [1] we were able to prove that fatty liver in diabetes is not a separate disease, but rather a symptom of the disturbance in carbohydrate-lipid metabolism [3] (fig. 1). The triglyceride content of the liver is therefore above all a function of the concentration of free fatty acids in the blood. These findings, obtained more than 20 years ago, have been confirmed by the investigations of Björntorp et al. [2] with respect to the role of abdominal obesity in the pathogenesis of insulin resistance. This also corresponds with the importance of steatosis hepatica as an early symptom of diabetes, as is obvious from the examination of blood donors in whom a liver biopsy was performed to clarify elevated transaminases; the histological diagnosis resulting in a fatty liver (tab. 2). Every cryptogenic steatosis hepatica, which can be easily detected by sonogram, should therefore justify a gentle diagnostic

Tab. 1: Prevalence of fatty liver in diabetes, primarily NIDDM [3]

Authors	Number of diabetics	Fatty liver n	Fatty liver %
Robbers et al. (1968)	171	120	70
Leevy et al. (1952)	30	7	21
Kalk (1959)	102	49	48
Creutzfeldt (1959)	40	24	60
Tiszai et al. (1960)	68	34	50
Domenici (1963)	122	55	46.7
Kautzsch (1963)	60	17	28
Zschoch and Mohnicke (1963)	51	20	40
Dobrzanski (1963)	40	12	30
Rostlapil and Zrustova (1968)	100	47	47
Takac et al. (1965)	165	43	26
Thaler (1966)	396	185	46.7
Thoms (1966)	52	29	55
Haller et al. (1967)	161	79	49
Beringer et al. (1968)	100	58	58
Totals	1658	779	47

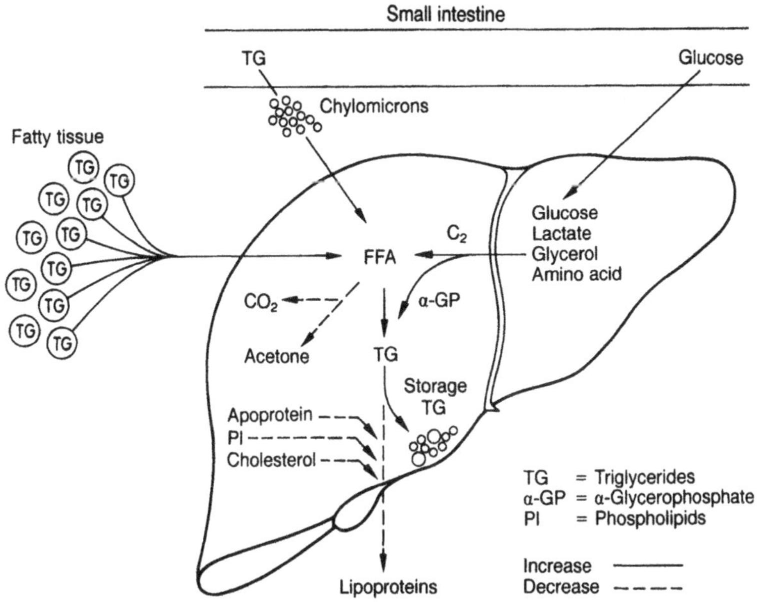

Fig. 1: Fatty liver as a problem of balance of complex metabolic processes [4].

Tab. 2: Analysis of etiological factors of fatty liver in 70 blood donors (ALAT 2 × > 2.5 μmol/l) [4]

Probable cause	n	%
Obesity (Broca ≥ 1.1)	24	35
Subclinical diabetes	17	24
Hyperlipoproteinemia*)	16	23
Manifest diabetes	10	14
Alcohol abuse	1	1
Unclear	2	3
Combined causes		
Diabetes and obesity	14	20
Hyperlipoproteinemia and obesity	13	19
Diabetes mellitus and hyperlipoproteinemia	0	0
Diabetes, hyperlipoproteinemia and obesity	11	16
Diabetes, hyperlipoproteinemia, obesity and alcohol	1	1

*) Hyperlipoproteinemia was assumed to be the primary cause with triglycerides ≥ 2.9 mmol/l and cholesterol ≥ 7.8 mmol/l.

search for diabetes or a lipid disorder. To what extent the fat deposition in the liver itself contributes to the insulin resistance is unknown. It is more likely that this only indirectly paves the path for chronic liver damage.

NIDDM is also accompanied by more frequent liver cirrhosis. In the DIS, the number of diabetic patients with liver cirrhosis was 7%.

Although clinically manifested liver cirrhosis was not included in the study, cirrhosis was the second most frequent cause of death in the first five years after the diagnosis. The number of reports is growing wherein hepatic diseases are gaining in importance for diabetic morbidity and mortality. There are in principle two possible scenarios for this:

1. Hepatic diseases, in particular fatty liver and liver cirrhosis increase insulin resistance and therefore the risk of NIDDM manifestation.

2. Diabetics do not metabolize alcohol and its toxic components well. The fatty liver, typical for diabetics, contributes to this effect. Liver cirrhosis therefore occurs more frequently with the same level of alcohol consumption. There is considerable evidence that these two processes negatively effect each other.

5.6.2 Gallstones and cholecystitis

Patients with NIDDM exhibit an increased risk of gallstones, because they are usually obese and frequently suffer anomalies of lipoprotein metabolism. A lithogenic bile results in both cases. In addition, the autonomic neuropathy may lead to delayed emptying of the gall bladder. This and the lower resistance to infection with increased tendency to pathogenic ascension of bacteria as a result of gastrointestinal motility disorders, favor the development of infectious processes in the gall bladder and the biliary tract.

5.6.3 Summary

Hepatic and biliary diseases occur more frequently in persons with NIDDM. The fatty liver and cholesterol stones are a partial aspect of the metabolic syndrome. Cryptogenic liver steatosis is an early symptom of diabetes. Liver cirrhosis increases the insulin resistance. Alcohol tolerance is on the other hand decreased with NIDDM, so that liver cirrhosis occurs more frequently and more severely.

References

[1] Beringer, A., H. Thaler: Zusammenhänge zwischen Diabetes und Fettleber. Dt. med. Wochenschr. 95 (1970) 836–840.

[2] Björntorp, P.: Obesity and diabetes. In: K. G. M. M. Alberti, L. P. Krall (eds.): The diabetes annual/5, 373–395. Elsevier, New York 1990.

[3] Hanefeld, M.: Untersuchungen zur Fettleberproblematik unter besonderer Berücksichtigung metabolischer Gesichtspunkte. Med. Habilitationsschrift, Medizinische Akademie Dresden 1973.

[4] Hanefeld, M.: Fettleber. In: H. Haller, M. Hanefeld, W. Jaroß (Hrsg.): Lipidstoffwechselstörungen. Diagnostik, Klinik und Therapie, 297–304. Fischer Verlag, Jena 1983.

[5] Knick, B., H.-J. Lange, K. Heckmann: Korrelationen zwischen latent-diabetischer Stoffwechsellage, Adipositas und Steatosis hepatis. Dtsch. med. Wschr. 90 (29) (1965) 1286–1289.

6 Diagnostics

6.1 Clinical diagnostics

J. Schulze

The diagnosis of diabetes mellitus can be made by means of detailed history-taking, clinical examination and simple paraclinical findings. It has proved practical to distinguish between

- detection methods and
- methods for evaluating the course

in the diagnostic measures.

Regular screening or check-ups are very important for determining the risk bearer > 35 years of age, because organ-pathological findings are detected in a great number at the time of diagnosis of a bland type II diabetes (tab. 1), [1].

Tab. 1: Important clinical findings in newly detected, diet-controllable type II diabetics (frequency in%) [1]

– Hepatomegaly		33%
– Xanthomas		4%
– Achilles tendon reflexes absent		7%
– CAD* (resting ECG) (n = 1126)	men	8.9%
	women	21.6%
– CAD* (ergometry) (n = 796)	men	14.6%
	women	32.0%
– Left ventricular hypertrophy (X-ray of thorax)		4.2%
– Pulmonary congestion (X-ray of thorax)		0.4%

* CAD = Coronary artery disease

Diagnosis, treatment and consultation of diabetics should be understood to be a life-long "close-to-home rehabilitation", whereby the majority of patients will be cared for by their general practitioners. Patients with diabetic complications and problem cases should be treated in "specialized" practices with trained internists, working closely with ophthalmologists, nephrologists, cardiologists, neurologists, gynecologists, and stomatologists. A prerequisite for a successful patient-physician relationship is the trusting partnership-like cooperation in the consulting team with the objective of encouraging and assisting the patient in self-monitoring of the metabolism. After thorough training and instruction, the patient is in the position to continually assess important metabolic parameters and bodily functions and if necessary, correct them (section 6.2):

- general condition
- body weight
- metabolic state (blood glucose and possibly urinary glucose)
- blood pressure, pulse
- skin assessment.

The medical monitoring consists of a thorough initial investigation and repeated determinations of clinical status every 1–2 years to be able to detect secondary or concomitant illness promptly (tab. 2). For more detailed clarification and improved assessment, a series of modern medical-technical possibilities have joined the standard examination procedures in the last few years, possibilities which allow for earlier and more differentiated treatment measures (tab. 3).

Tab. 2: Where should attention be paid in the clinical examination?

Head:	Rubeosis, hyperostosis, hirsutism in women, xanthelasmas,
Throat:	Struma, carotid bruits
Thorax:	Dry skin, furuncle, sebaceous gland abscess
Abdomen:	Hepatomegaly, positive Murphy sign, android obesity (WHR), costovertebral angle tenderness, bladder filling
Extremities:	Sensory neuropathy with decreased temperature perception and deep tendon reflexes, trophic disorders, possibly mycoses, lowered/absent foot pulse

Tab. 3: Physical examinations for NIDDM (once yearly)

Ocular fundus:	Ophthalmoscopy, if necessary fluorescence angiography, fundus photography
Kidney morphology:	Sonography possibly CT, cave i.v. pyelography
Nerve function:	Autonomic neuropathy tests: heart rate measurement with Valsalva and inhalation and exhalation. BP measurement while lying, sitting, standing
Vascular status:	Doppler sonography, if necessary digital subtraction angiography
Feet:	Tuning fork test, velocity of nerve conduction and possibly pedography
Heart and circulatory function:	ECG, ergometry, 24-hour profile of BP and ECG
Lung evaluation:	Chest X-ray, pulmonary function test

BP = Blood pressure

Summary

The clinical diagnostics for early detection of the diabetic metabolic state is very important with respect to the frequency of complications and excess mortality. Along with the detection of individuals who are endangered by either genetic or environmental factors, metabolic diseases should be diagnosed to a greater degree in the course of screening or check-ups by family doctors or company physicians.

References

[1] Fischer, S., M. Hanefeld, J. Schulze et al.: Die Diabetesinterventionsstudie (DIS), eine multizentrische Multiinterventionsstudie bei Typ-II-Diabetikern, 2. Mitteilung. Z. Klin. Med. 42 (1987) 1613–1616.

6.2 Laboratory diagnostics and self-monitoring

M. Weck

In any discussion of the diagnostic criteria of NIDDM a distinction must be made between those which are suited for (routine) tests for detecting and classification of diabetic subjects and those which appear necessary for the course and therapeutic control.

6.2.1 Blood glucose

Diabetes mellitus must be diagnosed if the fasting blood glucose (FBG) is over 6.7 mmol/l (120 mg/dl) in more than one assay and/or the blood glucose is found to be above 11.1 mmol/l (200 mg/dl) two hours after a 75 g glucose load (tab. 1).

Tab. 1: Diagnostic criteria for the diagnosis of diabetes mellitus (capillary blood)

	Fasting BG mg/dl mmol/l	BG 2 hours after glucose load (75 g oGTT) mg/dl mmo//l
Diabetes mellitus	≥120 ≥6.7	≥ 200 ≥ 11.1
Impaired glucose tolerance	> 100 < 120 > 5.6 < 6.7	> 140 < 200 > 7.8 < 11.1
No diabetes	< 100 < 5.6	< 140 < 7.8

BG = Blood glucose

The fasting blood glucose of healthy subjects is between 3.3 and 5.6 mmol/l (60 and 100 mg/dl). These values are valid for capillary whole blood, which is generally employed for blood glucose determinations, especially in the case of self-monitoring. If venous blood is examined the blood glucose is always a bit lower, meaning that the interpretation may be particularly difficult, especially in the threshold range. Even the interpretation of an apparently simple laboratory value such as fasting blood glucose requires care. At this point it should be mentioned that the maintenance of the fasting conditions is of the utmost importance (the patient should fast for 10 to 16 hours). A normal fasting blood glucose does not necessarily guarantee normal values in the oral Glucose Tolerance Test (oGTT). Because the diagnosis diabetes mellitus has far-reaching consequences for the patient, extreme caution is absolutely necessary in the diagnosis. Blood glucose values, which are not clear or are threshold values, require an oGTT. In assessing the fasting blood glucose attention must be paid, as in the oGTT, to intercurrent diseases, nutritional status and influences of drug therapy.

The assessment criteria for the diagnosis "diabetes mellitus" are summarized in table 1. The conversion factor from mmol/l to mg/dl is 18 and should be well known in a country and continent which currently has two different systems of measurement. In case of doubt it has been proven wise to perform an oral Glucose Tolerance Test, using the WHO recommendations of 75 g glucose. The following conditions should be maintained so as to make the oGTT, with its poor reproducibility, as standardized as possible:

- three-day carbohydrate-rich diet: no oGTT following a hunger period!
- a definitive Diabetes mellitus, diagnosed from the fasting and postprandial blood glucose measurements, need not be "guaranteed" by means of an oGTT; the patients will more likely only be endangered by massive hyperglycemia
- no oGTT with acute illness
- beware of falsification of the test results through medication (glucocorticoids, diuretics, ß-blockers, etc.)
- no excessive physical activity beforehand.

Procedure: fasting blood glucose sample is drawn. The patient then drinks 75 g glucose, dissolved in 250 – 300 ml water or tea. The glucose should be consumed within 5 minutes. The second blood sample is taken two hours later.

In addition, the blood glucose is often determined at other times (30, 60 minutes). This is not necessary for the diagnosis, but may serve to substantiate it. The blood glucose assay in oGTT should always be conducted by normal laboratory methods and not with test strips. Table 2a shows the constellation of the possible oGTT results [4].

Somewhat different guidelines with respect to the diagnosis and evaluation of the oGTT are used during pregnancy and in the detection of gestational diabetes. These are shown in table 2b.

Not only the fasting blood glucose values should be used for the follow-up examinations of the glycemic status, but also the pre- and postprandial values, i. e. 0.5 hours before and 1 – 2 hours after meals.

Blood glucose self-monitoring has become an essential component of metabolic control for many highly motivated diabetics, and NIDDM patients as well. Such monitoring also allows these patients to detect blood glucose imbalances and a worsening tendency of the metabolic status at an early stage.

Tab. 2a: Classification criteria for the test results of the oGTT (Bibergeil [4])

	Capillary BG concentration (mmol/l) during a 75 oGTT			
	0 min	30–90 min	120 min	
Normal GT	<5.6	<11.1	<7.8	
Non-classifiable GT (NC GT)	5.6–6.6	<11.1	<7.8	
	≥6.7	<11.1	<7.8	
	<5.6	≥11.1	<7.8	
	5.6–6.6	≥11.1	<7.8	R_1
	≥6.7	≥11.1	<7.8	R_1
Impaired Glucose Tolerance (IGT)	<5.6	<11.1	7.8–11.0	
	<5.6	≥11.1	7.8–11.0	
	5.6–6.6	<11.1	7.8–11.0	
	5.6–6.6	≥11.1	7.8–11.0	
	≥6.7	<11.1	7.8–11.0	R_1
	≥6.7	≥11.1	7.8–11.0	R_1
Diabetes mellitus	<5.6	<11.1	≥11.1	R_2
	5.6–6.6	<11.1	≥11.1	R_2
	≥6.7	<11.1	≥11.1	R_2
	<5.6	≥11.1	≥11.1	R_2
	5.6–6.6	≥11.1	≥11.1	R_2
	≥6.7	≥11.1	≥11.1	

BG = blood glucose
GT = glucose tolerance
R_1 = test repetition in the near future due to the risk of progression to diabetes
R_2 = test repetition within a short period of time to confirm the diagnosis of diabetes; classification according to the 2nd oGTT results

We recommend the Haemoglucotest 20–800R (Boehringer-Mannheim) or Glucostix strips (Bayer Diagnostica) to our patients. The blood required for the sugar determination is best drawn with the aid of a very small caliber needle by the patient him/herself from the side of the finger pad, because this region is relatively pain-free. Many diabetics who are afraid of the pinprick use pricking devices (Autoclix, Autolet, Autolance). The physician should examine the finger pad during outpatient visits so as to ensure that the blood samples are being properly taken.

The proper use of the test strips is of primary importance. When using the Haemoglucotest the blood should be wiped with a swab. With Glucostix on the other hand the blood should be dabbed. The ExacTech device (MedSense) measures blood glucose (capillary) within 30 seconds. The advantage is the quickness of the measurement. The lack of an optical control is, however, a great

Tab. 2b: Diagnostic procedure for suspicion of gestational diabetes (Lowy [12])

All pregnant women screening in the 28th week of pregnancy	High risk patients screening at the first examination and in the 28th week of pregnancy
FBG > 6mmol/l (108 mg/dl) and/or BG > 8mmol/l (148 mg/dl) 1 hour after 75 g oral glucose	– Obesity – Excessive weight gain during the pregnancy – Fetal macrosomia – Hydramnion – Glucosuria – Previous gestational diabetes – Diabetic first-degree relatives

75 g oGTT

FBG > 5.2 mmol/l (94 mg/dl)
2 hour BG > 9mmol/l (162 mg/dl)

Gestational diabetes

BG = blood glucose
FBG = fasting blood glucose

disadvantage. It is particularly important to explain the use of the test strips to the patient at the beginning. The physician should also be skilled in the method and ensure that the personnel in the practice are well-trained and able to explain the method properly.

Self-monitoring of the blood glucose in stable NIDDM patients should be performed at least twice weekly, fasting and postprandial. Situations which lead to or predispose to acute metabolic deterioration demand frequent controls. When changing to an additional insulin or insulin monotherapy, a blood glucose daily profile per week will also be required (tab. 3).

In general, the visual semi-quantitative blood glucose assessment by means of color comparison of test strips and comparator is sufficient. For certain patients (defective color vision, visual impairments, particularly motivated patients) additional measurements and digital display by means of a blood measurement device have proven themselves helpful (Reflolux, Glucometer II, ExacTech, among others).

Tab. 3: Frequency of self-monitoring in NIDDM

Type of monitoring	Body weight	UG	BG	AC
Type of treatment				
Diet alone	1 – 3 x wk	3 x wk pp	–	–
OHA	1 – 2 x wk	3 x wk pp	2 x wk fs + pp	upon worsening
Insulin in combination with OHA or fixed dosis	1 x wk	3 x wk fs	2 x fs 1 x 5 pt. monitoring	upon complica- tions

OHA = oral hypoglycemic agents
wk = weekly
fs = fasting
pp = postprandial
UG = urine glucose
BG = blood glucose
AC = acetone
5 point monitoring = mornings fasting, before all 3 main meals, 9:00 PM

6.2.2 *Urinary glucose*

As soon as the blood glucose values reach 8.9 to 10.0 mmol/l (160 to 180 mg/dl), glucose is excreted from the kidneys into the urine. This limit value, which may differ greatly between individuals, is called the kidney threshold. An elevated kidney threshold with a failure to excrete glucose is frequently found in elderly type II diabetics or patients with nephropathy. On the other hand, a reduced kidney threshold, i. e. glucose detected in the urine with normal blood glucose, may also be found. For this reason, some authors have completely abandoned blood glucose measurements for diabetes diagnostics. *But*: the individual kidney threshold can be determined if glucose is measured a number of times in the blood and fresh urine. Then blood glucose monitoring as a follow-up examination and treatment check of the NIDDM makes sense, because it is so simple.

A distinction is made between urinary glucose determination in fresh urine (also called spot urine), the spontaneous urine and the 24-hr urine. Only fresh urine is suitable for drawing conclusions about the current blood glucose situation. If, for example, the metabolic situation is to be checked one hour before or after a meal, the patient should empty his/her bladder 15 – 30 minutes before the actual check is made, drink about ¼ l of fluid, empty the bladder for the examination and the urinary glucose is measured by means of test strips.

Various test strips are offered for urinary glucose determinations: Glukotest, Clinitest, Clinistix, Diastix or Diabur 5000. As the attending physician in either the practice or the clinic, it is necessary to assure that the patient is not offered the entire spectrum of strips, but rather a single test strip should be recommended for the purpose of improved comparability and reproducibility.

If the metabolism is well-adjusted and the kidney threshold is normal, the postprandial urine should be free of glucose. With poor metabolic control, especially with an infection, a positive urinary glucose can be helpful, diagnostically speaking.

The spontaneous urine usually consists of a period of three to four hours, whereby glucose excretion over a period of several hours, for example following a meal, can be determined. The total glucose excretion during a day can be determined from the 24-hr urine, but not the time of the peak blood glucose. This is more readily determined from partial portions.

6.2.3 Ketone bodies

If a urinary glucose test offers positive results, an examination of the urine for ketone bodies should be conducted to assess the extent of the metabolic disorder. Ketone bodies occur with increased lipolysis: acetoacetate acid, ß-hydroxybutyrate and acetone. Ketone bodies are excreted more frequently with ketosis or ketoacidosis and can indicate the threat of a coma. There are also a number of test strips available for detecting acetone (Ketur, Keto-diabur 5000, Ketostix, Ketodiastic, Acetest).

6.2.4 Hemoglobin A_1 – glycosylated hemoglobin

The name "glycosylated" hemoglobin refers to a number of hemoglobin variations which occur as a result of the binding of glucose or glucose metabolic products to the adult hemoglobulin (HbA_0). These variations – HbA_{1a}, HbA_{1b}, HbA_{1c} – are also collected under the term HbA_1. The glucose molecule is attached to the N-terminals valie portion of the B-chain of the hemoglobin by means of an aldimine bond (Schiff's base). A stable irreversible ketoamine results from a so-called Amadori-conversion (fig. 1).

The level of the glycosylated hemoglobin (either HbA_1 or HbA_{1c}) reflects the integrated blood glucose course over a period of about half the life of the erythrocyte (about 4–6–8 weeks). Vice versa a significant drop in glycosylated hemoglobin in poorly adjusted diabetics should only be expected about 4 weeks after the improvement of the glycemia, at the earliest.

The measurement of HbA_{1c} is therefore a good control parameter for metabolic adjustment, but not for the diagnosis of diabetes. The HbA_{1c} represents about 4–6% of the total hemoglobin in normal blood glucose concentrations. Thus the HbA_{1c} value nowadays should be a part of every diabetic check-up, because

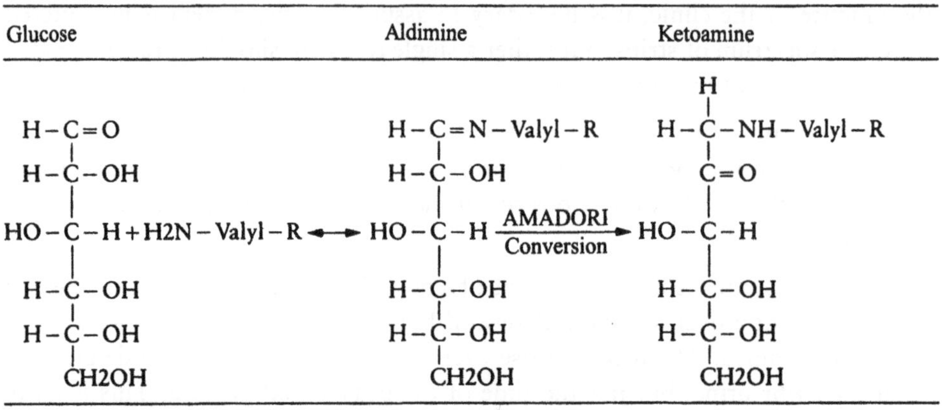

Fig. 1: Glycosylation of hemoglobin: reaction between glucose and the amino terminal valine of the hemaglobin b chain with the intermediate product aldimine.

it is the criterion for quality of the metabolic adjustment. The value for every patient can be entered on the "HbA_1 ruler" and the quality of the metabolic adjustment made visible (fig. 2). It is therefore recommended to perform a determination of the glycosylated hemoglobin every 3 to 4 months fo NIDDM patients as well. The determination of the HbA_{1c} should be given preference over the HbA_1 as a result of its higher specificity.

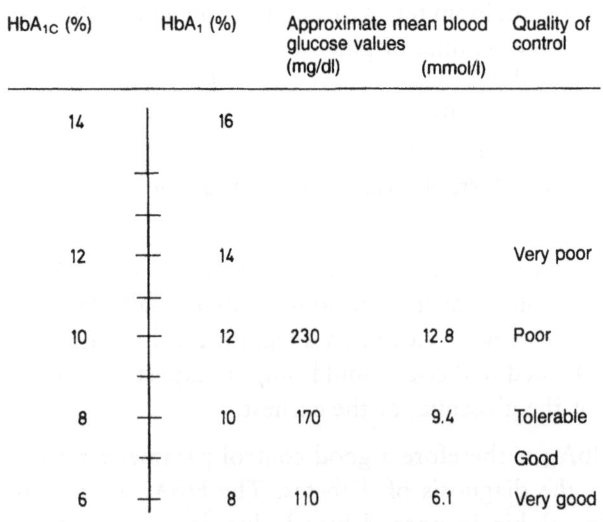

Fig. 2: The HbA_{1c} measurement. HbA_{1c} (HbA_1) and the quality of metabolic control.

The following factors may influence the HbA_1 values:

- Acute and chronic blood loss reduces the erythrocyte life span and thereby that of glycosylated hemoglobin. Caution is therefore recommended with iron deficiency anemia, gastrointestinal bleeding, hemochromatosis, hemolysis, etc.!
- With chronic renal insufficiency the glycosylated hemoglobin can, on the one hand, be subjected to a carbonylation (increased HbA_1 values) or, as already mentioned, lead to reduced HbA_1 values through hemolysis and gastrointestinal blood loss.
- The certainly rare hemoglobinopathies of course also influence the HbA_1.

There are problems with clear discrepancies between the other parameters of glycemic control (above all the blood glucose data, especially the self-determined blood glucose values) and the glycosylated hemoglobin. Assuming that the HbA_1 test procedure is precise and the possibilities of error have been considered, the HbA_1 value can be viewed as the valid index of the glycemic state.

6.2.5 *Glycosylated albumin and serum proteins*

Like hemoglobin, albumin and other serum proteins have amino acid residues which are predisposed to glycosylation. The in vivo glycosylation of albumin is responsible for about 90% of the glycosylation of the total serum protein. As a result of the short half-life of the serum protein, the measurement of the glycosylated proteins reflects the integrated course of the glycemia over a much shorter time than with HbA_1 (7–14 days). This opens up the possibility of making therapeutic influences more quickly apparent and controllable than is possible with glycosylated hemoglobin.

The fructosamine test uses the ability of ketoamines to act as a reduction medium in alkaline solutions. This method is simple, fast and easily reproduced. The strong influence of fluctuations in serum protein levels is a disadvantage.

6.2.6 *Serum insulin and C-peptide*

Insulin and C-peptide are generally detected by means of radioimmunoassays or enzyme immunoassays. Both methods are reserved for diagnostically difficult cases. Knowledge of the physiology of insulin secretion and degradation is necessary for the assessment of insulin and C-peptide levels. The so-called "Starling Curve" of the pancreas deserves special note in this context. According to this, insulin levels of the same degree in diabetics are possible in early stages of NIDDM with still compensatorily elevated insulin secretion as in a later stage with previously exhausted insulin secretion (see Chapter 2). The connecting peptide (C-peptide, human C-peptide, HCP) is secreted along with proinsulin from the B-cells of the pancreas as connective element between the A and B chain of the proinsulin and is excreted, almost unchanged, via the kidney (fig. 3). HCP is therefore a marker of the insulin secretion.

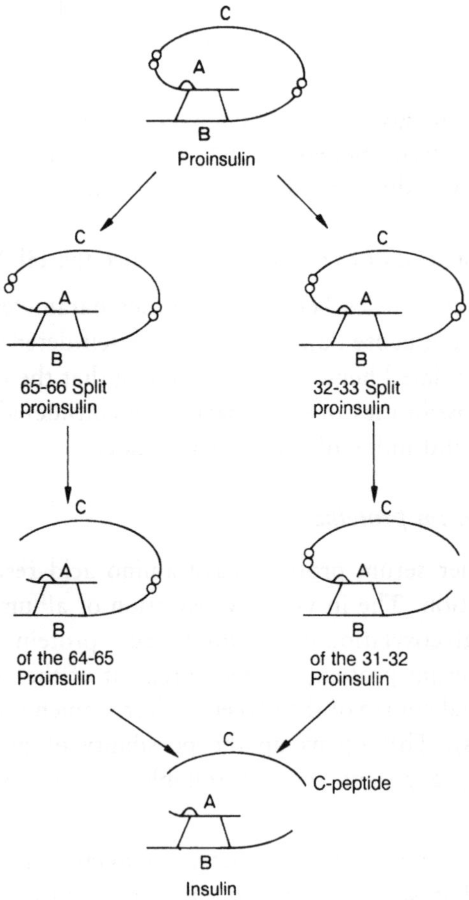

Fig. 3: From proinsulin to insulin.

By contrast, insulin is partially metabolized in the liver and it may be dependent, among other things, on the number and affinity of the insulin receptors which reduce or increase the hepatic clearance of the hormone. Hyperinsulinemia in the peripheral blood results. This makes it clear that elevated insulin values in serum do not allow for any conclusions to be drawn about the secretion of the pancreas.

The C-peptide can be detected in serum and urine. C-peptide urine excretion correlates well with the integrated plasma C-peptide level, but the excretion exhibits a high level of inter- and intra-individual variability. For these reasons the measurement of the C-peptide excretion in urine is considered a less precise marker of B-cell function. The C-peptide can be detected in serum under both fasting and stimulatory conditions. The fasting C-peptide shows a "soft" correlation to the blood glucose and an inverse correlation to the creatinine clearance. C-peptide values should therefore be interpreted with caution in cases of disturbed renal function.

The C-peptide determination has still not been standardized internationally, so comparisons with literature should only be made as proviso. The C-peptide measurements after a standard meal or glucose stimulation are valid for the B-cell function test. The maximum C-peptide secretion is reached about 60–90 minutes after a test meal, already about 6 minutes after i.v. administration of glucagon.

Procedure: Administration of 1 mg glucagon i.v. while fasting, obtain blood sample 6 minutes later for C-peptide determination. This so-called postglucagon C-peptide is considered the most certain discriminator between IDDM and NIDDM. The absolute lack of C-peptide is considered to be a definitive indicator of unstable IDDM. A serum C-peptide < 0.32 nmol/l indicates, with a 90% specificity, IDDM and a C-peptide > 1.1 nmol/l indicates, with 90% specificity, NIDDM (tab. 4), [8]. The exact classification of C-peptide data and especially the comparison of such values between different patients, as well as before and after therapeutic manipulation is only permitted with the same blood glucose ratios!

Tab. 4: Discrimination between NIDDM and IDDM on the basis of postglucagon C-peptides

		Serum C peptide postglucagon
0	0,32	1,1
With 90% specificity IDDM	Threshold range, classification not safely possible	With 90% specificity NIDDM

Making therapeutic decisions only on the basis of a C-peptide value can lead to grave treatment errors. The clinical picture and the specific stage of NIDDM must always be part of the calculation (tab. 5).

6.2.7 *Protein excretion in the urine*

6.2.7.1 *Control of microalbuminuria*

The kidney damage in diabetes is not only a consequence of diabetic nephropathy, but is usually caused by a combination of glomerulosclerosis in renal vessels and pyelonephritis. The frequency and severity of nephropathy correlate with the

Tab. 5: Typical case studies of the classification of NIDDM employing clinical data and C-peptide

Case A
58-year old male, BMI 31 kg/m^2, duration of diabetes 3 years, HbA_{1c} 10.3%, fasting blood glucose 210 mg/dl (11.7 mmol/l), postglucagon C-peptide 1.9 nmol/l, previous therapy : "diet".

Diagnosis: NIDDM with suspected, clear insulin resistance, clearly still in the phase of compensatory hyperinsulinemia with only short duration of diabetes.

Therapy: Weight reduction

Case B
61-year old female, BMI 29 kg/m^2, duration of diabetes 11 years, HbA_{1c} 11.2%, fasting blood glucose 260 mg/dl (14.4 mmol/l), postglucagon C-peptide 1.0 nmol/l, previous therapy : glibenclamide.

Diagnosis: NIDDM with prevailing secretory disorder.

Therapy: Combined glibenclamide/insulin treatment, possible following previous weight reduction, alternative: insulin alone.

Case C
52-year old male, BMI 27 kg/m^2, duration of diabetes 6 months, HbA_{1c} 9.9%, fasting blood glucose 220 mg/dl (12.2 mmol/l), postglucagon C-peptide 0.6 nmol/l, previous therapy : glibenclamide.

Diagnosis: Suspected slowly manifesting IDDM.

Therapy: Insulin

duration of diabetes and the quality of the metabolic control. In NIDDM even a slight increase in physiological albuminuria correlates with increased risk of nephropathy and cardiovascular disease. The determination of microalbuminuria (30 – 300 mg/die = 20 – 200 mg/l) is therefore of special importance in prognosing the course of the disease. Only with early proof of a microalbuminuria can therapeutic interventions still favorably influence the course of the disease. The Micral test allows a specific, semi-quantitative assessment of the albumin concentration in the urine.

Proteinuria is usually defined as a protein excretion of more than 0.5 g/die. Patients with proteinuria have a poor prognosis. The normal method to date for the total protein excretion in urine should be replaced by the albumin excretion. A proteinuria of 0.5 g/die corresponds to a microalbuminuria of 300 mg/die. The predicative value of the microalbumin assay for diabetic nephropathy is, however, often significantly impaired in type II diabetics. Primarily in older patients, a series of other factors (urinary tract infections, hypertension, coronary insufficiency, prostate hypertrophy, poor diabetic adjustment) may cause albuminuria.

6.2.7.2 *ß₂-microglobulin*

The $ß_2$-microglobulin is another essential parameter for the determination of renal function. Both glomerular and the tubular function can be estimated by measuring it in serum and urine. $ß_2$-microglobulin belongs to the small molecular proteins, is glomerularly filtered and resorbed or metabolized for the most part in the proximal tubulus. Correspondingly, $ß_2$-microglobulin is only present in small amounts in urine. Generally an increase of the serum concentration of this protein indicates an impairment of the glomerular function, while an increase of the renal excretion indicates a tubular defect.

$ß_2$-microglobulin can be detected with the help of a commercially available radioimmunoassay. With the development of global renal insufficiency the $ß_2$-microglobulin increases in the "creatinine blind" range. The special value of the $ß_2$-microglobulin determination, however, lies more in its ability to differentiate between primary tubulointerstitial and primary glomerular kidney diseases. With interpretation of the findings it is necessary to take into account the fact that, for example, during pregnancy and some malignant diseases, to some extent dramatically elevated $ß_2$-microglobulin values in the serum may occur.

6.2.8 *Other follow-up examinations*

The clarification of other parameters, especially of the other components of the metabolic syndrome (blood pressure, lipids, coagulation data, uric acid) are a part of the complete diagnosis, especially the diagnosis of the course of NIDDM. Intact renal function is of particular importance for the life expectancy of the patient. For that reason semi-annual examinations of the protein excretion in the urine (strip test or quantitative determination) and of the creatinine as well as the creatinine clearance are required to be able to be therapeutically effective at an early date. Table 6 offers an overview of the strategy of these follow-up examinations.

Tab. 6: Monitoring examinations for NIDDM performed by the physician

- At every visit to a clinic (every 6 – 8 weeks)
  Body weight (BMI)
  Blood glucose (postprandial BG)
  Urine glucose
  Blood pressure
  HbA_{1C}
  Monitoring of the skin and feet as well as possible injection sites
- Twice yearly
  Microalbuminuria
  Lipid status (chol., TG, HDL chol.)
  Urine status

6.2.9 *Self-monitoring*

Metabolic self-monitoring has been an integral part of diabetic therapy for years. Modern examination methods are now available to the patient, methods in which all of their essential metabolic parameters can be examined with sufficient accuracy. Because the patient can determine these in the course of his normal daily activities, they are much more valuable than the "momentary pictures" that the physician is able to take. It has been proven that patients who regularly monitor themselves are better controlled. This is particularly true for type II diabetes. Self-monitoring should be introduced immediately upon diagnosis of the disease and is not aimed only at the paraclinical data, but symptoms mentioned by the patient as well (tab. 7). The patients should know diabetes-specific symptoms and be informed of the importance of inspecting their feet.

Tab. 7: Self-monitoring by the diabetic as a requirement for an effective therapy

- Patient and physician are partners in the treatment – more than with other chronic diseases
- Self-monitoring begins upon the discovery of the disease
- Self-monitoring orients itself on symptoms both recognized by the patient and hidden.
- Self-monitoring is: requirement for a therapy which overcomes disease symptoms and prevents late complications

The maintenance of the (reduced-calorie) diet in the overweight NIDDM should certainly be a part of the self-control. The patient should regularly measure weight, blood pressure, blood glucose and urinary glucose and be familiar with the methods for determining acetone and microalbumin (tab. 8).The equipment and materials needed for monitoring are shown in tab. 9. In the framework of training the patient and at least once a year the accuracy of the patient's values, should be checked. Thus, errors in reading test strips can be detected at an early date and corrected.

The patient should enter the values in his/her diabetes diary. These form the basis for adjusting therapy and for discussion of the results at the next visit.

6.2.10 *Summary*

The diagnosis diabetes mellitus should be made if the fasting blood glucose is above 6.7 mmol/l (120 mg/dl) at more than one measurement and/or the blood glucose is over 11.1 mmol/l (200 mg/dl) 2 hours after an oral Glucose Tolerance Test (75 g oGTT). Blood glucose determinations are preferable to urinary glucose measurements to estimate the course of the disease and the therapy follow-up. Examination of the urine for ketone bodies should always be a part of the diagnostic repertoire in metabolic compensation. All these methods can be per-

Tab. 8: Self-monitoring for NIDDM

Self-monitoring

↙ ↘

Clinical symptoms	Paraclinical parameters	
		NIDDM
	Body weight	+
	Blood pressure	+
	Urine glucose postprand.	(+)
	Blood glucose	(+)
	Acetone	(+)
	Microalbuminuria	

↓

Maintaining the diet

Tab. 9: Aids in self-monitoring

Scale
Test strips for blood and urine glucose
Mirror for foot inspection (plantar)
Blood pressure measuring device desirable

formed by the patient by means of test strips in the course of the self-monitoring. The determination of the HbA_1 (HbA_{1c}) is certainly a decisive parameter for the control of the metabolic adjustment, because it reflects the integrated blood glucose concentration over a period of 4–8 weeks. In comparison, fructosamine indicates a short term imbalance.

The microalbumin excretion in the urine should be part of every diabetes check-up, because it offers the opportunity for an early diagnosis of nephropathy and as a result early therapeutic intervention.

Self-monitoring is an important component for optimizing diabetotherapy. It is not only directed at paraclinical data, but at symptoms pointed out by the patient as well.

References

[1] Baker, J. R., R. N. Johnson, D. J. Scott: Serum fructosamine concentrations in patients with type II diabetes mellitus during changes in management. Br. Med. J. *228* (1984) 1484–1486.

[2] Bennett, P. H.: Classification and diagnosis of diabetes mellitus and impaired glucose tolerance. In: J. C. Pickup, G. Williams (eds.): Textbook of Diabetes, 37–46. Blackwell, Oxford 1991.

[3] Bennett, P. H.: Albuminuria and diabetes: A critique assessment of urinary albumin excretion and its role in screening for diabetic nephropathy. Am. J. Kidney Dis. *13* (1989) 29 – 34.

[4] Bibergeil, H., D. Michaelis, B. Schulz: Diabetes mellitus. In: G. Brüschke (Hrsg.): Stoffwechselerkrankungen und Erkrankungen des endokrinen Systems, 35 – 120. Band 2, Teil 1. Fischer, Jena 1991.

[5] Cobelli, C., G. Pacini: Insulin secretion and hepatic extraction in humans by minimal modeling of C-peptide and insulin kinetics. Diabetes *37* (1988) 223 – 231.

[6] Diabetes mellitus. Report of a WHO Study Group. WHO Technical Report Series, No. 727. Genf 1985.

[7] Faber, O. K., C. Binder: C-peptide: an index of insulin secretion. Diabetes Metab. Rev. *2* (1986) 331 – 345.

[8] Gjessing, H. J., E. M. Damsgaard, L. E. Matzen: Reproducibility of β-cell function estimates in non-insulin-dependent diabetes mellitus. Diabetes *10* (1987) 558 – 562.

[9] Horwitz, D. L., J. Starr, M. E. Mako et al.: Proinsulin, insulin and C-peptide concentrations in human portal and peripheral blood. J. Clin. Invest. *55* (1975) 1278 – 1283.

[10] Hother-Nielsen, O., O. Faber, N. Schwarz-Sorensen et al.: Classification of newly diagnosed diabetic patients as insulin-requiring or non-insulin-requiring based on clinical and biochemical variables. Diabetes Care *11* (1988) 531 – 537.

[11] Johnson, R. N., O. A. Metcalf, J. R. Baker: Fructosamine: a new approach to the estimation of serum glykosylprotein. An index of diabetic control. Clin. Chim. Acta *127* (1982) 87 – 95.

[12] Lowy, C.: Pregnancy and diabetes mellitus. In: J. C. Pickup, G. Williams (eds.): Textbook of Diabetes, 835 – 850. Blackwell, Oxford 1991.

[13] Lefébvre, P. J., G. Paolisso, A. J. Scheen et al.: Pulsatility of insulin and glucagon release: physiological significance and pharmacological implications. Diabetologia *30* (1987) 443 – 452.

[14] Mogensen, C. E.: Microalbuminuria as a predictor of clinical diabetic nephropathy. Kidney Int. *31* (1987) 673 – 689.

[15] Schmitz, A., M. Vaeth: Microalbuminuria: A major risk factor in non-insulin-dependent diabetes. A 10-year follow-up study of 503 patients. Diabetic Med. *5* (1988) 126 – 134.

7 Therapy

The motto of the World Health Organization "Full life despite diabetes", which was formulated for the 50th anniversary of the isolation of insulin for therapeutic purposes by Banting and Best, first of all with respect to the insulin-dependent type I diabetes, is equally valid for NIDDM. In contrast to IDDM, it is rare that these patients are in acute danger of a coma at the beginning of the disease.

Tab. 1: Monitoring standards according to the "Euro-Norm"

		Good	Acceptable	Poor
Blood glucose				
– fasting	mg/dl	80 – 120	≤ 140	> 140
	mmol/l	4.4 – 6.7	≤ 7.8	> 7.8
– post-prandial	mg/dl	80 – 160	≤ 180	> 180
	mmol/l	4.4 – 8.9	≤ 10.0	> 10.0
HbA_1	%	< 8.5	8.5 – 9.5	> 8.5
HbA_{1C}	%	< 7	7 – 8	> 8
Urine glucose	%	0	≤ 0.5	> 0.5
Cholesterol	mg/dl	< 200	< 250	250
	mmol/l	< 5.2	< 6.5	≥ 6.5
HDL-cholesterol	mg/dl	> 42	≥ 35	< 35
	mmol/l	> 1.1	≥ 0.9	< 0.9
Fasting triglycerides	mg/dl	< 150	< 200	≥ 200
	mmol/l	< 1.7	< 2.2	≥ 2.2
Body Mass Index	kg/m^2	men < 25	≤ 27	> 27
		women < 24	≤ 26	> 26
Blood pressure	mmHg	≤ 140/90	< 160/95	≥ 160/95

Nevertheless, the adjustment of the blood glucose to at least acceptable values, as they are described by the Euro-Norms (tab. 1), is an important measure for guaranteeing freedom from symptoms and age-related performance. An antidiabetic therapy which is directed only at the prevention of coma will not also be acceptable for the very aged and should be the exception only in desolate cases. One should always keep in mind that many acute complications which limit the quality of life of elderly diabetics and those diabetics who have had the disease for many years, such as gangrene, pyelonephritis and other infections, are dependent on the quality of glycemic control.

In middle-aged persons with NIDDM, as well as for a vivacious seventy year-old who has a life expectancy of another 15 years, the Euro-Norms for good control are in principle the goal. This is above all true for blood pressure and – within limits in the very aged – the blood lipids.

Caution should be used when implementing drastically low fat diets above age 55–60. The prevention of macro- and microangiopathy, in the sense of primary and secondary prevention, should be given the same importance as the control of the diabetes in middle-aged patients. The two goals form an inseparable unit. Only by means of an integrated therapy concept can the complex disease NIDDM be successfully combated in the long run. Every decision is in the end individual and should be based on thorough cost/risk/benefit analysis. The therapy can only be successful if the patient accepts it and if possible, no drop in motivation should occur. Finally, a "good" therapy must guarantee the best possible quality of life and in the overall balance the lowest costs and the least amount of effort. The following chapter should serve as a guide as to how the goal can be attained using an individualized approach.

7.1 Health education and instruction

U. Julius

7.1.1 Health education

The efficacy of non-drug measures in the therapy of type II diabetes framework was impressively shown in the Diabetes Intervention Study [4]. Over the course of 5 years, it was possible, on average, to attain a better glycemic state with the use of fewer anti-diabetics. This comparison was done with a randomly selected control group in which the use of anti-diabetics was not limited. Life-style regulation makes sense in many cases for the reduction of high lipid concentrations [6]. Positive effects on high blood pressure could also be registered, especially with a reduction in weight, a limitation of salt consumption, and a reduction of stress.

The results of the Lifestyle Heart Trial are remarkable [9]. Patients in the therapy group were given a normal calorie, reduced cholesterol, ovolactovegetarian diet with nicotine abstinence. Regular stress management training in the form of stretching and breathing exercises, meditation, and concentrated relaxation for one hour per day made up the mental part of the intervention. Depending on the initial values of their physical fitness, the patients were subscribed an individual program of physical activity of 3 hours per week with a minimum in 30 minutes per training period. The change of lifestyle resulted in a decrease in total and LDL cholesterol, a noticeable reduction in the frequency and seriousness of angina pectoris attacks, and after one year a regression of coronary stenoses was observed by means of angiography.

Simply passing on knowledge – as clever as it may be and appropriately fitted to the age and intelligence of the patient – is completely insufficient. It especially depends on the motivation of the patients to lead a healthier lifestyle. This is in no way possible with the threat that diabetes complications will occur later. The discovery of diabetes is psychologically traumatic for many patients. The latter can, in individual cases, be eased by following the recommendations of the therapist. Emotional support of the patient is essential.

All recommendations offered must also truly be realizable by the patient. Secondary illnesses are to be considered. A family doctor often knows the social conditions of his/her patients and can, if necessary, include family members in the change in lifestyle.

It is important that type II diabetes patients are informed in the following areas, are advised and directed (more specific explanations follow below):

1. Diet
2. Physical exercise
3. Blood pressure management
4. Non-smoking
5. Reducing alcohol consumption
6. Avoidance of maximal stress
7. Sleep, regularity in the daily schedule
8. Social issues
9. Sexuality (for the target group of this book, only rarely on questions of wanting children and pregnancy)
10. Uncontrolled drug abuse

In addition to these, problem areas are to be discussed that specifically relate to diabetes and its resulting diseases (see subjects of diabetic instruction below).

ad 1. Diet

Today's requirements for the diet of a type II diabetic are shown in the respective section (7.3). If you become aware of a dietary discretion on the part of the patient, you should not react angrily; instead, discuss with the patient which effects these discretions have and how one should behave in the future. Few patients behave ideally; you will hardly have success as a therapist without offering certain concessions and human understanding.

ad 2. Physical exercise

It was proven in a large-scale American study [2] that even light physical exercise, which can be done by most anyone, noticeably decreases the total mortality rate. This trend also remained after a statistical correction for other risk factors such as age, smoking, cholesterol level, systolic blood pressure, fasting blood sugar level, and family risk for coronary heart disease.

Aerobic exercise has wide-ranging usefulness for a type II diabetic. Encourage all your patients to be physically active. A measurable increase in performance is not important; activities started abruptly are to be absolutely avoided. A light physical activity can definitely be effective.

The activity should be fun. For most of your patients an appropriate form of activity will be walking, hiking, bike riding, swimming, and eventually gymnastics. Involvement in sports teams can serve the purpose.

You should complete the following examinations to test for physical capacity if you recommend regular exercise to your patient:

- General medical examination
- ECG at rest

- Ergometry
- X-ray of the thorax
- in the case of an abnormal ECG or hypertension: echocardiographic examination

Complete controls of the physical capacity at regular intervals (quarterly at the beginning). A blood pressure measurement by the patient is sensible. The medication for metabolic or blood pressure decreasing must be modified for patients in training, if necessary.

ad 3. Blood pressure management

Since hypertension is a particular danger, regular blood pressure measurements under day to day conditions are certainly recommendable. It is most practical when the patient does the blood pressure check on his/her own.

ad 4. Non-smoking

Due to the macroangiopathy often developed by type II diabetics, smoking is to be considered especially harmful for this patient group. Definitely discourage your patients from smoking. It could be recommendable to complete a stop-smoking program.

ad 5. Reduction of alcohol consumption

Type II diabetics often have a fatty liver as well as associated or secondary hyperlipoproteinemias. For this reason, alcohol consumption should be very limited and only allowed, if possible, at social functions.

ad 6. Avoidance of maximal stress

Type II diabetics are especially in danger with respect to the development of coronary heart disease. Psychosocial risk factors play a vital role in the etiopathogenetic concept of coronary heart disease. With respect to careers, the constant willingness for competition, the ambitious striving for success, domination, and recognition are of importance. Outside of the workplace, social isolation and the impression of having lost the security of family and friends can occur. These factors must in no way be considered as questions of fate, and can be eliminated through the use of appropriate measures.

ad 7. Sleep, regularity in the daily schedule

Sufficient rest overnight is just as essential for a type II diabetic as for a non-diabetic. A nightly polyuria can be bothersome. Pain, fear, worries, or depression can lead to sleeplessness. Advise your patients to be active in fresh air, to take a rest in the evening, or to take other non-drug measures that have been proven practical. Sedatives or hypnotics should only be used with reservation. The nightly intake of a heterocyclic anti-depressives is indicated for sleeplessness due to depression. Nightly blood pressure increases which can be recorded with a 24-hour measurement are to be considered for a differential diagnosis.

ad 8. Social issues

Jobs with a certain amount of physical activity are favorable for type II diabetics. If a patient must constantly eat while working (e.g., degustating at regular intervals), problems with the metabolism and especially with body weight may arise. The patients who take sulfonyl ureas or inject insulin must not be endangered by hypoglycemia at work. Special directions for motorists are necessary to avoid hypoglycemia. Type II diabetics are generally just as professionally capable as non-diabetics. A night-shift or shift work should, however, not be recommended.

ad 9. Sexuality

Diabetic men often have potency problems. Both vascular and neurogenic causes are to be considered in this case. Psychological factors can, however, also be of importance. Remember that beta-blockers and fibrates can have a negative effect on sexual function. A loss of libido for female type II diabetics is possible.

ad 10. Uncontrolled drug abuse

A variety of drug groups can have direct negative effects on the metabolism, e.g., glucocorticoids, diuretics, drugs containing sugar. Other medications can interfere with oral hypoglycemic agents or inhibit the reaction of the organism to a hypoglycemia. You should always have a good overview of the medication that you subscribe the patient or that he/she takes on his/her own.

7.1.2 *Instruction*

Problems of health education are an integral part of the instruction programs for type II diabetics. Group instruction has been proven to be advantageous (group dynamics), rational, and effective [7]. It can be completed with mid-level personnel (physician's assistant, diabetic advisor, dietician) under the direction of a physician. The attendance of appropriate training (in Germany advised by the Central Institute for Medical Insurance Care Cologne, Project Office for Instruction Programs; publishing of materials by the German Physicians' Publishing House) for the entire instruction team is a prerequisite for the introduction of such programs in a practice. Such teams can also be effective in the framework of specialized departments in hospitals or university clinics. The Association of Diabetic Patients should be involved in the instruction.

The demand exists that every diabetic, independent of his/her age, should complete such instruction (exceptions: non-educable and psychiatric patients).

The following didactically excellent, well-constructed, and well-structured instruction programs are available for type II diabetics:

1. Instruction for type II diabetics not treated with insulin
2. Instruction of older insulin-dependent diabetics
3. Instruction program "Living well with diabetes" (German language)

The program named in point 2 is to be performed in a hospital setting; the one named under point 1 can be performed on an out-patient basis.

The instruction programs for type II diabetics who do not inject insulin (ad 1.) includes the following instruction units ($1^1/_2$ hours each; completion in 4 weeks in one-week segments):

First Class
- General information on diabetes
- Metabolic control

Second Class
- Reasons for blood sugar increase
- Pills to reduce blood sugar
- Diet

Third Class
- Foot care
- Physical activity and diabetes

Fourth Class
- Behavior for concomitant diseases
- Late complications

In addition to oral instruction, special emphasis is put on working with written material that can be taken home by the patient: self-monitoring techniques (here: urine self-monitoring), a repetition of the contents of the last instruction unit and the evaluation of the knowledge of the patients at the beginning and the end are vital elements of the program. The patients are encouraged to turn to the instructors with any questions dealing with their disease or affecting their daily life.

In the course of the program a "sulfonyl urea withdrawal trial" is performed on the patients who were previously given the appropriate preparation. It is suggested, along with the expectation of a noticeable weight reduction (the most important goal of the program), that the preparation be no longer taken. The danger of a metabolic imbalance is limited by the glucosuria self-monitoring learned parallel and the detailed knowledge of the symptoms of hyperglycemia. An adaptation of the dose should also occur for acarbose and metformin.

This instruction program (ad 1.) is especially oriented towards the therapeutic objectives for elderly type II diabetics:

- Freedom from symptoms
- Avoidance of diabetic coma
- Prevention of the diabetic foot
- Identification and combatance of hypoglycemia.

For the program mentioned under point 3 (Toeller et al., German Physicians' Publishing House, 1992), the aim of treatment must be determined for the individual patient. To attain these goals, the active involvement of the patient is encouraged. The instruction is conceived to be continual, begins at the first visit, is completed systematically and structurally, and is individually tailored [10]. As with the program described in point 1, it has been created for application in the physician's practice and is based on an evaluated motivation and contractual concept. Depending on the individual patient's risk profile and the willingness to change unfavorable behavior, agreements are made with the physician and patient on health-related activities. The patient receives special motivation brochures. A time commitment of 15 to a maximum of 45 minutes is intended for one instructional unit; the appointments should be made in about a 4-week cycle.

Seminars are also offered for physicians and assistants for the latter instructional program. In the long run, however, reinforcement of health education is essential to maintain the improved health behavior.

7.1.3 Summary

Structured instruction programs give type II diabetics knowledge of the disease symptoms, performing self-monitoring techniques, therapy completion, as well as avoiding complications. It is desirable that all still-active patients complete such a course, even at an older age. The programs allow for group instruction in which the physician's assistant has the decisive role of the teacher. Every physician who treats a diabetic should be concerned with the lifestyle of his/her patient. Health education is a life-long task.

References

[1] Assal, J. P., I. Mühlhauser, A. Pernet et al.: Patient education as the basis for diabetes care in clinical practice and research. Diabetologia *28* (1985) 602–613.

[2] Blair, S. N., N. H. Kohl, R. S. Pfaffenbarger et al.: Physical fitness and allcause mortality. A prospective study of healthy men and women. J. Amer. med. Assoc. *262* (1989) 2395–2401.

[3] Diabetes Education Study Group of the European Association for the Study of Diabetes: The Teaching Letter. Geneva 1985.

[4] Hanefeld, M., S. Fischer, H. Schmechel et al.: Diabetes Intervention Study. Multi-Intervention Trial in Newly Diagnosed NIDDM. Diabetes Care *14* (1991) 308–317.

[5] Hasche, H.: Fehler in der Diabetestherapie – Zwangsläufig oder vermeidbar? Schulung. Akt. Endokr. Stoffw. *10* (1989) 212–217.

[6] Julius, U., M. Hanefeld: Environmental factors and serum lipoproteins. Current Opinion in Lipidology *1* (1990) 255–261.

[7] Kronsbein, P., I. Mühlhauser, A. Venhaus et al.: Evaluation of a structured treatment and teaching programme on non-insulin-dependent diabetes. Lancet *II* (1988) 1407–1411.

[8] Mühlhauser, I.: Die Bedeutung der Patientenschulung in der Behandlung chronischer Krankheiten: Diabetes mellitus, Hypertonie, Asthma bronchiale. Intern. Welt *8* (1987) 1–14.

[9] Ornish, D. et al.: Can lifestyle changes reverse coronary heart disease? The Lifestyle Heart Trial. Lancet *336* (1990) 129–133.

[10] Toeller, M., W. Schumacher, A. Klischan: Patientenschulung: Standbein für den Therapieerfolg. Diabetes Praxis (1992) 57–64.

7.2 Weight reduction

M. Weck

7.2.1 Introduction

If one consistently follows the main points of the pathogenesis of NIDDM and the metabolic syndrome presented in the previous chapters, it is clear that, with the presence of a metabolic disorder and especially with NIDDM, weight reduction and normalization present an essential and pathogenetically-oriented therapy concept. Weight reduction does not only have a cosmetic effect, but also produces profound improvements in the cardiovascular risk factor profile: reduction of hyperglycemia, lowering of the elevated insulin level, normalization of lipids and blood pressure, improvement of hemo-rheological factors. In cases of obese NIDDM, it is known that, through the reduction of (especially abdominal-visceral) fat mass, hyperinsulinemia is reduced, hepatic glucose production is lowered, peripheral insulin sensitivity is improved and, of course, blood glucose is lowered. The patients who benefit most from weight reduction are those whose disease process is in an early phase, who still show sufficient insulin secretion and whose blood glucose drops drastically during therapeutic weight reduction.

In other words: early weight reduction and normalization is a therapeutic imperative in cases of obese NIDDM. Even more desirable is combating obesity *before* the manifestation of NIDDM, especially in persons with a high risk for diabetes (first-degree relatives of NIDDM patients). As mentioned at the beginning, these recommendations are oriented on the pathogenesis of NIDDM. It should be mentioned that until now there have been no long-term studies which show a positive effect for early weight reduction on the long-term prognosis or life expectancy of NIDDM patients. This can only be indirectly concluded from the improvement of the cardiovascular risk factor profile.

7.2.2 Weight reduction – a problem of balance

The energy balance of the body is shown in fig. 1. Body weight can be held constant, if the intake and energy release side of the balance remain equal. Weight reduction is only possible when the energy intake is reduced or the energy release is increased. Vice versa, weight gain can result from excessive calorie intake or a reduction in energy release. This manner of presentation suggests that effective weight reduction must *always* be accompanied by a reduction of calorie intake and should be combined with an increase in physical activity. It should also not be forgotten that permanent weight reduction only succeeds through the addi-

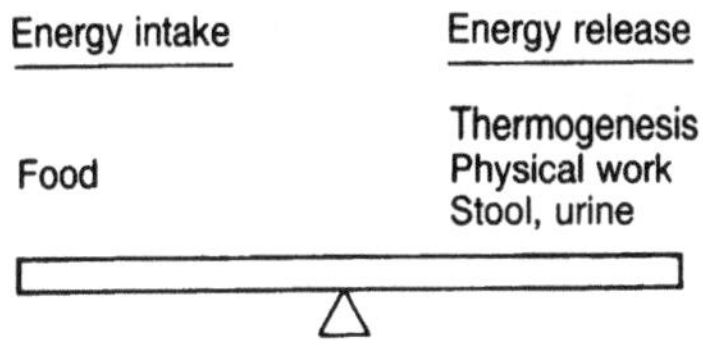

Fig. 1: Weight reduction – a problem of balance.

tional change of eating habits. Calorie restriction, physical training and behavior therapy are essential components of a weight reduction program.

At this point it must be noted that certainly not all obese people are over-eaters, but rather, that a small portion of these patients also show a reduced energy release. These diabetics are characterized by reduced fasting basal metabolic rate and/or lowered postprandial thermogenesis. The farmers' saying about an animal which is an "easy keeper", finds its scientific verification in a small portion of obese individuals (ca. 20 %). For these patients, a weight reduction is only possible by a drastic calorie restriction. Pharmaceutics, which stimulate the energy release side of the energy balance, the so-called "thermogenic pharmaceutics", are in development.

7.2.3 *What is obesity, how is it measured?*

The measurement of obesity is an old problem. In general, one tends to define obesity today as the deviation from the desired weight. The desired weight or ideal weight have been calculated by American insurance companies with millions of insurance holders as being the weight with the highest life expectancy. In the tables provided by this effort, one can see the ideal weight for 3 body types, separated by sex. Recently, the easy-to-use body mass index (BMI, also Quetelet index, i. e. body weight (kg)/body height (m^2)) has come to be preferred. The so-called Euro-Norm for the BMI states that in cases of obese NIDDM, a BMI < 25 (men) and < 24 (women) should be aimed for. Simplified, a < 25 should be aimed at for patients with metabolic diseases. With a height of 170 cm, a BMI of 25 would require a body weight of 72.5 kg.

Because we now know that the cardiovascular and metabolic risks, brought on by obesity are essentially dependent on the regional depositing of the fat, the BMI alone is not sufficient for the characterization of obesity. As an additional parameter for evaluating the risks, the WHR (waist-to-hip ratio) has proven itself:

$$\text{WHR} = \frac{\text{waist circumference}}{\text{hip circumference}}$$

The waist circumference is measured in the mid-point between the lower edge of the rib cage and the upper edge of the illiac crest; in slim persons this is the waist, in obese persons the point of the largest belly girth. The hip circumference is measured at the height of the greater trochanter or at the point of greatest hip girth.

The WHR in women should not be > 0.85 and in men not > 1.0. Crudely simplified: if the women loses her typical feminine proportions, and if the man shows the so-called "beer belly", then one can already assume prima vista an android obesity with the related metabolic and cardiovascular consequences. The goal of weight reduction is primarily the prevention of the fat mass in the abdominal region. Accordingly, not only a BMI < 25, but also a WHR of < 1.0 in men and < 0.85 in women is to be aimed for (tab. 1).

Tab. 1: Weight classes and risk ranges

Weight class		Risk ranges
Underweight	BMI <20	
Target weight	BMI 20–25	
Overweight	BMI 25–30	BMI 25–30 WHR > 0.85 (w) WHR > 1.0 (m)
Obese	BMI 30–40	BMI 30–40 WHR > 0.85 (w) WHR > 1.0 (m)
Morbid obesity	BMI >40	BMI > 40

7.2.4 *Methods of weight reduction*

The essential methods of weight reduction available are listed in tab. 2.

Tab. 2: Methods of weight reduction

Behavioral therapy
Dietary regime for weight reduction
- total fasting (zero diet)
- hypocaloric mixed diet (energy content 800–1500 kcal/day)
- very low calorie diets (VLCD, "protein-supplemented, modified fasting", energy content 400–800 kcal/day)

Gastroplasty among other invasive procedures

Of primary interest are the dietary procedures:

- Many authors see a *hypocaloric mixed diet*, as the therapy of choice, especially since the greatest learning curve for the patient is thought to occur with this variant. According to our experience, such hypocaloric mixed diets are definitely appropriate for patients with moderate obesity (BMI 25–30) where weight reduction is targeted over a longer time span. These patients must be clearly told how much weight loss is possible per time interval with this diet (average 0.5 kg/week), as exaggerated ideas often exist. Realistic therapy goals should be set by the physician and patient together. Meal plans for a hypocaloric mixed diet are presented in tab. 3.

In our opinion, however, this form of diet is not suited to the majority of very obese type II diabetics. These patients should lose weight rapidly and effectively for two reasons:

1. A quick breakthrough of the ever present insulin resistance is indicated for excessive obesity and decompensated metabolism.
2. With significant obesity, a drastic weight loss of 10–15 kg in 4–6 weeks seems advisable, in order to motivate the patients to further weight reduction.

- The *zero diet* always has a large loss of water and proteins, i. e. of active body mass, as a consequence and can lead to severe keto-acidoses. This form of diet/fasting is therefore no longer acceptable today. The so-called outsider diets always cause publicity, but due to their unbalanced nature, lack of long-term effect and many complications they have not withstood serious scientific examination.
- The *very low calorie diets* (in the form known as protein-substitution fasting), the origins of which go back to the 1930s, combine the advantages of total fasting – effective weight reduction of between 300 and 400 g per day – and the low calorie diets – extensive sparing of the lean body mass and high safety. A whole series of commercially available VLCDs (very low calorie diets) are on the market, with the energy content and nutrient relations differing only somewhat. In Germany, Modifast® and the Cambridge Diet® have been successful. Most use low-fat milk powder or egg white as a protein source. We use the so-called "Dresden slim drink" for the treatment of obesity in diseases of the metabolic syndrome (tab. 4, tab. 5.1, tab. 5.2). The essential difference to the industrially produced diets lies in the fact that the "Dresden slim drink" is based on a recipe system with natural food stuffs, which the patient personally prepares in the first days of the weight reduction during a stay at the clinic. In this way, the diabetic is actively shaping his/her energy balance and gathers the necessary know-how for the production and calculation of a VLCD. A not unimportant advantage over the commercial instant products is the lower price. A further, for us very essential, advantage of the VLCD lies in the fact that after 6–10 days, hunger largely disappears through the re-orientation of the metabolism to ketobodies and the patients experience an emotional "high".

Tab. 3: Meal plan for a hypocaloric mixed diet

1. *Breakfast (250 kcal)*
   40 g bread (whole wheat or multi-grain) or
   25 g rye crisp or
   25 g oatmeal or similar or
   40 g whole wheat roll or similar

   10 g lowfat margarine

   100 g lowfat quark or
   50 g lowfat cheese or
   50 g lean meat or
   25 g cheese or farmer's cheese or
   25 g lean cold cuts or
   15 g salami or liverwurst or pate or
   1 egg
2. *Breakfast (100 kcal)*
   250 ml buttermilk or low-fat yogurt or
   180 ml milk or
   200 g fruit or fruit juice or
   20 g rye crisp and 5 g diet margarine or
   400 g vegetables
3. *Lunch (325 kcal)*
   100 g potatoes or
   25 g rice/noodles (uncooked weight)
   100 – 200 g vegetables
   50 – 100 g lean meat/poultry or
   100 – 150 fish or any sort or
   100 – 150 g lowfat quark or
   1 egg
   5 – 10 g diet margarine or oil

   (instead of the pre-meal soup, one cup of lowfat broth)
4. *Tea/snack (75 kcal)*
   150 g fruit or
   20 g rye crisp or whole wheat crackers or
   10 g rye crisp and 10 g honey/jam

(Jams and jellies, cakes, cookies or ice cream with artificial sweeteners are to be chosen for diabetics)

5. *Dinner (250 kcal)*
   40 g bread
   5 g lowfat margarine
   100 g lowfat quark or see breakfast
   100 – 200 g vegetables (fresh vegetables/salads)

Daily beverage intake at least 1½ liters of tea, mineral water, 2 – 3 cups of coffee

Tab.4: Self-made VLCD ("Dresden slim drink")

440 kcal per day
100 g nonfat powdered milk
20 g wheat bran
100 g vegetables
2 g sunflower seed oil

= 40 g protein
58 g carbohydrate
4 g fat

550 kcal per day
130 g nonfat powdered milk
20 g wheat bran
100 g vegetables
2 g sunflower seed oil

= 51 g protein
73 g carbohydrate
4 g fat

The weight loss consists of approximately equal parts fat and water. In contrast, body protein is essentially not consumed or else only in very small amounts.

Differing opinions exist in the literature regarding the optimal composition of a VLCD. An expert commission of the British Ministry of Health has recommended that only VLCDs with the following minimal portions of calories and proteins should be used:

- for moderately obese women: 400 kcal/day and 40 g protein/day
- for men and large or particularly obese women: 500 kcal/day and 50 g protein/day.

In addition, the USRDA (recommended daily allowances) should be adhered to for vitamins and minerals. Other authors have recommended the composition of the VLCD proposed in tab. 6. It has been legally established in Germany that the protein content of a commercial diet for weight reduction not fall below 50 g/day and that this protein must be of high biological value.

In massive obesity ("morbid obesity", BMI > 40), which is accompanied by a significant reduction of life expectancy, the indication for invasive procedures for weight reduction is to be considered. For this, these patients should be transferred to a specialist center.

Behavioral therapy techniques should be a component of every weight reduction plan.

Tab. 5.1: Partial fasting (VLCD) Dresden Slim Drink (440 kcal/day): Practical performance – 28 day meal plan

Preparation/Use

1. Keep a diary of the 28-day plan (morning/ noon /evening /weight/ comments) and present it at weekly consultations with the physician.
2. Purchase 3 – 4 packages of nonfat powdered milk and 1 – 2 packages of wheat bran (bran flakes) as basic provisions. In addition: different types of tea and mineral water. Additional daily beverage amounts on all days: 2 liters as soda water, mineral water, tea, 1 – 2 cups of coffee, vegetable broth. No other food or calorie-containing beverages during this time!

Morning: daily

300 ml nonfat milk (30 g nonfat powdered milk, l warm water)
10 g bran flakes or 5 g rye crisps
1 cup of coffee or hot chocolate made with water or tea
for flavoring: artificial sweetener, lemon, aromas
tea or soda water or similar
milk, bran or coffee are each to be offered separately, mixed or flavored

Noon: Monday, Tuesday, Thursday, Friday

300 ml nonfat milk (30 g nonfat powdered milk, l warm water) or
300 ml buttermilk or 300 ml nonfat yogurt and 100 g fresh vegetables (tomatoes, cucumbers, lettuce, cabbage, cauliflower) in a salad – spiced with pepper, salt, cayenne pepper, artificial sweetener, vinegar, herbs and 2 g sunflower seed oil.

Wednesday, Saturday

100 g lowfat quark – mix to a smooth consistency with water, flavor with herbs and spices and add 2 g sunflower seed oil, and 50 g fresh fruit (small apple or similar), tea and/or mineral water.

Sunday

70 g lean meat/poultry/fish (cook/grill/bake or roast) and
100 g vegetables or 50 g fruit. All spices are allowed, including salt and pepper. Tea and /or mineral water or similar.

Evening: daily

300 ml nonfat milk (30 g nonfat powdered milk, ¼l warm water) or
300 ml buttermilk or 300 ml nonfat yogurt and 10 g bran flakes
tea and /or mineral water or similar
flavoring with herbs, aroma, artificial sweetener, cocoa, coffee, rose hip tea

Preparation tip:
If desired, each portion of milk can be solidified – ¼l is made "eatable" with 7 g gelatin. (Dissolve and mix according to directions).

7.2.5 Indications for weight reduction in NIDDM

As has already been discussed, every patient with a metabolic disease should aim to reach the ideal weight as per the Euro-Norm in connection with the appropriate WHR. The scope of the obesity determines the diet form. Here, of course, a weight reduction should only be undertaken when one can expect a substantial improvement of the metabolic condition, the risk factor profile, the physical and

Tab. 5.2: Partial fasting (VLCD) Dresden Slim Drink (550 kcal/day): Practical performance – 28 day meal plan (general points as in Tab. 5.1)

Morning: daily

400 ml nonfat milk (40 g nonfat powdered milk, ¼l warm water)
10 g bran flakes or 5 g rye crisps
1 cup of coffee or hot chocolate made with water or tea
for flavoring: artificial sweetener, lemon, aromas
tea or soda water or similar
milk, bran or coffee are each to be offered separately, mixed or flavored

Noon: Monday, Tuesday, Thursday, Friday

400 ml nonfat milk (40 g nonfat powdered milk, l warm water) or
400 ml buttermilk or 400 ml nonfat yogurt and 100 g fresh vegetables (tomatoes, cucumbers, lettuce, cabbage, cauliflower) in a salad – spiced with pepper, salt, cayenne pepper, artificial sweetener, vinegar, herbs and 2 g sunflower seed oil.

Wednesday, Saturday

150 g lowfat quark – mix to a smooth consistency with water, flavor with herbs and spices and add 2 g sunflower seed oil, and 50 g fresh fruit (small apple or similar), tea and/or mineral water.

Sunday

70 g lean meat/poultry/fish (cook/grill/bake or roast) and
100 g vegetables or 50 g fruit. All spices are allowed, including salt and pepper. Tea and /or mineral water or similar.

Evening: daily

400 ml nonfat milk (40 g nonfat powdered milk, ¼l warm water) or
400 ml buttermilk or 400 ml nonfat yogurt and 10 g bran flakes
tea and /or mineral water or similar
flavoring with herbs, aroma, artificial sweetener, cocoa, coffee, rose hip tea

Tab. 6: Recommendations for the protein composition of a VLCD

1. Protein quality: Excellent biological value
2. Protein contents per day:
   - 55 g: women of small or average size with moderate obesity
   - 70 g: obese men and large or significantly obese women
   - 100 g: massively obese men

psychological performance capabilities, i. e. ultimately of the sense of well-being. In elderly obese diabetics with good metabolic control, a stringent weight reduction is naturally not indicated.

7.2.6 *Contraindications*

The contraindications for a weight reduction by means of VCLD are documented in tab. 7. In each case, the risks and benefits should be weighed. In contrast, contraindications for a hypocaloric mixed diet are only seen in infrequent cases of severe acute and chronic diseases. In the maintenance of the inclusion and exclusion criteria referred to, we have observed no essential imbalances of the electrolyte and acid-base households, especially no ketoacidosis. Using Holter ECG registration we found only occasional benign arrhythmias. We have concluded therefore that during a VLCD an ECG – or with special indications a Holter ECG – should be performed every 2 weeks. In patients with known coronary artery disease or elevated risk of thrombosis (past history, fibrinogen, hematocrit, plasma viscosity), we recommend low-dose heparinization in addition.

Tab. 7: Contraindications for the use of a very low-calorie diet (VLCD) in NIDDM

- Diabetes-specific contraindications:
  severe late syndrome (retinopathy > 1st degree, significant nephropathy, autonomic neuropathy, pronounced polyneuropathy, diabetic gangrene).
- Unstable angina pectoris or documented coronary atherosclerosis stenosis
- Coronary insufficiency
- High grade arrhythmias
- Psychiatric disorders
- Widespread diseases, including diseases of the hematopoietic system
- Gout
- Severe liver and kidney insufficiency
- Unreliable patients

In the end, the indication is therefore always an individual one, made upon weighing of the risks and advantages. The variable self-made VLCD described above is preferred over commercial instant products by our patients. Through the self-monitoring of weight, blood glucose and blood pressure, the patients quickly experience the beneficial aspects of VLCD themselves. In uncomplicated cases, an out-patient continuation of this diet form is possible after a hospital run-in phase of 5 - 8 days.

7.2.7 *Practical application*

Before every weight reduction, along with the indications, the patient's motivation is to be examined and the principles, application and goals are to be discussed with him/her. Group therapy with a maximum of 10 people is well-suited to this purpose. The time length of the VLCD phase should last between 4 and 6 weeks and can be extended to 8 weeks for particularly motivated patients. We usually initiate this treatment with a ca. 3–4 day in-hospital phase, in which the patient is thoroughly examined and the preparation of the diet learned. This is followed by out-patient group therapy. A prerequisite for the successful completion of the reduction diet is the preparation of the diet plan together with the dieticians. A further basic condition is the maintenance of a liquid intake of 2.5 l per day including the volume of the "Dresden slim drink". The monitoring examinations to be performed weekly are listed in tab. 8. As a result, it may become necessary to substitute potassium. We first prescribe allopurinol with uric acid values over 600 µmol/l. Over the past few years we have not observed an acidosis which required treatment. Oral hypoglycemic agents can be quickly stopped or drastically reduced in dosage. The long half-life of, for example, glibenclamide should definitely be included in the considerations. The effect of most medications is reinforced or changed by partial fasting treatment. In general, therefore, they must be reduced or stopped during the diet phase. The drug therapy can often be reduced over the long-term after the completion of the fast.

Tab. 8: Control parameters in VLCD treatment

Before the start of the diet phase:
Clinical examination, blood pressure, ECG, possibly extended ECG, Chest X-ray, CBC, Na, K, Ca, Fe, creatinine, uric acid, ALAT, BG, HbA_{1C}, Astrup analysis
Daily:
Body weight, acetone in urine, blood glucose
Weekly:
Clinical controls, blood pressure, Na, K, creatinine, uric acid, ALAT, BG, Astrup analysis
After no more than 4 weeks:
Additional Ca, Fe, HbA_{1C}, extended ECG Additional controls may be necessary for problem cases

Regular light exercise activity during the diet period is useful in order to counteract the drop in the resting energy metabolism.

After the conclusion of the dieting phase, a very slow and step by step readjustment of the organism to a higher food intake is necessary. The patients should consume a mixed diet of 600 kcal for 1 week, 800 kcal for 1 week, 1,000 kcal for 1 week, and then retain this calorie intake for another 5 weeks.

Duration/target parameters: The VLCD should be conducted for at least 6 weeks. According to recent findings, better results regarding weight behavior and metabolic parameters can be achieved if the VLCD phase is further extended under strict monitoring.

Results: We have successfully administered this form of diet to over 200 type II diabetics without significant incidents. The short-term results have been particularly successful, but the long-term results have also been considerable given the less than ideal selection of patients (mostly so-called "sulfonyl urea failures") (tab. 9). In principle, as soon as patients with obese NIDDM manifest the disease they should be prescribed weight reduction (by means of a VLCD). This early phase of the diabetic process with pronounced insulin resistance and still present insulin secretion is the domain of weight reduction. The greatest experience with very low calorie diets has been reported by Kirschner with over 3000 patients [7]. These impressive results are documented in tab. 10.

How can the reduced weight be maintained?

The main problem with forms and methods of weight reduction lies in the maintenance of the reduced weight. The long-term results related to this are mostly poor. The altered energy balance is often not taken into consideration in fasting or partial fasting. The following patho-physiological viewpoints should be considered in the phase after the weight reduction, in so-called restorative diets. Weight reduction is connected to the reduction of metabolically active mass, i. e. the non-fat mass. The basal or fasting basal metabolic rate, i. e. the release side of the energy balance (fig. 1), is significantly lowered. As a result, after a VLCD or also a hypocaloric mixed diet, the calorie intake can only be raised very slowly and in a step-by-step fashion. The patients should continue to weigh themselves regularly and introduce some days with renewed calorie restrictions. In this way, a new steady-state can be established and, in the course of many weeks, the individually possible calorie intake for the maintenance of the reduced weight can be titrated. For women, this is often in the region of 800 – 1000 kcal/day. Physical training takes on particular significance in this phase, because increased activity can compensate a portion of the drop in the basal metabolic rate.

7.2.8 Summary

Weight reduction, aimed at the depletion of the abdominal fat depot, has profound metabolic effects on obese NIDDM patients and is the therapy of choice in the early phases of this form of diabetes with prevailing insulin resistance.

Treatment with a very low calorie diet (VLCD) in particular presents an effective, safe and cost effective method of becoming slim and eumetabolic. This diet results in a drastic improvement of the glucose and lipid metabolism, as well as the blood pressure. There is increased success the more the patient actively shapes his/her treatment. Through the self-monitoring of weight, blood glucose and

Tab. 9: Sample of a VLCD treatment

Patient data

W. G. 57 years old	male
Duration of diabetes	5 years
Treatment	5 mg glibenclamide/day
BMI 28.1	
WHR 1.01	
Percentage body fat	28.1%

VLCD treatment: 8 weeks 500 kcal "Dresden Drink", thereafter 6 weeks of dietary build-up to 1200 kcal mixed diet

Results

Anthropometric data and metabolic parameters before the VLCD and after dietary build-up

	before VLCD	after VLCD and dietary build-up
Body weight (kg)	85.0	73.3
BMI	28.1	24.3
BP (mmHg)	155/100	130/85
FBG (mmol/l)	13.1	5.9
postprand. BG (mmol/l)	16.4	8.3
HbA_{1C} (%)	8.8	5.2
euglycemic glucose-clamp investigation		
M-value (mg/kg/min)	2.3	7.8
Cholesterol (mmol/l)	7.3	5.2
Triglycerides (mmol/l)	3.2	1.7

Tab. 10: Results of a VLCD treatment (Optifast®) with 3020 patients (from Kirschner [8])

1. *Hypertension (41% of the patients)*	
blood pressure normalized, medications stopped	71%
blood pressure normalized, medications continued	12%
blood pressure further raised after weight reduction	17%
2. *Hypercholesterolemia (41% of the patients)*	
cholesterol normalized through the diet	73%
cholesterol reduced	27%
3. *Hypertriglyceridemia (29% of the patients)*	
TG normalized	77%
TG reduced	23%
4. *Diabetes mellitus*	
oral hypoglycemics stopped	100%
insulin stopped	87%
insulin dose reduced	10%

blood pressure, he/she experiences the advantages of the treatment. Additional physical conditioning, behavioral-therapeutic guidance and the described procedure for the post-fasting period are significant in determing long term success.

References

[1] Ferner, R. E., M. D. Rawlins, K. G. M. M. Alberti: Impaired β-cell responce improved when fasting blood glucose concentration is reduced in non-insulin-dependent diabetes. Quart. J. Med. *66* (1988) 137 – 146.

[2] Hanefeld, M., M. Weck: Very low calorie diet therapy in obese non-insulin dependent diabetes patients. Int. J. Obesity *13* (suppl. 2) (1989) 33 – 37.

[3] Henry, R. R., T. A. Wiest-Kent, L. Schaeffer et al.: Metabolic consequences of very-low-calorie diet therapy in obese non-insulin-dependent diabetic and non-diabetic subjects. Diabetes *35* (1986) 155 – 164.

[4] Henry, R. R., P. Wallace, J. M. Olefsky: Effects of weight loss on mechanisms of hyperglycaemia in obese non-insulin-dependent diabetes mellitus. Diabetes *35* (1986) 990 – 998.

[5] Henry, R. R., B. Gumbiner: Effects and limitations of very-low-calorie diet therapy in obese NIDDM. Diabetes Care *14* (1991) 802 – 823.

[6] Howard, A. N.: The historical development of very low calorie diets. Int. J. Obesity *13* (suppl. 2) (1989) 1 – 9.

[7] Kirschner, M. A., G. Schneider, N. H. Ertel et al.: An eight-year experience with a very-low-calorie formula diet for control of major obesity. Int. J. Obesity *12* (1988) 69 – 80.

[8] Uusitupa, M., M. Laakso, H. Sarlund et al.: Effects of a very-low-calorie diet on metabolic control and cardiovascular risk factors in the treatment of obese non-insulin-dependent diabetes. Am. J. Clin. Nutr. *51* (1990) 768 – 773.

[9] Wadden, T. A., T. B. VanItallie, G. L. Blackburn: Responsible and irresponsible use of very-low-calorie diets in the treatment of obesity. JAMA *263* (1990) 83 – 85.

[10] Weck, M., S. Fischer, M. Hanefeld et al.: Loss of fat, water and protein during very low calorie diets and complete starvation. Klin. Wochenschr. *65* (1987) 1142 – 1150.

[11] Weck, M., M. Hanefeld, K. Schollberg et al.: Die Behandlung des Typ-II-Diabetes mit sehr-niedrigkalorischen Diäten (VLCD) – ein pathogenetisch orientiertes Therapiekonzept. Z. klin. Med. *43* (1988) 15 – 19.

[12] Weigle, D. S., K. J. Sande, P. H. Iverius et al.: Weight loss leads to a marked decrease in nonresting energy expenditure in ambulatory human subjects. Metabolism *37* (1988) 930 – 936.

[13] Wing, R. R., L. H. Epstein, M. Paternostro-Bayles et al.: Exercise in a behavioral weight control programme for obese patients with type II (non-insulin-dependent) diabetes. Diabetologia *31* (1988) 902 – 909.

[14] Wing, R. R.: Behavioral strategies for weight reduction in obese type II diabetic patients. Diabetes Care *12* (1989) 139 – 144.

7.3 Health promoting nutritional management

U. Julius

7.3.1 *Dietary fundamentals for type II diabetic patients*

Every effective treatment of type II diabetes includes recommendations to optimize nutrition. This is particularly understandable when considering the fact that for the inhabitants of the industrialized countries:

- the intake of calories often exceeds the need,
- the amount of fat is too high and it's composition is not optimal (too much animal fat),
- a considerable portion of mono- and disaccharides are consumed,
- the intake of certain nutritional components (for example fiber, vitamins, minerals) often does not meet requirements.

With the Diabetes Intervention Study, it has been proven that an intensified health education can provide a better glycemic level with less anti-diabetic medication after five years. Diet is a significant part of the non-drug therapy. During the study, the intervention patients increased their intake of polyunsaturated fatty acids (increase of the P/S ratio). However, on an average neither the total calorie intake nor the high fat content could be reduced. One has to bear in mind that the food supply after 1990 has changed significantly in the areas which were included in the study. However, high fat contents in the diet of diabetic patients have been documented by other groups both in the former West German states and outside Germany.

As a matter of principle, the diabetic diet is to be applied to every patient and is never contraindicated. Its function is essentially the preservation of the working and living standards.

Which goals are to be achieved with the diet?

The main emphasis is placed on

- the improvement of body weight (often: weight reduction), prevention of a high increase in postprandial blood glucose.
- the reduction or elimination of concomitant dys- and hyperlipoproteinemia (anti-atherogenicity)
- the reduction of the risk of late complications
- providing a sufficient amount of essential nutrients, vitamins and minerals.

The current recommendations concerning the diet for type II diabetics include the following fundamental rules:

a) restricted calorie intake
b) consumption of several small meals (5 – 6 daily)
c) general restriction in the consumption of monosaccharides and disaccharides
d) low cholesterol intake (<300 g daily)
e) restriction in the consumption of alcohol (<30 g daily)

The following proportions of daily calorie intake should be observed:

carbohydrates 50%   fats 35%   protein 15%

This roughly corresponds to a daily intake of:

150 – 200 (– 300) g carbohydrates
60 – 80 g protein (the equivalent of 0.8 – 1.0 g per kg of body weight)
60 – 80 g total fat (the equivalent of 1.0 g per kg of normal weight).

Individual wishes and preferences can be taken into consideration as long as they do not completely contradict the basic rules of the diabetes diet [15].

7.3.2 *Attaining the ideal weight*

The emphasis in the therapy of type II diabetes is weight reduction. Two approaches are:

a) gradual weight reduction through hypocaloric mixed diet or
b) limited periods of fasting therapy.

The simplest method to determine whether the calorie intake should be reduced is a regular documentation of changes in body weight. According to a recommendation of the German Nutrition Association (quoted in [11]), the daily calorie requirements for adults, depending on age and sex, lay between 2200 (9.20MJ) and 2600 kcal (10.88 MJ). For practical purposes, tables are suitable to determine individual calorie requirements, taking sex, ideal weight, age and physical activity into consideration (tab. 1).

If a reduction of weight is necessary, the daily calorie intake has to lie at least 500 kcal below the calculated needs.

Should you be confronted with unsuccessful weight reduction (adherence problems) you should increase your attention to this patient. Convincing proof of the superiority of a certain diet for weight reduction is not available. Patients who do not lose weight are to be supported by recommendations that they keep more exact records concerning calorie intake. Simple forms of behavioral therapy can be used. Especially when the goal of the treatment is not attained immediately, long-term care from a dietician has proven advantageous. Many diabetics can be convinced to change their eating habits as a result of suitable, comprehensible, and enthusiastically communicated instructions.

Tab. 1: Calculation of caloric needs

	Height [cm]	Weight [kg]	Energy requirements [kcal]									
			Light activity (age/years)					Increased activity (age/years)				
			up to 40	40 – 50	50 – 60	60 – 70	over 70	up to 40	40 – 50	50 – 60	60 – 70	over 70
Women	150	48	1600	1500	1400	1300	1200	2000	1900	1800	1600	1400
	155	51	1700	1600	1500	1400	1300	2100	2000	1900	1700	1500
	160	54	1700	1700	1600	1400	1300	2300	2200	2100	1900	1700
	165	57	1900	1800	1700	1600	1500	2400	2300	2200	2000	1900
	170	60	2000	1900	1800	1700	1600	2500	2400	2300	2100	2000
	175	64	2100	2000	1900	1800	1700	2600	2500	2400	2200	2100
	180	67	2200	2100	2000	1900	1800	2700	2600	2500	2300	2200
	185	72	2400	2300	2200	2000	1900	2800	2700	2600	2400	2300
Men	155	54	1900	1800	1700	1500	1400	2500	2400	2300	2100	2000
	160	58	2000	1900	1800	1600	1500	2600	2500	2400	2200	2100
	165	62	2100	2000	1900	1700	1600	2700	2600	2500	2300	2200
	170	66	2300	2200	2100	1800	1700	2900	2800	2600	2400	2300
	175	70	2500	2400	2300	2100	2000	3100	2900	2800	2600	2400
	180	74	2600	2500	2400	2200	2100	3200	3000	2900	2700	2500
	185	77	2800	2700	2500	2300	2200	3400	3200	3100	2800	2600
	190	81	3000	2800	2700	2500	2300	3600	3400	3200	3000	2800

7.3.3 Special aspects of the dietary recommendations for diabetics

7.3.3.1 First hints for patients with newly diagnosed diabetes mellitus

When you have discovered a new case of diabetes and can only start or arrange the dietary instruction in the days to come, the following preliminary recommendations should be made (modified after [13]):

- ▶ Quench thirst with calorie free drinks (mineral water or tea)
- ▶ Satisfy hunger with normal food items, eat smaller amounts at regular intervals
- ▶ The main components of meals should consist of vegetables, potatoes, fruits, bread or pasta
- ▶ Meat, sausages or cheese should only make up a small portion of the diet.

7.3.3.2 Diet categories for type II diabetes

Dependent on the severity of the diabetes, the age and intelligence of the patient, and concomitant diseases, the attending physician must decide between two categories of diet for type II diabetics.

▶ 1. Calorie defined diabetes diet ("Calorie Diet")

Definition:

- Recommendations concentrate on the calorie balance, fat modification, and avoiding quickly absorbed carbohydrates
- Foods are classified as suitable, less suitable and unsuitable
- Recommendations are given using normal portions of food (for example, one potato, one slice of bread).

Preferred use with:

- Type II diabetes not needing drug treatment
- Patients with whom weight reduction has the top priority
- Elderly patients
- Patients with limited mental capabilities
- Patients who have other life threatening diseases (for example, tumors) or with multimorbidity

Advantages:

- Easy to learn
- Simple and flexible implementation
- Use of scales not necessary

Disadvantages:

- Visual inspection provides an inaccurate assessment of food portions and composition.

► 2. Diabetes diet with defined amounts of carbohydrates

Definition:

- Maintains same basic principles as the above mentioned diet
- Meals are planned using units to measure carbohydrate portions (10 – 12 g carbohydrates)

Preferred use by:

- Younger, cooperative patients
- Patients that take oral hypoglycemic agents
- Patients that inject insulin

Advantages:

- More precise quantification of carbohydrate intake
- Use of a carbohydrate equivalents table allows replacing of carbohydrate-containing foods within the different food groups
- In certain situations, anti-diabetic medication can be adapted to the amount of carbohydrates to be eaten during a meal.

Disadvantages:

- More difficult to learn
- During the learning period the use of a scales is useful
- The amount of carbohydrates in a certain food may not be the same as stated on the table
- Tables are imprecise with respect to the calorie content.

7.3.3.3 *Quality of the main food types*

Carbohydrates

Results of experiments document that with an increase in the intake of carbohydrates the triglyceride level also increases. That would of course be an adverse event for a type II diabetic patient. For that reason it is important that high molecular, high fiber, carbohydrate containing food (whole wheat products) are preferred over quickly absorbed, "low molecular" low fiber foods. The large amount of carbohydrates required in the modern diabetic diet can only be attained through a comprehensive use of vegetables, fruits and cereal. Pasta can also be used.

Ice cream or regular Coca Cola can lead to high blood glucose peaks in patients who do not inject insulin with meals. This normally does not cause an immediate disturbance of condition but promotes the development of diabetic complications. The addition of glucose or saccharose can not be generally recommended. (compare section on sweeteners below).

Fats

The diabetic diet should always be designed so as to enable a positive effect on the lipid metabolism. The basic general elements of the lipid-lowering diet are especially important for type II diabetic patients (tab. 2).

Tab. 2: Basic principles of a lipid-lowering diet
(Recommendations of the European Atherosclerosis Society, to be found in [1])

Recommendation		Main sources
I.	Decreased total fat intake and	Butter, margarine, whole milk, cream, ice cream, hard cheeses, soft cheeses, visible fat in meat, common beef and
II.	Decreasing of saturated fatty acids	Pork, duck, goose, common types of sausage and cold cuts, pastries, common coffee cream, coconut, products with coconut and palm oils
III.	Increased use of foods with high protein content and few saturated fatty acids	Fish, chicken, turkey, game, veal
IV.	More complex carbohydrates, fiber from cereals, fruits and vegetables, especially legumes	All fresh and frozen vegetables, all fresh fruits, whole grain products of all sorts, legumes, rice
V.	Slightly raised intake of simple unsaturated and polyunsaturated fatty acids	Sunflower oil, germ oil, safflower oil, soy oil and products produced from them, olive oil
VI.	Decreased cholesterol intake	Brain, sweetmeat, kidney, tongue; eggs, (not more than 1 – 2 egg yolks per week); liver (not more than twice a month)

The allotment of fat should consist of:

⅓ saturated fats (mostly in animal products)
⅓ simple unsaturated fatty acids (vegetable oils)
⅓ polyunsaturated fatty acids (vegetable oils, fish)

The composition of fatty acids in fats and oils varies. All available vegetable oils, excluding coconut oil, are suitable for the diabetic diet. Fats are taken in the following forms:

- spreadable fats
- cooking fat
- hidden fat

When using fat the following points should be considered:

1. Read product labels and consider presence of hidden fats
2. Use low fat products
3. Prepare food with oil, avoid butter or lard
4. Use low fat cooking methods (foil, grill, modern pans)
5. Do not overheat fat (overheated fats can be unhealthy)
6. Store cooking fats in a dark, cool place

Protein

Plant products and fish are valuable sources of protein. Protein from meat is often connected to saturated fats and cholesterol.

7.3.3.4 *Dietary planning in the practice*

▶ a. *Determination of the daily energy requirement*

With a calorie-defined diabetic diet ("Caloric Diet"): Teach the use of the calorie control tables (compare section 7.3.2).

▶ b. *Information concerning preferred foods, or foods to be avoided*

Concerning the above mentioned "Caloric Diet", the patients can be instructed with simple illustrations if necessary. These illustrations are a part of the training program for type II diabetic patients that do not perform insulin injections. A classification according to the degree of suitability of foods is helpful (tab. 3).

▶ c. *Determination of the portion of carbohydrates, fats and protein*

In order to determine the daily recommended quantities in grams, based on the total calorie intake, a table is provided (tab. 4).

▶ d. *Realization in terms of foodstuffs*

Food tables are used for this. Normally for a subtle introduction, a dietitian or diabetes counselor is necessary. For type II diabetics who do not inject insulin, simple demonstration cards are used.

▶ e. *Submitting a carbohydrate equivalents table (in as far as carbohydrates should be calculated)*

Basis of the computation is one unit:
carbohydrate portion (10–12 g carbohydrate)

Tab. 3: Classification of foods according to their suitability to a diabetic diet (taken in a modified form from [16])

Vegetable varieties especially well-suited for diabetics			
Eggplant	Fennel	Brussel sprouts	Spinach
Bamboo shoots	Green beans	Red beets	Tomatoes
Celery	Cucumbers	Red cabbage	White cabbage
Cauliflower	Kohlrabi	Sauerkraut (low-salt)	Savoy cabbage
Broccoli	Leeks	Celery root	Zucchini
Chicory	Green or red peppers	Asparagus	Onions

Vegetables and legumes suitable for diabetics	
Artichokes	Pumpkin
Dried white beans	Lentils, dried
Beans	Corn on the cob
Peas	Horseradish

Drinks suitable for diabetics	
Apple wine	Mineral water
Beer (diabetic pilsner)	Dry champagne
Diet cola	Diet tonic water
	Dry wine

Binding substances well-suited for diabetics
Gelatin, pectin
Products from carob meal

Unsuitable and suitable fish and shellfish varieties			
Unsuitable	*Suitable*		
Eel	Perch	Cod	Salmon
Salmon in oil	Trout	Crab	Sole
Matje herring	Pike	Mussels	Tunafish
Smoked haddock	Herring	Shellfish	Pike-perch
	Lobster	Tench	Mackerel
	Shrimp	Summer flounder	Turbot

Tab. 3: (Continued)

Unsuitable and suitable side dishes		
Unsuitable	*Suitable*	
Dumplings	Buckwheat	Potatoes
Croquettes	Glass noodles	Potato puree
French fries	Unripe grain	Noodles } whole grain
	Millet	Rice } if possible

Unsuitable and suitable meats to be given preference			
Unsuitable	*Suitable*		
Mutton	Poultry	Veal	Beef
– Breast	– Breast	– Shoulder	– Filet
– Cutlet, fat	– Leg	– Breast	– Haunch
– Shoulder	Mutton	– Filet	– Roast beef
Pork	– Filet	– Haunch	Pork
– Shank	– Haunch	– Cutlet	– Breast
– Shoulder ham		– Schnitzel	– Filet
			– Schnitzel, lean
			Game

Unsuitable and suitable soups		
Unsuitable	*Suitable soup bases*	*Suitable soup ingredients**
Soups, thickened	Vegetable soup, clear	Vegetables
with semolina	Meat broth, fat removed	Dropped egg
flour or starch	Bone broth, fat removed	Meat cubes, lean

* not counted in the diet plan

Unsuitable and suitable fruits		
Unsuitable	*Suitable with limitations*	*Well-suited*
Chestnuts	Bananas	Pineapple
Dried fruit	Lichee	Apples
– Apricots		Apricots
– Dates		Berries
– Figs		Pears
Grapes		Grapefruit
		Watermelon
		Fruit juices, freshly squeezed

Tab. 4: Distribution of nutrients in the diet of an adult diabetic

Calories	Fat g Total	Fat g of which is butter or margarine	Protein g	CH Portion	1st Breakfast	2nd Breakfast	3rd Breakfast	Lunch	Afternoon snack	Dinner	Evening snack
					Distribution of the portions in the daily meals 1 Portion = 10 – 12 g Carbohydrates						
1000	40	–	40	8	2	1	–	1	1	2	1
1100	40	–	40	9	2	1	–	2	1	2	1
1200	45	10	45	10	2	2	–	2	1	2	1
1300	50	10	50	11	2	2	–	2	2	2	1
1400	55	10	50	12	2	2	–	3	2	2	1
1500	60	20	55	13	2	2	–	3	2	3	1
1600	60	20	60	14	2	2	–	3	2	3	2
1700	65	20	65	15	2	2	1	3	2	3	2
1800	70	20	70	16	2	3	1	3	2	3	2
1900	75	20	70	17	2	3	1	4	2	3	2
2000	80	20	75	18	2	3	1	4	2	4	2
2100	80	20	80	19	2	3	2	4	2	4	2
2200	85	20	80	20	3	3	2	4	2	4	2
2300	90	30	85	21	3	3	2	5	2	4	2
2400	95	30	90	23	4	3	2	5	2	5	2
2500	95	30	95	24	4	3	2	5	3	5	2
2600	100	30	95	25	4	3	2	6	3	5	2
2700	105	30	100	26	4	3	2	6	3	6	2
2800	110	30	105	27	4	4	2	6	3	6	2
2900	115	30	110	28	5	4	2	6	3	6	2
3000	115	30	110	29	5	4	2	6	4	6	2
3100	120	40	115	30	5	4	3	6	4	6	2
3200	125	40	120	31	5	4	3	6	4	6	3
3300	130	40	125	32	6	4	3	6	4	6	3
3400	130	40	125	33	6	4	4	6	4	6	3
3500	135	40	130	34	6	4	4	6	5	6	3

Example:

The carbohydrate content of one 25 gram slice of bread equals one carbohydrate portion.

The following food groups are to be considered in these calculations:

1. Grains, grain products, bread, cake, and pastries
2. Fruits

3. Potatoes
4. Milk and milk products
5. Vegetables (only fresh pods and corn are considered; other types of vegetables can be consumed in normal quantities without being calculated).

Groups 1 – 4 can be varied internally using an equivalents table. To insure the proper relationship of nutrients and the supply of essential minerals, fiber and vitamins, an exchange of bread for fruit or potatoes for milk is to be avoided.

7.3.3.5 *Consideration of concomitant diseases*

When planning the diet, the attending physician must take present concomitant diseases into proper consideration. Tea and soups are recommended for acute gastrointestinal disturbances (vomiting, diarrhea). The supply of sugars (glucose! – sucrose is not absorbed when disaccharidase inhibitors are used) should be withheld for patients with hypoglycemia. An actual protein restriction is considered for type II diabetics should a renal insufficiency appear.

7.3.3.6 *Conducting the dietary counseling*

All diabetics are to be repeatedly instructed (verbally and in writing) on nutritional matters after the manifestation as well as after, for example in case of a worsening of the glycemic level (see 7.1). The inclusion of dieticians in this regard has proven very well. Professionally put together meal plans can illustrate the desired nutrition. It is important that the patient himself is allowed to be active in the diet counseling (for example with food models or cooking in a training kitchen). Inviting the spouse to the dietary counseling is recommended. Suggestions and positive motivation should take precedence and restrictions should be kept to an absolute minimum.

7.3.3.7 *Instructions for other elements of the diet*

Drinks

Mineral water, especially those that contain electrolytes, are especially recommended. Tea and coffee are allowed without restriction, with use of artifical sweeteners can be permitted. Processed sugar-free drinks with low calorie content, usually containing sweeteners, can be used by many diabetics.

Alcohol

Keeping the calorie count in mind, diabetics can drink carbohydrate-free alcoholic beverages in limited amounts. These carbohydrate-free drinks include cognac, brandy, whisky, and all clear spirits. Also low carbohydrate beverages such as diabetic beer and dry wine may be consumed in limited amounts. Beer (check malt content!) often stimulates the appetite so that more food is consumed than should be. Naturally it must be additionally taken into consideration that alcohol consumption can be expected to have a negative effect on other illnesses (for example hypertriglyceridemia, hypertension, gout/hyperuricemia, fatty liver).

Dietetic foods

Nutrition experts do not consider dietetic foods to be necessary for supplementing or varying the diet. Some are not recommended due to a high fat content. Foods that are produced with the use of artificial sweeteners are low in calories and can be useful for overweight patients.

Vitamins

The vitamin requirement for diabetics is the same as that for non-diabetics. Especially when storing, conserving and preparing fruits, vegetables and potatoes, a considerable loss of vitamins should be taken into account. Resorption difficulties should be considered. Especially in older people, indications of vitamin deficiency, also in sub-clinical form, can be countered by means of guaranteeing a mixed variety of foods, including fresh foods. Milk and fish liver oil are valuable sources of lipid-soluble vitamins. Through vitamin enhancing, certain products, such as margarine can cover part of the requirement.

Minerals and trace elements

The elements in foods include calcium, phosphorus, magnesium, sodium, potassium, and chloride. Of these elements the supply of calcium, due to the frequency of osteoporosis, is of special importance. Calcium is especially present in milk and milk products, in fruits and grain products. The recommendations of the German Nutrition Association take into account higher requirements in old age. The danger of a magnesium deficiency is especially possible with insufficient intake of whole-wheat products and vegetables in combination with excess consumption of protein, fat, or alcohol. Potassium is supplied in vegetables.

Trace elements are those nutrients that are consumed in only relative small amounts with the daily food intake. A regular intake of iodine is necessary to ensure the normal functioning of the thyroid. Seafood is a good source of iodine and should be regularly consumed (1 – 2 times weekly). A zinc deficiency can occur with very small consumption of meat and dairy products (vegetarian diet). The requirement for manganese is provided primarily by cereal products, legumes, and black tea. Selenium is mostly taken from meat, fish and grain products. A selenium deficiency can result from long-term parenteral nutrition as well as in areas with low selenium content in the soil.

Fiber

High fiber foods have a low calorie content and for that reason are well-suited for type II diabetics. The use of fiber as adjuvant therapy will be discussed in section 7.5.5.

Sweeteners

One makes a distinction between:

Sweeteners: Aspartame, saccharin, cyclamate

These have a low calorie content and need not be counted in the dietary plan. These substances are harmless when consumed in normal amounts and are recommended due to taste and calorie considerations.

Sugar substitutes: fructose, mannitol, sorbitol, xylose

These have a higher calorie content, like glucose (1g = 4 kcal) and must be counted in the dietary plan.

At this time they are mainly used in industrial processing of food.

The intake of sugar substitutes has to be limited. Diarrhea frequently occurs with the consumption of more than 30 grams of sorbit or xylit per day. This is to be considered especially in the presence of the alpha glucosidases inhibitors!

Natural fructose (fruits) is permitted however, where carbohydrate units are counted in limited quantities (not over 50 g/day, distributed among several meals). The immediate glycemic effect of fructose is slight; can, however, pose problems to patients who are not well-controlled. Consumption of large amounts of fructose can have an undesired effect, since hypertriglyceridemia, hyperuricemia, lactacidemia have been observed.

Isomalt can be used by diabetics in small amounts (<30 g/day). It has only about half the calories of sugar and does not promote dental caries.

Salt, spices

Due to the common combination of hypertension with diabetes, the daily consumption of salt should be kept under five grams. Adding salt to food is undesirable since many foods already contain it. All spices can be used in the diabetic diet. One should use herbs and spices to supplant the ever-popular taste of salt. It is recommended that no spice be allowed to overpower the normal flavor of a food. Processed spices or condiments (for examples tomato paste or ketchup) should be avoided due to their sugar content.

Fish, fish oil capsules

Fish contains large amounts of biologically high value protein, valuable minerals such as phosphorus, potassium, iodine, and vitamins A, B_1, B_2, niacin and vitamin D. The fat content is normally low. Fatty fish such as herring, mackerel, salmon and others are high in polyunsaturated fats. According to the nutritional recommendations of the German Nutrition Association, fish, preferably ocean fish, should be eaten once to twice a week. This also insures the iodine requirements. Fish contain little connecting tissue, is for that reason tender, wholesome and easily digestible. While the consumption of fish is recommended without limitations, the taking of fish oil capsules is not universally recommended. At any rate, diabetics should not take large doses (>4 g daily).

7.3.4 Summary

For most type II diabetics, the establishment of a “calorie diet” of 50% carbohydrates, 35% fat and 15% protein should be considered. The high portion of carbohydrates is to be met by utilizing whole wheat products, fruits, vegetables, cereal, or pasta. Reduction of the fatty portion is important and with that the reduced consumption of animal fats. Plant oils with monounsaturated or polyunsaturated fatty acids are useful. The regular consumption of fish is recommended. Patients should be provided with simple calorie tables for food. These include summaries that classify foods as being suitable/not suitable for diabetics. The patient should record his weight several times a week and through that coordinate total calorie need with frequently needed weight reduction.

References

[1] Assmann, G.: Fettstoffwechselstörungen und koronare Herzkrankheit. MMV Medizin Verlag, München 1991.

[2] Beebe, C. A., J. G. Pastors, M. A. Powerset et al.: Nutrition management for individuals with noninsulin-dependent diabetes mellitus in the 1990s: a review by the Diabetes Care and Education dietetic practice group. J. Am. Diet. Assoc. *91* (1991) 196 – 202, 205 – 207.

[3] Bruns, W., K. Vetter, H. Bibergeil: Diabetiker-Kost heute – 50 Jahre nach Veröffentlichung der „Grazer Thesen“. Z. Klin. Med. *43* (1988) 261 – 265.

[4] Bruns, W.: Neue Erkenntnisse zur Diättherapie des Typs 2 (non insulin dependent)-Diabetes. Z. gesamte inn. Med. *45* (1990) 290 – 294.

[5] Canzler, H., H. Kasper, R. Kluthe et al.: Rationalisierungsschema 1990 der Deutschen Arbeitsgemeinschaft für klinische Ernährung und Diätetik geV für die Ernährung und Diätetik in Klinik und Praxis. Akt. Ernährungsmedizin *15* (1990) 97 – 102.

[6] Deutsche Diabetes-Gesellschaft: Grundlagen der Ernährung und Diätempfehlungen für Diabetiker. Akt. Ernährungsmedizin *15* (1990) 27 – 38.

[7] Diabetes and Nutrition Study Group of the European Association for the Study of Diabetes: Nutritional recommendations for individuals with diabetes mellitus. Diab. Nutr. Metab. *1* (1988) 145 – 149.

[8] Haller, H., M. Hanefeld, W. Jaroß: Lipidstoffwechselstörungen – Diagnostik, Klinik und Therapie. VEB Gustav Fischer Verlag, Jena 1983.

[9] Hanefeld, M., G. Crepaldi: Diabetes and glucose intolerance. In: A. G. Olsson (Ed.): Atherosclerosis – Biology and Clinical Science, 445–452. Churchill Livingstone, Edinburgh, London, Melbourne, New York 1987.

[10] Hanefeld, M., S. Fischer, H. Schmechel et al.: Diabetes Intervention Study. Multi-Intervention Trial in Newly Diagnosed NIDDM. Diabetes Care *14* (1991) 308–317.

[11] Kasper, H.: Ernährungsmedizin und Diätetik. Urban & Schwarzenberg, München, Wien, Baltimore 1987.

[12] Ketz, H.-A.: Grundriß der Ernährungslehre. Gustav Fischer Verlag, Jena 1990.

[13] Lean, M. E. J., J. I. Mann: Dietary Management of Non-Insulin-Dependent Diabetes Mellitus. In: J. Pickup, G. Williams: Textbook of Diabetes, 453–461. Blackwell Scientific Publications, Oxford 1991.

[14] Mehnert, H.: Diabetes mellitus. In: H. Mehnert (Hrsg.): Stoffwechselkrankheiten. Grundlagen, Diagnostik, Therapie, 115–261. Georg Thieme Verlag, Stuttgart, New York 1990.

[15] Petzoldt, R.: Grundlagen der Diabetesdiät: ernährungswissenschaftliche Aspekte. Ernährungs-Umschau *38* (1991) 395–399.

[16] Rosak, C.: Diabetes mellitus und Ernährung. Der Feinschmecker für Ärzte 1990, Heft 6, 19–21.

[17] Use, G. (unter wissenschaftlicher Beratung von W. Bruns und H. Mehnert): Diabetes-Therapie heute. Ein praktischer Leitfaden in Tabellen. Aktuelles Wissen Hoechst, Reihe Diabetes, 1991.

7.4 Physical exercise

M. Hanefeld

7.4.1 Introduction

Physical exercise has already been recommended by G. Katsch as a cornerstone of diabetes treatment. However, to date, it has led a Cinderella-like existence in the therapy concept of NIDDM. This is a quite unwarranted position, given that the musculature is the most important organ in glucose utilization and that aerobic training influences metabolism and hormonal regulation in a complex fashion (tab. 1) [5].

Tab. 1: The effects of physical training on metabolism, hormonal regulation and the circulatory system

Metabolism and coagulation	
– Glucose tolerance	↑
– Triglycerides	↓
– HDL cholesterol	↑
– LDL cholesterol	=
– Uric acid	=
– Fibrinolytic activity	↑
– Whole blood viscosity	↓
– Fibrinogen	↓
– Thrombocyte aggregation	↓
Hormonal regulation	
– Insulin resistance	↓
– Hyperinsulinemia	↓
– Stress hormones	↓
– Endorphins	↑
– Testosterone	↑
Circulatory system	
– Cardiac efficiency	↑
– Electrical stability	↑
– O_2 requirement of the heart	↓
– Blood pressure	↓
– Circulation in the muscles	↑

Physically active persons, not only endurance athletes, have lower insulin values and improved glucose tolerance when compared with inactive control groups, something that can only be explained by a elevated insulin sensitivity in the muscle and liver [4]. They also indicate a better cardiovascular risk factor profile. When previously inactive middle-aged persons begin an endurance training program of an average of 20 – 30 minutes per day at 60 – 80% VO_2max, the whole body glucose utilization and the insulin sensitivity of the musculature improve within 3 – 6 weeks [1].

A first direct proof of the preventative effect of physical training is provided by a longitudinal study by Frisch [2], according to which, college students active in sports later developed diabetes less frequently than their passive co-students.

7.4.2 *The therapeutic effects of physical exercise*

As is the case with healthy subjects, regular endurance training influences insulin effect and glucose tolerance in NIDDM.

Insulin-dependent glucose utilization rises during exercise and the insulin level drops. Both the peripheral as well as the hepatic insulin effect remain elevated 12 – 16 hours after an intensive endurance workout. A diminished triglyceride production and an accelerated breakdown of triglyceride lipoproteins via an increase in muscle lipoprotein lipase activity are associated with this.

Whether elevated blood pressure can be lowered in this way is unclear. Another effect of exercise is also important: the improvement in the overall health condition and an improved self-confidence.

7.4.3 *The application of physical exercise in NIDDM*

It is essential to state that the positive effects of physical exercise are only applicable to aerobic (i. e. endurance) sports. In view of the limited duration effect of an exercise bout (12 – 16 hours), one training session of middle intensity should take place daily. In order to prevent hypoglycemia in patients who receive sulfonyl ureas or insulin daily, the best time is 1 – 2 hours after a meal. In obese NIDDM patients, one should begin with exercises that constitute less static strain, such as swimming, bicycling, rowing, or similar sports. The transition from a movement-poor lifestyle to regular physical exercise must be carefully planned, monitored and developed (tab. 2) [3]. The appropriate forms of exercise and intensities are summarized in table 3. A daily walk of 30 – 45 minutes is sufficient for elderly people. Dangers lie above all in the circulatory system. The most dangerous complications are cardiac arrhythmias, which are the most frequent cause of death during sports. Therefore, before the start of a exercise program, an ECG is always prescribed. Warning symptoms are crescendo angina during the exercise, arrhythmia and unusual shortness of breath. In each case this should be cause for an observation with a 24-hour Holter ECG. Good exercise shoes (Adidas Torsion, Nike Air), socks made from absorbent natural substances with good heat distribution and careful warm-up and stretching exercises before the

Tab. 2: Guidelines for physical conditioning in NIDDM

Requirement:	Medical examination, training, motivation
Selection and organization:	Exclusion of medical and psycho-social contraindications, group training with 10 – 15 persons of similar performance capacity, age and social situation, attractive program, *one* therapist
Preferred forms of exercise:	Hiking, swimming, bicycling, light jogging, cross-country skiing, rowing
Controls:	Blood glucose, pulse, blood pressure, lipids, weight

Tab. 3: Training recommendations for NIDDM

Intensity		
	Age (years)	Pulse/minute
	20 – 29	130 – 155
	30 – 39	120 – 145
	40 – 49	110 – 135
	50 – 59	100 – 125
	60 – 69	80 – 110
	over 70	80 – 100
	Frequency/week	Minimum duration (min)
	daily	12 – 15
	3 ×	25 – 30
	2 ×	> 45
	1 ×	> 90

Basic rules

- Train daily or every other day, according to possibility
- Longer and with lower intensity is preferred
- In case of chest pain, arrhythmia and heavy exhaustion – consult a doctor
- Do not train in hot or humid weather or with acute infections

start of training, protect the limbs and tendons from over-exertion. Strenuous work-outs which raise blood pressure should be avoided during warm, humid weather.

7.4.4 *Summary*

Aerobic physical exercise is an integral part of therapy in NIDDM. Regular exercise improves glycemic control and insulin effect. 20 – 30 minutes of exercise should take place daily with pulse rates of 150 – age of patient/minute. Exercises appropriate to patient weight, careful exercise programming, foot care and circulatory monitoring help prevent complications.

References

[1] DeFronzo, R. A., R. S. Sherwin, N. Kraemer: Effect of physical training on insulin action in obesity. Diabetes *37* (1987) 1379 – 1385.

[2] Frisch, R. E., G. Wyshak, T. E. Albright et al.: Lower prevalence of diabetes in former college athletes compared with nonathletes. Diabetes *35* (1986) 1101 – 1105.

[3] Hanefeld, M., J. Huttunen: Exercise. In: A. G. Olsson (ed.): Atherosclerosis. Biology and clinical science, 481 – 486. Churchill Livingstone, Edinburgh 1987.

[4] Koivisto, V. A., H. Yki-Jarvinen, R. DeFronzo: Physical training and insulin sensitivity. Diabetes Metab. Rev. *1* (1986) 445 – 451.

[5] Vranic, M., M. Berger: Exercise and diabetes mellitus. Diabetes *28* (1979) 147 – 167.

7.5 Oral hypoglycemics

7.5.1 Alpha glucosidase inhibitors

M. Hanefeld

7.5.1.1 Introduction

More than 30 years had passed since the introduction of sulfonyl ureas and biguanides, before the licensing of acarbose in several European countries in 1991 introduced a new working principle in diabetes therapy, the optimization of glucose release and mono-saccharide absorption in the small intestine. It is worth mentioning that within one year of the introduction, already over one hundred thousand people with NIDDM in Germany had been placed on acarbose.

Alpha glucosidases are important enzymes in the plant and animal worlds, which cause the release of glucose from di- and polysaccharides in the human small intestine. Their inhibition can thereby slow the tempo of carbohydrate digestion and dampen the postprandial glucose rise, which provides an advantage, when one considers the sluggish release of endogenous insulin in NIDDM. In IDDM with exogenous insulin administration, acarbose can be useful to overcome rapid postprandial glucose increase.

In the systematic search for potent inhibitors of the glucosidases in the natural substance pool, two effective substances, in the form of acarbose and miglitol were finally isolated. The licensing of miglitol, which differs from acarbose in its range of action, pharmacokinetics and side effects, is expected in 1994/95.

7.5.1.2 Clinical pharmacology

Acarbose is isolated from the culture of a strain of the actinoplanacea bacteria. Chemically, acarbose resembles a tetrasaccharide (fig. 1) as it appears naturally in food. Through this resemblence, this pseudo-tetrasaccharide binds to the alpha glucosidases in the small intestine and thereby suppresses the carbohydrates of the food (fig. 2). The affinity of acarbose is 10 – 100,000 times greater than that of carbohydrates. With X-ray crystallographic methods a French research group has recently been able to provide direct proof that acarbose actually locates itself at the active center of the alpha-amylase. The binding is reversible and lasts only minutes. In a manner of speaking, acarbose is an externally effective, competitive inhibitor, which works exclusively in the small intestine. The resorption of monosaccharides, like glucose and fructose, is not suppressed. Less than 1% of the ingested acarbose appears in the blood. However, only 79% of the ad-

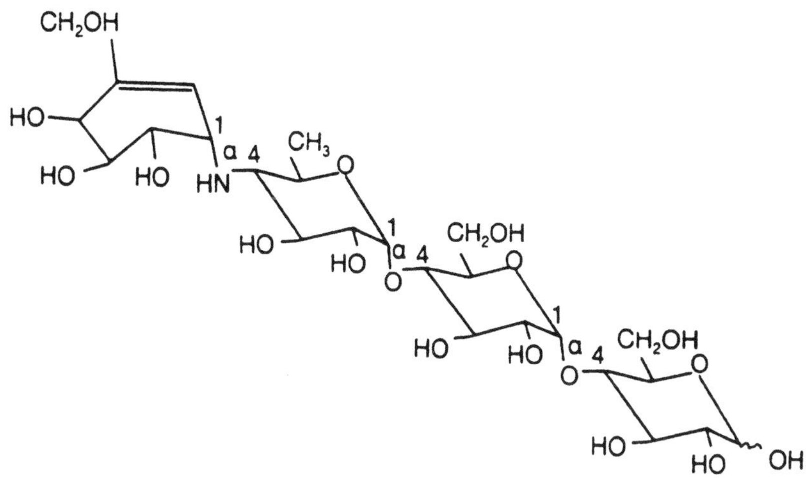

Fig. 1: Structural formula of the pseudotetrasaccharide acarbose.

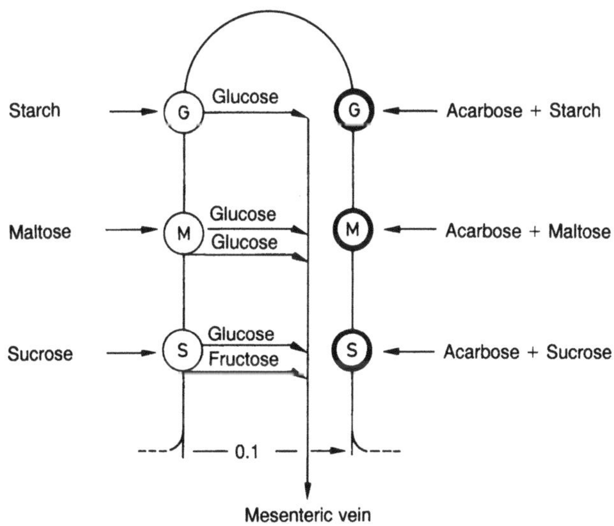

Fig. 2: Sites of action of acarbose on the small intestine, break-down of starch, maltose and sucrose by glucosidases (left) and their blocking by acarbose (right). G = glucoamylase; M = maltase; S = saccharase; ○ active enzyme; **O** blocked enzyme

ministered dose is excreted in the feces, 14% in the urine and only a small amount of C_{14} – acarbose fragments appear in the breath. This shows that about 20% of the ingested acarbose is broken down in the intestinal tract and these degradation products are also processed. In chronic toxicity studies in dogs, no damage of the gastroenterone or the liver was registered. To date there is no evidence that the transitory transaminase increase witnessed in a few cases in the USA and Israel are the result of liver-toxic effects from acarbose. This is substantiated by the fact that, miglitol, which is largely reabsorbed, has to date shown no hepatotoxic side effects. The use of acarbose is therefore largely independent of an intact liver and kidney function. This is particularly important regarding the administration in multi-morbid elderly diabetics.

In therapeutic doses, acarbose suppresses the various glucosidases of the small intestine with varying intensities: glucoamylase 82%, saccharase 68%, maltase 31.2%, isomaltase 8%, trehalase 3.6% and lactase 0% [1]. Because acarbose is only reabsorbed in an unchanged form in minimal concentrations, an effect on intracellular lysosomal enzymes and the excessive glycogen storage associated with this have not been noted up to now and are also not expected. Interactions with most of the other medications, especially sulfonyl urea, digitoxin and beta blockers, have not occurred.

7.5.1.3 *Mechanism of action*

Like metformin, acarbose is primarily an anti-hyperglycemic drug. Via the competitive suppression of the alpha glucosidases, carbohydrate digestion is largely delayed to the lower small intestine, such as is still the case today in traditional rural populations with a high portion of complex carbohydrates in their diet. A chain of events is thereby initiated (fig. 3), which, through a reduction of the postprandial hyperglycemia and lowered insulin, leads to an improvement in peripheral insulin effect. This is the only explanation for the 10 – 20% drop in

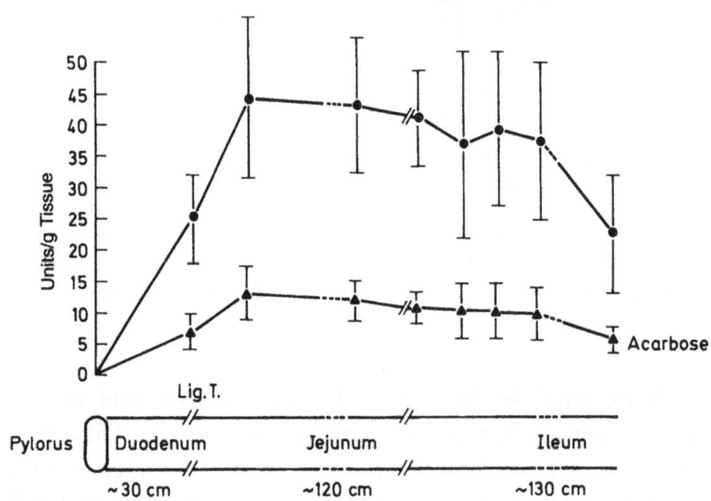

Fig. 3: Resorption delay by alpha glucosidase inhibitor [8].

the fasting blood glucose level after monotherapy of NIDDM [4]. Insulin secretion, measured by the C-peptide, is essentially not influenced by acarbose. The degree to which a long-term improvement of the insulin secretion dynamics can be achieved by perfect glucose control in mild to moderate diabetes cases, in terms of the glucose toxicity theory, still needs clarification. Additional effects on the gastrointestinal tract are a delayed stomach emptying and secretion of the gastric inhibitory peptide (GIP). The suppression of carbohydrate digestion in the upper gastrointestinal tract does not, however, lead to malabsorption, thus keeping the body weight constant at therapeutic doses. Long-term observations of rats have shown that it leads to enzyme adaption in the lower small intestine. An analogous adaptation in humans is assumed, as 4–8 weeks after the start of therapy, gastrointestinal side effects such as flatulence, bloating and diarrhea largely subside. In subtle investigations, W. F. Caspary was able to show that the carbohydrates, to the degree they reach the large intestine as a result of ingestion of acarbose, are there broken down by bacteria hydrolases and disaccharidases to monosaccharides, which are in turn transformed to short-chain fatty acids, hydrogen, carbon dioxide and methane. The results of this are a drop of the pH and rise of the osmolarity in the colon, which can lead to the above-named effects. To what extent the colon flora adapt to this long term has not yet been definitively clarified. A further remote effect of acarbose relates to the metabolism of triglyceride-rich lipoproteins. The postprandial rise in triglycerides is dampened after a carbohydrate-rich meal. As Nestel et al. [4] were able to prove, a lowered hepatic triglyceride synthesis can be considered the cause of both the action of acarbose on hyperglycemia as well as the action on hyperinsulinemia.

7.5.1.4 *Monotherapy with acarbose*

Due to its mode of action, acarbose can be viewed as a first-line drug for obese NIDDM patients with hyperinsulinemia. This is essentially true as well for the early phases of the slender type IIa, as long as insulin resistance and consecutive hyperinsulinemia are still present. An important indication is also the combination of NIDDM with mild hypertriglyceridemia [3]. Acarbose is particularly effective as monotherapy for NIDDM with low fasting and high postprandial blood glucose levels (tab. 1).

Tab. 1: Indications for therapy with acarbose in NIDDM

- Dietetically no longer controllable NIDDM
- Sulfonyl urea failure with sufficient insulin secretion
- Insufficient effect from metformin
- Dietetically controlled NIDDM with hypertriglyceridemia (?)
- Weight stabilization after a successful weight reduction treatment
- Massive postprandial blood glucose increase despite best effort with insulin adaptation
- Insulin reduction in insulin-requiring NIDDM

The pooled data from controlled studies of patients whose NIDDM was no longer controllable by means of diet, show a drop in the fasting blood glucose of ca. 10% and in the postprandial values of 20 – 30%. This effect can be shown longer than 5 hours after a carbohydrate-rich test meal.

Dependent on the initial state, the HbA_1 and/or HbA_{1c} drops 0.6 – 2.5 percentage points after 12 – 24 weeks. Further therapeutic effects are the reduction of the postprandial hyperinsulinemia and hyper-triglyceridemia. This result is of particular significance, because the triglyceride-rich lipoproteins in diabetics contribute not only to insulin resistance, but also represent an independent coronary risk factor.

Because acarbose does not cause any malabsorption, the body weight is not influenced. There is clinical experience which shows that acarbose assists in the maintenance of a new weight after a successful weight-reduction program. Alpha-glucosidase inhibitors do not significantly change food absorption. In patients who barely responded to the medication, the cause was repeatedly shown to be a very narrow portion of complex carbohydrates in the diet and instead large amounts of meat, milk and milk product, as well as a high alcohol consumption. The pre-condition for an optimal therapeutic effect from acarbose is a diet which is rich in complex carbohydrates, such as is recommended by the European Diabetes Society. Acarbose is, however, not a dietary replacement, rather it requires a health-promoting diet and enhances its maintenance.

Side effects

Bloating, flatulence and diarrhea are the most common complaints associated with acarbose use (tab. 2). They occur primarily in the first 4 – 6 weeks after treatment start. Through explanation to the patients about the cause and harmlessness of these complaints, they are mostly controlled. The drop-out rate is less

Tab. 2: Side effects of acarbose

Flatulence
Bloating
Diarrhea
Transaminase increase
Decrease in serum iron

than 3%. A great advantage of the drug, especially for the elderly, is that there is no hypoglycemia with acarbose monotherapy. Excretion is also essentially independent of liver and kidney function. In cases where gastrointestinal complaints still exist after a few months, it should be determined through a subtle diet history whether too much simple sugar or diet food with sugar alcohols are being taken. An additional cause of diarrhea can be latent gastro-intestinal illness, especially of the colon. In studies in the USA and Israel transaminase increases were observed in isolated cases, and these increases were reversible after the discontinuation of the medication. In Germany, there have been no reports of liver enzyme imbalances or hepatotoxic effects. Negative effects on kidney function and the hematopoietic system have thus far not been described. In two studies, a drop in the serum iron level under acarbose was observed.

Contraindications

For the most part, gastrointestinal diseases, which lead per se to diarrhea and bloating, are to be considered contraindications. Another problem is gastroparesis in patients with autonomous neuropathy.

Practical aspects

Tolerance and compliance are dependent to a decisive degree on the method of approach. This includes, on the one hand, the complete informing of the patient about the mode of action and resulting consequences for the diet, in order to minimize side effects. On the other hand, it is important to begin with a low dosage of 50 mg in the morning and to climb in intervals of 2 – 3 weeks to a maximum of 3 x 200 mg per day. In general, 50 – 100 mg at breakfast, lunch and dinner are sufficient in order to provide a good metabolic control in mild to moderate NIDDM.

7.5.1.5 Combination therapy

Acarbose can be used for the smoothing of the glucose profile and for insulin dosage reduction in IDDM as well as in insulin-requiring NIDDM. In practice, however, the most important combination is that connected to other oral antidiabetics, in the event monotherapy is not sufficient or – more infrequently – in order to reduce side effects or to primarily use complementary effects. The first controlled studies to this last possibility are now available.

Sulfonyl urea and acarbose

Several controlled studies related to this have been reviewed to by Clissold and Edwards [2] and Willms [9]. In cases with insufficient glucose control under sulfonyl ureas, glibenclamide comes up most frequently, the HbA_1 was able to be reduced by 1 – 2 percentage points and the circadian glucose level lowered by 10 – 20%. In general, a dosis of 3 x 100 mg acarbose is given with a maximal sulfonyl urea dosis. Interactions with the glibenclamide pharmacokinetics did not appear. In the opinion of Willms [9], along with intensification of the diet and physical exercise, the combination of acarbose and glibenclamide is the last chance to control the diabetes without insulin in elderly diabetics with metabolic imbalances. Metformin is here largely rejected as an alternative, due to its long list of contraindications.

It is an extension of the logic of the therapy concept for NIDDM which we present, that we view the reversed procedure, the addition of sulfonyl ureas upon insufficient efficiency of acarbose, as the meaningful future next step for obese patients with NIDDM. The available experiences show that, as in monotherapy, within a few days of discontinuing acarbose, glycemia returns to the level at the start of the therapy.

Metformin and acarbose

This combination has been tested in a large study in Canada, which showed a similar effectiveness as the combination acarbose – sulfonyl urea . Surprisingly, the side effects, also regarding the gastroenterone, with this combination were essentially no more frequent than with monotherapy.

Insulin and acarbose

An improvement of the glycemic control and reduction of insulin requirement were consistently achieved in insulin-treated NIDDM by the administration of acarbose. Acarbose is particularly useful when the postprandial blood glucose rise cannot be controlled with combination insulin in elderly diabetics.

7.5.1.6 *Summary*

The alpha glucosidase inhibitors (acarbose, miglitol) lead to delayed release of glucose from di- and polysaccharides in the small intestine and thereby to a flatter and delayed rise in the blood glucose. Furthermore, they lead to a reduction in postprandial hyperinsulinemia and hypertriglyceridemia, and probably in insulin resistance as well. Acarbose has proven itself as a first-line drug for NIDDM, which can no longer be controlled by diet. Further indications are the combination treatment upon sulfonyl urea failure, the breaking of insulin resistance through combination with metformin and the insulin dosage reduction in insulin-requiring NIDDM. The most important side effects are flatulence and diarrhea at the beginning of treatment. To date, serious side effects have not been observed.

References

[1] Caspary, C. W.: Inhibitors influencing carbohydrate absorption. In: W. Creutzfeldt, P. Lefebvre (eds.): Diabetes mellitus: Pathophysiology and Therapy, 172 – 196. Springer Verlag, Berlin 1988.

[2] Clissold, S., C. Edwards: Acarbose. A preliminary review of its pharmacodynamic and pharmacokinetic properties and therapeutic potential. Drugs 35 (1988) 214 – 243.

[3] Fölsch, U. R., B. Lembcke: Inhibition der intestinalen Alpha-Glukosidasen in der Therapie des Diabetes mellitus. Internist *32* (1991) 699–707.
[4] Hanefeld, M., S. Fischer, J. Schulze et al.: Therapeutical potentials of acarbose as first-line-drug in non-insulin dependent diabetes insufficiently treated with diet alone. Diabets Care *14* (1991) 732–737.
[5] Hanefeld, M.: Acarbose monotherapy in non-insulin dependent diabetes mellitus – the german experience. In: P. Lefebvre, E. Standl. (eds.): New Aspects in Diabetes, 147. De Gruyter, Berlin 1992.
[6] Lefebvre, P. J., A. J. Scheen: Update on the treatment of NIDDM. In: P. Lefebvre, E. Standl (eds.): New Aspects in Diabetes, 71. De Gruyter, Berlin 1992.
[7] Nestel, P., J. Bazelmans, M. Reardon et al.: Lower triglyceride production during carbohydrate-rich diets through acarbose, a glycoside hydrolyse inhibitor. Diabet. Metab. *11* (1985) 316–317.
[8] Puls, W., U. Keup, H. P. Krause et al.: Glucosidase inhibition: a new approach to the treatment of diabetes, obesity and hyperlipoproteinemia. Naturwissenschaften *64* (1977) *536–537.*
[9] Willms, B.: Therapie des Typ-II-Diabetes – Alpha-Glukosidasehemmer (Acarbose). Akt. Endokr. Stoffw. *13* (1992) *51–56.*

7.5.2 Biguanides

M. Hanefeld

7.5.2.1 *Introduction*

Biguanides have been employed for oral diabetic therapy for over three decades [3]. Metformin (dimethyl biguanide) (fig. 1) is the only biguanide which is registered in Germany. Phenformin (phenylaethyl biguanide) and buformin (butylbiguanide) were taken off the market in Germany in 1978 because an increased number of deaths from lactic acidosis were observed in the USA and Europe under phenformin. The number of biguanides used in oral diabetic therapy was subject to considerable fluctuation as a result of changes in the indications and developments in the pathophysiologic perspective of diabetes. These differences still hold true for Europe. The percentage of use in monotherapy in Romance countries is about 25%. Metformin is the most frequently used oral hypoglycemic in France. In Germany, it is only recommended for use in combination with a sulfonyl urea. In principle, however, monotherapy is permissible with a proper indication and observation for contraindications.

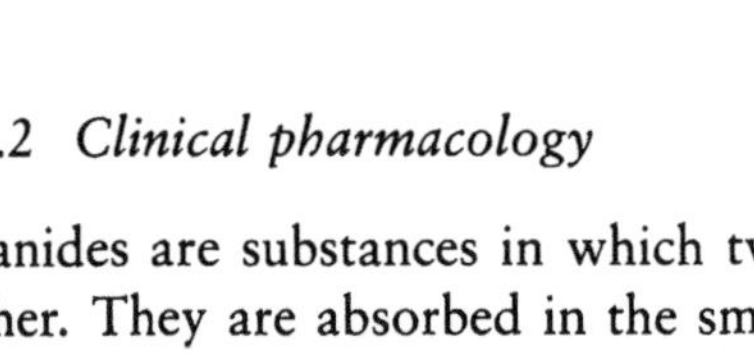

Fig. 1: Structural formula of metformin

7.5.2.2 *Clinical pharmacology*

Biguanides are substances in which two guanidine molecules are bound to one another. They are absorbed in the small intestine. The half-life of metformin is 2–4 hours. It is not metabolized, but is excreted via the kidney in unaltered form. Intact renal function is therefore an essential prerequisite for safe therapy. Two cellular mechanisms are important for potential dangers: biguanides inhibit cellular respiration and stimulate the anerobic glycolysis, whereby lactate formation increases. This is particularly critical if hypoxic conditions are present, e.g. in advanced atherosclerosis and cardiac failure. A central mode of action appears to be the improvement of the adenylcyclase inhibitory action on endogenous insulin via a G-protein. The binding to the lipophilic membrane elements and the accumulation in the liver, which is associated with this, are important for the toxicity of biguanides. This increases the longer the carbohydrate side chain becomes from metformin, to buformin, to phenformin, respectively. This is apparently an important reason for the low toxicity of metformin in comparison to phenformin [1, 8].

7.5.2.3 Mechanism of action

Metformin, like acarbose, has a blood glucose reducing effect only in diabetics. It is, in the narrower definition of the term, an anti-hyperglycemic substance. The medication intervenes at a number of points in glucose metabolism. The main difference to sulfonyl ureas is that it does not significantly affect insulin secretion in a direct manner, but acts only extra-pancreatically. It has been known for some time that there is an intial weight loss of 2 – 3 kg under biguanide treatment [3]. A mild anorexic effect has been shown to be the explanation for this. Biguanides inhibit intestinal glucose absorption and delay postprandial hyperglycemia, without creating malabsorption. Metformin's most important antidiabetic actions are the inhibition of hepatic gluconeogenesis and the increase of peripheral glucose utilization in muscle and adipose tissue [1]. Metformin reinforces the insulin effect on the glucose transport of muscle cells and adipocytes. It is therefore dependent on sufficient quantities of insulin being secreted. The activity of tyrosine-kinase, as the key enzyme of the insulin signal transmission in diabetic rats could therefore be normalized following the administration of metformin. The inclusion of glucose in glycogen in rat liver cells increases under therapeutic doses of metformin. The study results from Jackson [9] in NIDDM are clinically relevant. These show that hepatic gluconeogenesis, probably as a result of an improved insulin effect, decreases significantly under metformin, which is reflected in an especially effective correction of fasting hyperglycemia. To what extent the decrease in triglycerides and the therapeutic effects on coagulation and fibrinolysis are a direct effect or an indirect consequence of the improved diabetic metabolic state is not clear.

7.5.2.4 Monotherapy with metformin

On the basis of the mechanism of action, metformin is indicated, above all, in the early phases of NIDDM, because at this point in time the patients are, for the most part, hyperinsulinemic. This is especially true for the obese type IIb diabetic. Its use is limited by a number of contraindications in higher ages so that patients above the age of 70 are de facto out of the question. The therapeutic effects which are to be expected are summarized in tab.1. Metformin is particularly effective in patients with high fasting blood sugar, as a result of the

Tab. 1: The therapeutic effects of metformin

- Improvement in peripheral insulin effect
- Improvement in hepatic insulin effect and reduced gluconeogenesis
- Inhibition of glucose absorption in the small intestine
- Decreased appetite
- Triglyceride reduction
- Increased fibrinolysis (PAI ↓)
- Inhibition of platelet aggregation

suppression of the excessive hepatic gluconeogenesis described above. In the review by Schernthaner [11] the mean drop in fasting blood glucose in 15 controlled studies was 25%. The number of cases were, however, sometimes small and the observation period short, so the long-term drop in glycemia may be 20% or less. The mean HbA_{1c} drop was 1.5%. This corresponds to approximately the same therapeutic effect of sulfonyl ureas. The weight reduction of 1–3 kg associated with the anorexic effect is an advantage [3]. In view of the long-term prognosis, the additional effects on the coronary risk factor profile are important (tab. 1). In many studies, but not all, the triglycerides were lowered significantly and the HDL cholesterol increased [11]. This was associated with a decrease in plasminogen activator inhibitor (PAI) [12]. This was confirmed in animal experimental models on the antithrombotic properties of metformin. The insulin level is hardly influenced by metformin.

There are still no solid, long-term controlled studies on possible antiatherogenic properties. According to the present state of knowledge, secondary failure occurs less often than with a sulfonyl urea. A subtle reevaluation of metformin, which is currently starting, is absolutely necessary.

Side effects

The most important side effect (tab.2) is lactic acidosis. Lactic acidosis is diagnosed with a lactate > 5 mmol/l and pH values < 7.25. The danger is, however, usually overestimated. The metformin-associated mortality rate in England, for instance, was 0.017/1,000 patient-years between 1976 and 1986, in Canada 0. In contrast, with phenformin there were 0.3 fatal cases in Sweden and even 0.48 fatal cases per 1,000 years in Switzerland. Warning symptoms are unexplained lack of appetite, vomiting, weakness and nausea. The mortality is still as high as 50% [11].

Treatment consists of supplying large quantities of fluids, glucose and insulin. The use of hemodialysis in severe cases helps to eliminate metformin and lactate. Gastrointestinal side effects are relatively frequent. In 15 to 20% there is initially

Tab. 2: Side effects of metformin

Gastrointestinal complaints (pressure, nausea, vomiting, metallic taste, diarrhea)	5–20%
Lack of appetite	common
Lactic acidosis	very infrequent
Skin allergies	infrequent
Abnormalities in the blood count	very infrequent

a loss of appetite, vomiting, stomach pain and diarrhea [4]. This can be avoided by gradually increasing the dosage. It is necessary to discontinue the drug in less than 5% of the cases.

Contraindications

The contraindications (tab.3) are above all, all types of hypoxia, which prohibit its use in elderly, multimorbid patients. Alcoholism and renal functional disorders (creatinine > 140 μmol/l) are also definite contraindications. The same is true for liver damage. The cases of lactic acidosis associated with metformin which have been published occur almost exclusively in this group of patients.

Tab. 3: Contraindications for metformin therapy

All hypoxic conditions
– respiratory insufficiency
– coronary insufficiency
– arteriosclerotic ischaemic vascular diseases (IHD, PVD, CAD)
– anemias
Liver diseases (except fatty liver)
Impaired kidney function [creatinine > 140 μmol/l (1.4 mg/dl)]
Advanced age
Multi-morbidity

7.5.2.5 Combination therapy

Metformin and sulfonyl ureas

As early as 1958 Mehnert and Seitz [10] suggested treating patients, who had not been satisfactorily controlled with sulfonyl ureas, in combination with biguanides. This treatment has become widespread. However, there have still been only a few controlled studies [6] in which the efficacy of this combination has been compared to that of insulin alone and insulin plus sulfonyl urea. Due to the fact that the two medications differ in their mechanisms of action and point of action, a complementary effect is well likely even with sulfonyl urea failure. The inverse has hardly been pursued to date. It is not known whether the effect is simply additive, synergistic or even potentiating. Even the direct medication interactions have been hardly analysed. In a prospective, open study of 200 normal weight NIDDM patients with sulfonyl urea failure, 50% were still successfully treated after 3 years with chlorpropamide plus metformin [2]. The success rate (64.6%) was highest in the age group 60 – 74 years. If the data of the few controlled studies is extrapolated, it can be seen that the combination is most effective in elderly patients who exhibited only moderately imbalanced NIDDM with monotherapy. The mean additional fasting blood glucose reduction is 18 – 40% [11]. In a randomized double-blind study Hermann [7] obtained an additional HbA_{1c}-drop of 29% after 6 months therapy after the addition of metformin to glibenclamide. The most extensive investigation in this field was recently presented by Haupt [5] who took 1833 consecutive patients, who despite maximum sulfonyl urea therapy, were poorly controlled, and lowered their HbA_1 from 11% to 9.1%. Gastrointestinal complaints occurred in 7% following metformin, in 4.2% the metformin intake had to be discontinued due to side effects. Well-founded data about the side effect rates under combined therapy are not available for the vascular system. One possible indication for combination therapy is to reduce of the side effects of monotherapy by means of dose reduction with combination.

With sulfonyl urea failure the maximum metformin dosage (2500 mg) should be given in stages, keeping the contraindications in mind. If, however, the HbA_1 is $> 8.5\%$ and the C-peptide value after glucagon stimulation is below 1.1 nmol/l, insulin treatment should not be delayed.

We would like to express our support for Schernthaner's opinion that the use of metformin with sulfonyl urea failure, when the insulin reserves are often exhausted and the patients are multimorbid, is considerably more dangerous and less reasonable than early monotherapy with metformin.

Metformin and acarbose

The first results available in this connection indicate that this therapy is similarly effective to the combination sulfonyl urea plus biguanides. Benefits and side effects of this combination must be investigated further. It appears to be very promising in insulin resistance with hyperinsulinemia, which can not be sufficiently compensated with the individual monotherapies.

Metformin and insulin

This combination has shown itself to be of little or no effect and should no longer be employed.

7.5.2.6 *Summary*

Biguanides improve peripheral insulin effect and inhibit hepatic gluconeogenesis. They are therefore antihyperglycemic substances which should be used especially in cases of obese NIDDM with hyperinsulinemia and hypertriglyceridemia, which show a high fasting blood sugar. Due to the numerous complications, their use is not recommended for multimorbid elderly NIDDM patients. As a rule, monotherapy is reasonable after the exclusion of contraindications following failure of the diet control in obese NIDDM patients with sufficient insulin reserves. Due to the danger of lactic acidosis, above all in renal and hepatic disease, creatinine, transaminases and – in appropriate symptoms – lactate should be monitored. Their combination with sulfonyl ureas after failure of monotherapy has proven itself to be positive. The initial results of controlled studies are positive for their combination with acarbose, but their use in insulin requiring NIDDM is not sensible.

References

[1] Bailey, C. J.: Metformin revised: Its actions and indications for use. Diabet. Med. *5* (1988) 315–320.

[2] Clarke, B. F., L. J. Duncan: Comparison of chlorpropamide and metformin treatment on weight and blood glucose response of uncontrolled obese diabetics. Lancet *1* (1968) 123–126.

[3] Haller, H., S. E. Strauzenberg: Orale Diabetestherapie. Thieme Verlag, Stuttgart 1966.

[4] Gerich, J. T.: Oral hypoglycemic agents. New Engl. J. Med. *321* (1989) 1231–1245.

[5] Haupt, E., B. Knick, H. Koschinsky et al.: Oral antidiabetic combination therapy with sulfonylureas and metformin. Diab. Metab. *17* (1991) 224–231.

[6] Hermann, L.: Biguanides and sulfonylureas as combination therapy in NIDDM. Diabetes Care *13* (suppl. 3) (1990) 37–42.

[7] Hermann, L., T. Kjellström, P. Nilson-Ehle: Effect of metformin and glibenclamide alone and in combination on serum lipids and lipoproteins in patients with non-insulin-dependent diabetes mellitus. Diab. Metab. *17* (1991) 174–179.

[8] Hermann, L. S.: Metformin. A review of its pharmacological properties and therapeutic use. Diab. Metab. *9* (1983) 148–163.

[9] Jackson, R. A., M. Hawa, J. Jaspan et al.: Mechanism of metformin action in non-insulin-dependent diabetes. Diabetes *36* (1987) 632–640.

[10] Mehnert, H.: Sulfonylharnstoffe oder Biguanide in der Behandlung des Typ 2 Diabetes. Deutsch. Med. Wschr. *114* (1989) 1086–1088.

[11] Schernthaner, G.: Kritische Analyse der antidiabetischen Therapie mit Metformin: Stoffwechselwirkungen, antiatherogene Effekte und Kontraindikationen. Akt. Endokr. Stoffw. *13* (1992) 44–50.

[12] Vague, P., J. Juhan-Vague, M. Alessi et al.: Metformin decreases the high plasminogen activator inhibition capacity, plasma insulin and triglyceride levels in non-diabetic obese subjects. Thromb. Haemost. *57* (1987) 326–328.

7.5.3 Derivatives of sulfonyl urea

U. Julius

7.5.3.1 Introduction

The era of oral hypoglycemics therapy was ushered in, at least experimentally in animals, with the accidental discovery in 1942 by Janbon and Loubatiéres that certain sulfonamides have a hypoglycemic action as a side effect. Franke and Fuchs are credited with introducing derivatives of sulfonyl urea to the treatment of human diabetes mellitus in the year 1954. Thorough clinical investigations of this group of drugs were performed in the 50s and 60s in Dresden (Haller and Strauzenberg 1966). Amongst the preparations available, glibenclamide, which was first introduced in 1967, has become most popular. The portion of type II diabetics who receive sulfonyl urea drugs is generally estimated as being over 40%. In the Diabetes Intervention Study as well as in the control patients, glibenclamide (Maninil®) was the most often used as oral treatment. According to study criteria, the patients had to be treatable by diet alone at the beginning of the study. While oral hypoglycemic drugs were used in 28.2 or 34.0% (groups with and without clofibrate) of the intervention patients after 5 years, 47.4% of the control group were prescribed this medication. Interestingly, despite this treatment, the mean glycemic level was worse in the control group than in the intervention group. From basic knowledge of the pathogenesis of type II diabetes, it is possible to deduce that it is desirable to reduce the number of sulfonyl urea-treated patients in favor of non-drug treatment or anti-diabetic agents with another profile of action. It is viewed as particularly inappropriate to further stimulate a hyperinsulinemia, which is already present, with the addition of a sulfonyl urea compound.

7.5.3.2 Mechanism of action

The main effect of sulfonyl urea drugs is the stimulation of insulin secretion [12]. The synthesis of insulin is apparently not increased. There is no evidence to indicate that the mechanism of action of the various substances that constitute this group is different. Sulfonyl urea-receptors have been found on the insulin-producing beta-cells of the islets of Langerhans. The order of the binding strength of the sulfonyl urea compound to these receptors is parallel to its potential to release insulin. The most potent representatives of the 2nd generation sulfonyl ureas, glibenclamide and glipizide, bind to the receptors in nanomolar concentrations [2]. Sulfonyl ureas appear to be dependent on the additional effect of modulating factors. The most important of these is glucose, which potentiates the insulin-releasing effect of the sulfonyl uric drug.

Evidence of the extrapancreatic influence of sulfonyl ureas has been gained from experiments. These effects do not, however, have any clinical relevance. Sulfonyl ureas are ineffective in type I diabetics.

The following factors influence the efficacy of sulfonyl ureas [9]:

1. Presence of an endogenous insulin production

The initially-elevated insulin secretion decreases over the course of years (see Chapter 3).

2. Duration of the diabetes

As a rule, the highest efficacy can be expected from the lowest dosages of sulfonyl uric compound following manifestation.

3. Concomitant illness

Concomitant illness can elevate the peripheral insulin resistance to the level where sulfonyl ureas are practically ineffective.

4. Accompanying medication

The glucose tolerance (tested with 75g oGTT) in type II diabetics treated with glibenclamide deteriorated under propranolol medication, the insulin level decreased.

Antidiabetic agents are often employed too early (before all the possibilities of non-drug treatment have been exhausted) and discontinued too late (when they are no longer effective) [11].

7.5.3.3 *Pharmacokinetics*

The sulfonyl urea preparations available (fig. 1) differ under the following aspects:

- Bioavailability
- Dosage employed
- Half-life
- Potency
- Breakdown, excretion

Glibenclamide has proven itself to be the most effective preparation. It can be used in very low dosages (in preparations with good bioavailability).

The plasma binding of glibenclamide to albumin (90 – 99%) takes place by means of non-ionic forces. Glibenclamide is almost completely transformed to hydroxy-

Substance	Common	Preparation
Glibenclamide	1.75–10.5 mg	Daonil, Euglucon N, Maninil
	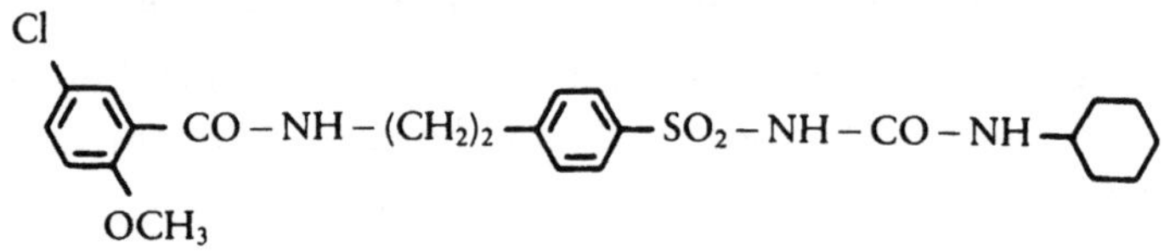	
Glibornuride	12.5–75 mg	Glutril, Gluboride
	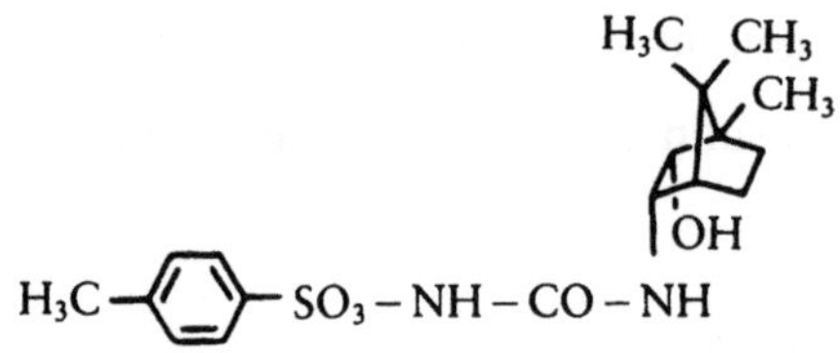	
Glipicide	5–30 mg	Glibenese
	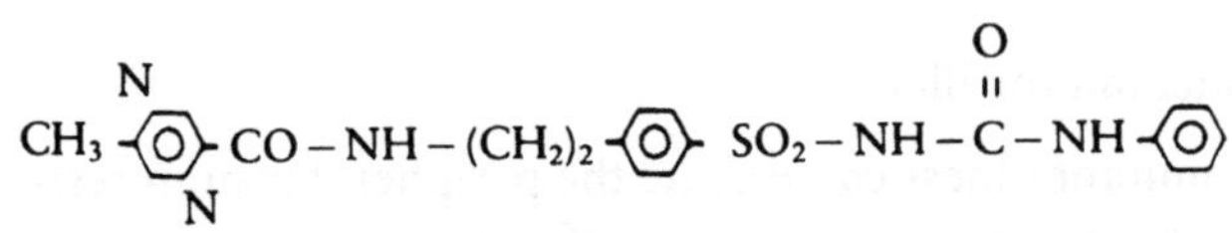	
Gliquidon	15–90 mg	Glurenorm
	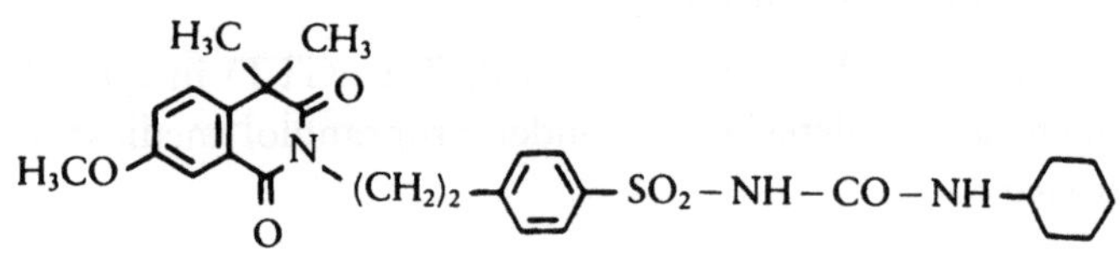	
Glisoxepide	2–12 mg	Pro-Diaban
	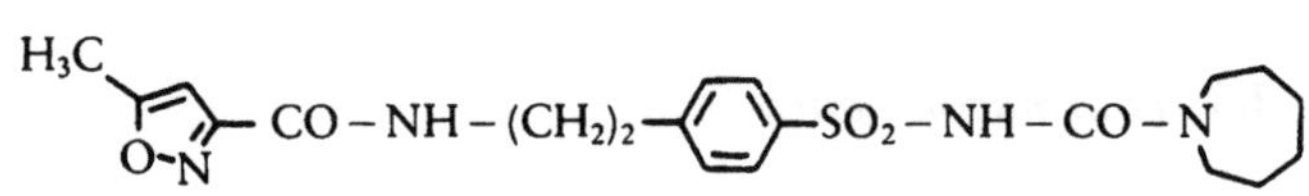	
Tolbutamide	0.5–1.5 g	Rastinon, Orabet
	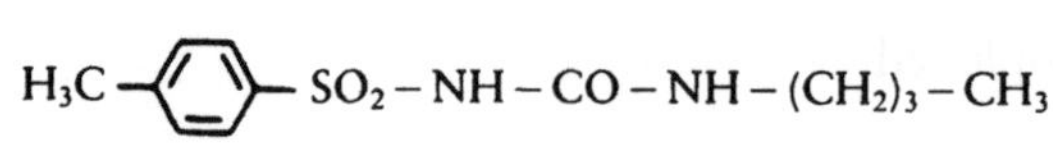	
Gliclacide	40–240 mg	Diamicron
	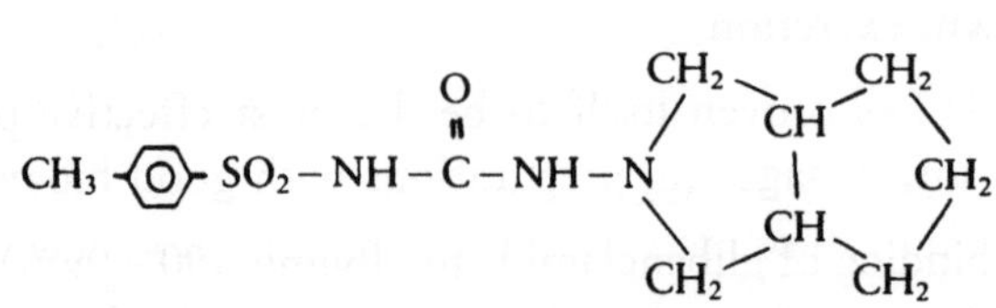	

Fig. 1: Selection of available SU preparations

derivates in the liver. A blood glucose reducing effect has also been demonstrated for the metabolites, it is, however, 5 – 10 times weaker. Only about 4 – 6% is excreted by the feces in unaltered form. The elimination of the metabolites occurs to the extent of about 50% via the gall in the feces and about 50% via the kidneys in the urine. The half-life of glibenclamide is listed as 6 – 12 hours (mean 10 hours) [8], longer elimination half-lives are, however, possible with long-term use. The peak effect is reached between 3 and 5 hours.

An increased excretion of the metabolites via the bite occurs, depending on the degree of the renal excretion disorder, in renally insufficient patients. A preparation with short half-lives, e.g. tolbutamide or glibornuride, are recommended for elderly diabetics or patients at hypoglycemic risk (see side effects of sulfonyl ureas).

7.5.3.4 Monotherapy with sulfonyl ureas

Indications for the use of sulfonyl ureas

Sulfonyl urea compounds are indicated in type II diabetics if,

- ▶ Diet and physical training are no longer sufficient in and of themselves
- ▶ Weight reduction and a regulation of lifestyle has been previously attained
- ▶ No acute or chronic secondary illness is present and no operation is planned which could have a negative effect on the metabolism
- ▶ Regular food intake is guaranteed.

The general attitude has to be:
Wait with sulfonyl urea therapy, as long as the non-drug measures have not been exhausted and hyperinsulinemia still exists.

There is no blood glucose concentration above which the prescription of sulfonyl ureas appears to be absolutely necessary. It is definitely possible to reduce even high blood glucose levels by introducing dietary measures after the manifestation of type II diabetes.

A change to glibenclamide may be successful with a very low insulin requirement in type II diabetics [13]. The blood glucose will be lowered over the course of several weeks by glibenclamide (fig. 2).

With a certain delay there is also a reduction in glycosylated hemoglobin (fig. 3).

Contraindications

- Type I diabetes mellitus (lack of endogenous insulin production)
- Pregnancy, nursing
- Acute ketoacidosis, precoma, hyperosmolor coma
- Metabolic decompensation in the course of infectious diseases

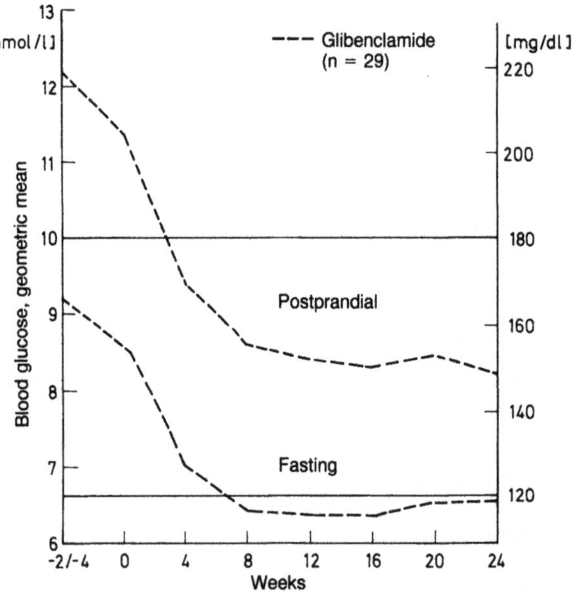

Fig. 2: Blood glucose levels (fasting and postprandial) of type II diabetics during 24-week glibenclamide treatment (taken in a modified form from [15]).

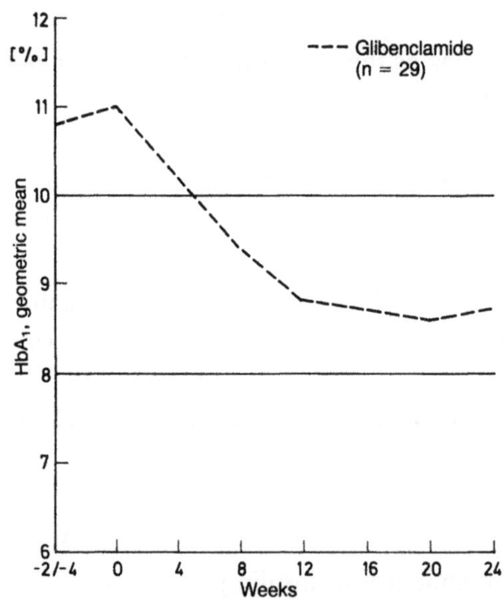

Fig. 3: HbA_1 levels of type II diabetics during 24-week glibenclamide treatment (taken in a modified form from [15]).

- Known hypersensitivity to sulfonyl ureas or sulfonamides
- Severe organ insufficiencies (e.g. liver, kidney)
- Major operations

Relative contraindications

- Cerebral performance disorders (e.g. cerebral arteriosclerosis, dementia)
- High fever infections
- Unreliable patient with respect to diet, e.g. advanced age or alcoholism
- History of sulfonyl urea-induced hypoglycemia

Practical approach

Starting treatment: The treatment begins with ½ to 1 tablet glibenclamide 1.75 mg before breakfast. This dosage is maintained for several days. After 3–5 days there is a metabolic check (generally out-patient). If necessary, the dosage is increased in steps of ½ to 1 tablet glibenclamide 1.75 mg until the metabolic situation is optimized. In no way should this increase take place too quickly, because the maximum effect is only to be expected after weeks. With daily doses of two tablets of glibenclamide 1.75 or more, it is also possible to use glibenclamide 3.5. Glibenclamide is taken with liquid, without chewing. Daily dosages up to 2 tablets are administered once up to 30 minutes before breakfast, the remaining dosage about 30 minutes before dinner. Administration of a partial dose is also possible before lunch. Punctual intake is important. Forgotten tablets should not be taken later than 1–2 hours after the proper time. Reaction time, and thereby driving ability, may be impaired during adjustment phases.

Long-term use: The maintenance dose (usually 3.5 to 7 mg daily) should be the lowest effective dose. In general, the maximum effect is reached with a daily dose of 3 tablets glibenclamide 3.5 mg; more should not be usea.

The following notes should be observed:
- If it is not possible to orally feed a diabetic treated with a sulfonyl urea preparation, it is necessary that the patient quickly receive medical treatment and consultation.
- In cases of extraordinary stress (e.g. accidents, operations, high-fever infections) it may be necessary to switch the patient to insulin for a period of time.
- The effect of sulfonyl ureas can be potentiated by alcohol (hypoglycemia): chronic alcoholism may lead to a worsening of the metabolic situation (hyperglycemia). The permissible amount of alcohol is to be arranged with the patient.

Therapeutic goal: Fasting blood glucose concentrations below 6 mmol/l (110 mg/dl) and postprandial blood glucose levels below 11 mmol/l (200 mg/dl) and hemoglobin A_{1c} concentrations below 6% should be the objective with younger and cooperative patients. Rigid metabolic control is often neither possible nor desirable for the elderly. In these cases, there is the danger of hypoglycemia due to altered elimination and unreliable eating habits. In every such individual case, it is necessary to check whether, with high postprandial blood glucose values (above 15 mmol/l; 270 mg/dl), insulin therapy should be used to supplement, or even replace, the oral antidiabetic therapy.

Withdrawal tests: If the fasting blood glucose level normalizes during treatment with glibenclamide, it may be worth attempting to stop the drug administration.

Change of preparation: Within the group of sulfonyl ureas, it only makes sense to change from a weaker preparation to glibenclamide.

Side effects of sulfonyl ureas

The following relevant side effects have been observed under glibenclamide:

- hypoglycemic reactions
- gastrointestinal reactions
- allergic skin reactions.

Hypoglycemia is the most important side effect and occurs, according to the literature, in over 1% of those treated. Systematic investigations prove that symptomless hypoglycemia occurs considerably more often. Factors which favor the occurrence of hypoglycemia are:

- lack of food intake (not enough carbohydrates)
- uncompensated disturbances of the endocrine system (e.g. adrenal insufficiency)
- extreme physical stress
- impaired kidney function
- alcohol consumption.

Between 1971 and 1982 over 57 cases of glibenclamide-induced hypoglycemia in elderly patients were reported in Sweden in over 300,000 patient-years. In 24 cases the hypoglycemia was prolonged (12–72 hours), 10 patients died.

In Switzerland, in a 10-year observation period – 100,000 patient-years – the following "order of risk" of hypoglycemia was determined: glibenclamide 38, chlorpropamide 34, glipicide 15, glibornuride 9, carbutamide 8, tolbutamide 7. In 25% of the patients there was an acute infection which may have been responsible for a lack of nutritional intake. Of the chronic concomitant diseases, renal insufficiency, which was present in not less than 21% of the patients, deserves particular note.

Clinical signs of hypoglycemia are an expressed sensation of hunger, as well as a lack of concentration, acute, often creeping weakness, sweating, headache, fatigue, nervousness, confusion or even unconciousness or convulsions.

Therapy of hypoglycemia: Mild hypoglycemia can best be combated directly by the patient by drinking tea with sugar or fruit juices. The patient must be carefully and properly educated in this respect. Diabetics being treated with glibenclamide must always carry several pieces of candy or sugar cubes with them. Persons living with the patient should be informed to contact a physician in cases of emergency.

In case of unconsciousness, intravenous application of glucose, if possible as a bolus (e.g. 50 g glucose in the form of 20% or 40% solution) and then as an indwelling infusion if necessary until the patient can be stabilized with oral carbohydrates. If necessary glucagon i.v., s.c. or i.m. may be applied. The follow-up period should not be too short and must frequently be combined with monitoring in the hospital.

In elderly patients (over 70) hypoglycemia is a particularly hazardous complication and has been observed at relatively low dosages of the preparation. An impending vascular or degenerative cerebral insufficiency can, on the one hand, mask this, but on the other hand be worsened as a result of it. In addition to this, is the fact that the physiological counterregulatory mechanism is dulled with increasing age.

On rare occasions there are other side effects: blood, hematogenic system: thrombocytopenia; nervous system: paresthesia, optic atrophy; alcohol intolerance.

Failure of sulfonyl ureas

If an optimal metabolic compensation cannot be attained with glibenclamide, the so-called primary failure, there is cause to suspect insufficient insulin supply by the pancreas.

Secondary failure: A secondary failure is present if, after at least three months of good metabolic control there is an increasing deterioration of the metabolic state, despite diet and optimal dosaging of the sulfonyl urea, with continuous imbalances of the mean postprandial blood glucose above 11 mmol/l (200 mg/dl). As glibenclamide is the most potent blood glucose reducing sulfonyl urea-derivate, it is only possible to speak of "secondary failure" after it has been used unsuccessfully.

The rate of failures is 5 – 10% per year, however, in previous evaluation patients were included who would no longer be considered suitable for oral antidiabetic therapy.

All possiblities for improving the non-drug antidiabetic therapy (diet, weight reduction, muscle training) should be exhausted first in cases of secondary failure. This is even more important because the failure is frequently not one of the sulfonyl uric compound, but rather that of the patient ("secondary failure" in sulfonyl urea therapy).

When there are no contraindications for biguanides (this must be carefully checked) a combination with a preparation from this group (metformin) may lead to an improvement in metabolism. A combination with an alpha glucosidase inhibitor (e.g. acarbose) is possible.

If these measures are not sufficient insulin therapy should be introduced, although some authors today prefer a combination therapy with glibenclamide.

7.5.3.5 Combination therapy

Combination with insulin

The continued presence of endogenous insulin secretion is also an important prerequisite for the combination of sulfonyl ureas with insulin injections [10, 13]. The following indications are possible:

1. Type II diabetics, who cannot be properly controlled with insulin monotherapy, where the failure cannot be attributed to dietary discretions, concomitant diseases or a, for the most part, lack of endogenous insulin secretion. If it is not technically possible to perform a necessary second insulin injection, it is possible to combine a single injection with oral sulfonyl urea therapy (psychosocial indication)
2. Sulfonyl urea secondary failure in which the sulfonyl urea therapy can be continued and supplemented by an additional insulin injection treatment.

Combination with biguanides or alpha glucosidase inhibitors

Due to the differing mechanisms of action, a combination of these preparations with glibenclamide may be quite positive.

Interactions with other drugs

Both undesired decreases and increases in blood glucose have been described with the simultaneous use of sulfonyl urea and other compounds. The relevance of some of this data for the practice is, however, not very great. Glibenclamide can be used in patients who are taking an anticoagulant. Beta blockers may mask the patients' symptoms of a decrease in blood glucose.

7.5.3.6 Summary

With metabolic decompensation (increase of the blood glucose) under diet therapy and despite weight reduction, the stimulation of endogenous insulin production with a sulfonyl urea may be reasonable. This is especially true if insulin secretion increasingly drops off. Amongst the sulfonyl urea preparations, glibenclamide has proven itself to be the most effective. It should be used in the lowest possible dosages. It is important – particularly in elderly diabetics, that hypoglycemia be avoided. In the case of a failure of the oral therapy, one should not wait too long before initiating insulin therapy (if possible as a combination therapy sulfonyl urea insulin).

References

[1] Althoff, P. H.: Das Sulfonylharnstoff-Sekundärversagen – Definition und Therapie. In: NOVO Industrie GmbH, Pharmaceutika Med.-wiss.-Abteilung, Neue Aspekte des Typ-II-Diabetes, 117–125. Berichtsband über den Workshop am 14. und 15. September 1987 in Leipzig.

[2] Ammon, H. P. T.: Molekularer Wirkungsmechanismus der Sulfonylharnstoffe. Dtsch. med. Wschr. *113* (1988) 864–870.

[3] Beck-Nielsen, H.: Treatment of NIDDM patients with peroral antidiabetic drugs – sulfonylureas, biguanides and new pharmacological approaches –. In: C. E. Mogensen, E. Standl: Pharmacology of Diabetes. Present Practice and Future Perspectives, 75–92. Walter de Gruyter, Berlin, New York 1991.

[4] Gerich, J. E.: Oral Hypoglycemic Agents. New England Journal of Medicine *321* (1989) 1231–1242.

[5] Haller, H., S. E. Strauzenberg: Orale Diabetestherapie. Thieme-Verlag, Leipzig 1966.

[6] Hanefeld, M., S. Fischer, H. Schmechel et al.: Diabetes Intervention Study. Multi-Intervention Trial in Newly Diagnosed NIDDM. Diabetes Care *14* (1991) 308–317.

[7] Holman, R. R., R. C. Turner: Oral Agents and Insulin in the Treatment of Non-Insulin-Dependent Diabetes Mellitus. In: J. Pickup, G. Williams: Textbook of Diabetes, 462–476. Blackwell Scientific Publications, Oxford, London 1991.

[8] Jackson, J. E., R. Bressler: Clinical pharmacology of sulphonylurea hypoglycaemic agents. Part 1. Drugs *22* (1981) 211–245.

[9] Julius, U.: Indikationen und Kontraindikationen der Sulfonylharnstoffe. In: NOVO Industrie GmbH, Pharmaceutika Med.-wiss.-Abteilung, Neue Aspekte des Typ-II-Diabetes, 99–109. Berichtsband über den Workshop am 14. und 15. September 1987 in Leipzig.

[10] Lotz, N., W. Bachmann, H. Mehnert et al.: Combining insulin with oral antidiabetic agents (including problems of secondary failure). In: C. E. Mogensen, E. Standl: Pharmacology of Diabetes. Present Practice and Future Perspectives, 113–133. Walter de Gruyter, Berlin, New York 1991.

[11] Mehnert, H.: Differentialtherapie mit oralen Antidiabetika. Medizinische Klinik *86* (1991) 521–525.

[12] Melander, A.: Clinical pharmacology of sulfonylureas. Metabolism *36* (1987) Suppl. 1, 12–16.

[13] Mezitis, N. E. E., S. Heshka, V. Saitas et al.: Combination therapy for NIDDM with biosynthetic human insulin and glyburide. Diabetes Care *15* (1992) 265–269.

[14] Ratzmann, K. P.: Das sekundäre Sulfonylharnstoff-Versagen. Dtsch. med. Wschr. *115* (1990) 1404–1407.

[15] Spengler, M., G. Hänsel, K. Boehme: Acarbose und Glibenclamid bei Typ-II-Diabetes. Zeitschrift für Allgemeinmedizin *66* (1990) 3–15.

7.5.4 Anorectics

U. Julius

7.5.4.1 *Definition of anorectics*

Anorectics (appetite suppressants) are supposed to reduce the food consumption by inhibiting the feeling of hunger and thereby contribute to weight reduction.

As already mentioned (section 7.2), the elimination of excess weight in type II diabetes has a high priority for the control of diabetes and risk factors.

Amphetamine-like substances were the most commonly used anorectics for a long period of time. As a result of their side effects and limited effectiveness, they are no longer recommendable. Fenfluramine, which is also chemically similar to amphetamines, is also important, but does not possess any central stimulating effects. Fenfluramine represents a racemic mixture of D- and L-stereoisomers.

The right-rotating D-form (*dexfenfluramine*, preparation Isomeride®) has shown itself to be the effective and low-side-effect component [1, 3]. As a result this substance is of increased or growing interest, because it also causes a direct positive effect on the insulin-sensitivity of obese type II diabetics, independent of the weight reduction.

7.5.4.2 *Effect*

Dexfenfluramine reduces the feeling of hunger, extends the postprandial time until hunger occurs and leads to a reduction in calorie uptake. The substance was tested against placebo and on average induced a larger reduction in weight [1, 2, 6]. Weight losses of about 3 kg in the month and 7 kg in 3 months have been described without the patient having been aware of a change in lifestyle. There was always detailed dietary instruction and patients were seen on a regular basis. The average slight weight increase in the period from 6 months to one year was slightly less in comparison to placebo in the international multi-center study (with one-year use of dexfenfluramine) [2]. The results of experiments on animals and humans which indicate a change of eating habits (reduction of the carbohydrate intake and spontaneous eating), are interesting. Dexfenfluramine inhibited an initial dysphoria after smoking cessation in one study [7]. These patients exhibited, in contrast to placebo, a weight loss while carbohydrate consumption was lower. Dexfenfluramine had a positive effect on women with premenstrual syndrome (tension, weariness, etc.). Here, too, excessive carbohydrate intake was slowed in this phase. [8].

Fenfluramine lowers the blood glucose level and improves insulin sensitivity, without impairing insulin secretion, in type II diabetics who are not optimally compensated. Even after a one week, placebo-controlled application of dexfenfluramine [5] a reduction in blood glucose and free fatty acids could be shown, by means of clamp examinations in overweight type II diabetics, despite constant weight. The glucose flow-off increased. The latter was not observed in the parallel examination of obese normal persons (without diabetes).

7.5.4.3 Indication and therapy

It has not been possible to determine which obese patients could profit most from dexfenfluramine. It should, however, only be used in those patients who have metabolic, degenerative or cardiopulmonary consequences from the obesity. Under these circumstances, its use in type II diabetics can be seen as sensible. It is imaginable that the substance can be viewed as a first-line drug in mild type II diabetes with obesity, if a satisfactory metabolic compensation can not be managed in a purely dietary manner.

Possible indications for the use of dexfenfluramine are:
1. Obesity which is resistant to non-drug therapies (e.g. type II diabetes)
2. Preventing weight gain after smoking cessation
3. Women with pronounced premenstrual complaints and disturbed eating habits (in the course of weight control programs)
4. Follow-up treatment after partial fasting to avoid renewed weight gain.
5. Obesity with compulsive hyperphagia, possibly stress-induced.

► This pharmacotherapy is not a general substitute for dietary therapy!

According to the present state of knowledge dexfenfluramine can be prescribed for up to one year. The daily dosage is 15 – 30 mg (1x1 or 2x1 tablets).

Side effects

The most important side effects are weariness, diarrhea, dry mouth, polyuria, and sleepiness. Beyond that sleep disorders, vision disturbances, hypotension, impotence, loss of libido, rashes, blood changes, and pulmonary hypertension have been occasionally reported.

Contraindications

The preparation should only be used with caution in patients with arrhythmia; pregnancy, renal and hepatic disorders, the presence of glaucoma or psychiatric illness (including alcoholism) are contraindications.

Comedication

Monoamineoxidase inhibitors must be discontinued several weeks before the use of dexfenfluramine. Dexfenfluramine can potentiate the effect of sedatives, antihypertensives and sulfonyl ureas, and the hypotensive effect of tricyclic antidepressives.

7.5.4.4 Summary

The serotonine agonist dexfenfluramine can contribute to blood glucose reduction and weight reduction in mild type II diabetes with obesity. It is important to keep the contraindications to the preparation in mind, especially during critical phases (imbalance of diet-controlled diabetes, smoking cessation, stabilization of the effect of fasting).

According to the present state of knowledge therapy should not be continued for more than a year.

References

[1] Editorial: Dexfenfluramine. Lancet *337* (1991) 1315 – 1316.

[2] Guy-Grand, B., G. Crepaldi, P. Lefebvre et al.: International trial of long-term dexfenfluramine in obesity. Lancet *II* (1989) 1142 – 1990.

[3] Lehnert, H., J. Beyer, H. K. Biesalski et al.: Bedeutung des zentralnervösen serotoninergen Systems für die Pathogenese der Adipositas. Akt. Ernährungsmedizin *16* (1991) 232 – 240.

[4] Pestell, R. G., P. A. Crock, G. M. Ward et al.: Fenfluramine increases insulin action in patients with NIDDM. Diabetes Care *12* (1989) 252 – 258.

[5] Scheen, A. J., G. Paolisso, T. Salvatore et al.: Improvement of insulin-induced glucose disposal in obese patients with NIDDM after 1-wk treatment with d-fenfluramine. Diabetes Care *14* (1991) 325 – 332.

[6] Schmülling, R.-M., D. Luft, U. Arnold et al.: Gruppentherapie bei Adipositias: Wirkung einer adjuvanten Pharmakotherapie mit Dexfenfluramin. Akt. Ernähr. *14* (1989) 221 – 224.

[7] Spring, B.: Smoking withdrawal, eating behaviors, body-weight control and dexfenfluramine treatment. Abstrakt. In: Overweight and dexfenfluramine: a perspective for the 90's. International symposium organized on the occasion of the IIIrd European congress on Obesity (EASO) by the Institut de Recherches Internationales Servier and Ardix Médical, France, Nice, May 30 – June 1, 1991.

[8] Wurtman, J., A. Brzezinski, R. Wurtman et al.: Premenstrual syndrome, eating behavior, body weight control and dexfenfluramine treatment. Abstrakt. In: Overweight and dexfenfluramine: a perspective for the 90's. International symposium organized on the occasion of the IIIrd European congress on Obesity (EASO) by the Institut de Recherches Internationales Servier and Ardix Médical, France, Nice, May 30 – June 1, 1991.

7.5.5 Fiber

U. Julius

7.5.5.1 *Definitions*

Fiber is an (almost exclusively vegetable) nutritional element, which is not hydrolyzed by the digestive enzymes and therefore not reabsorbed in the small intestine. Amongst others, the following groups of substances are counted amongst them:

- cellulose, hemicelluloses
- lignin
- pectin substances
- exudates and mucin
- starches
- various polysaccharides
- unresorbable di- and oligosaccharides
- lactose

For the most part these are framework and supporting substances from plant cells. Starches and lactose are generally split off, but to some extent do reach the colon. A distinction is made between soluble and insoluble fiber.

7.5.5.2 *Gastrointestinal effects of fiber intake*

Fiber has the following effects [4]:

- dilution of the energy and nutrient concentration in food
- effect on intestinal morphology and physiology and the transit (acceleration) of chymus
- binding of water, substances, enzymes and influence on digestion and resorption
- supply of substrate for the microorganisms of the intestinal flora
- aids in forming the stool.

Highly viscous hydrocolloidal fiber (e.g. pectin, guar) slows the rate of evacuation of the stomach considerably. It should be noted that a vegetable-rich diet may lead to the loss of minerals, e.g. calcium, zinc or iron. This is, however, not likely with moderate increases in fiber supply.

7.5.5.3 *Metabolic effects*

An increased fecal excretion of cholesterol supplied with food has been shown for fiber. A long-term reduction of the cholesterol concentration is with certain fibers (water soluble hydrocolloids) only possible to a limited extent.

The resorption of carbohydrates can be slowed by fiber. It has been proven in experiments that the postprandial increase of plasma glucose concentration following the uptake of various carbohydrate-containing foods (for instance, potatoes, macaroni, legumes) differs greatly. The glycemic index was defined in comparison to the course of plasma glucose following oral glucose intake (equivalent amount of carbohydrates). This value is low following the intake of fiber-rich carbohydrate carriers. The additional administration of pectin or guar may impair the elevation of plasma glucose.

Protein, fat, minerals and vitamins are in the germ and outer layers of grain. This is another reason for eating grain in the whole and not in the processed form.

7.5.5.4 *Recommendations*

The average fiber content of the foodstuffs eaten in industrialized countries is considered to be too low. The desired amount of total daily fiber is estimated to be between 30 to 40 g. Persons with sensitive stomachs may however, often have digestive problems (fullness, bloating, diarrhea) with such a quantity. Many dietary tables contain no or only very general information about fiber content. A precise calculation or determination of the fiber supply is generally neither possible nor necessary in the diabetological practice. The present state of knowledge does not allow for a minimum or optimum daily supply for diabetics. The dietary plans should, however, place considerable value on a "good" consumption of vegetable products.

▶ Advise your patients to eat whole grain, black bread, linseed breads, bran rolls and rye and oat cookies and cereals. Vegetables such as celery, brussel sprouts, broccoli, green beans, cabbage, leek and others guarantee fiber supply and are low in calories. If legumes are tolerated, peas, beans and lentils can also be recommended.

Guar (Glucotard®) is used by some diabetologists [2, 5]. This is a polysaccharide component (galactomannan), which forms a non-absorbable liquid. It is administered with 5 g in 250 ml water at meals. Rough bran (i. e. do not grind into small particles) can be used in cases of obstipation (3x1 tablespoon).

7.5.5.5 *Summary*

Fiber-rich food is highly recommended for the type II diabetic patient. Besides diluting the calorie content of the food, the stimulation of intestinal activity and a certain reduction in cholesterol concentration and postprandial blood glucose level are clinically important. Whole grain products and especially vegetables and legumes are valuable suppliers of fiber, and also promote a feeling of satiation. The quantity of the daily intake is however, frequently limited by digestive problems.

References

[1] Anderson, J. W., A. O. Akanji: Dietary fiber – an overview. Diabetes Care *14* (1991) 1126–1131.

[2] Bain, S. C., P. M. Dodson: The pharmacological treatment of obesity and diabetes mellitus. In: C. E. Mogensen, E. Standl: Pharmacology of Diabetes, 163–179. Walter de Gruyter, Berlin, New York 1991.

[3] Deutsche Diabetes-Gesellschaft: Grundlagen der Ernährung und Diätempfehlungen für Diabetiker. Akt. Ernährungsmedizin *15* (1990) 27–38.

[4] Friedrich, M., J. Schulze: Bedeutung der Ballaststoffe für die Ernährung. In: H.-A. Ketz (Hrsg.): Grundriß der Ernährungslehre, 149–165. VEB Gustav Fischer Verlag, Jena 1990.

[5] Mehnert, H.: Diabetes mellitus. In: H. Mehnert (Hrsg.): Stoffwechselkrankheiten. Grundlagen, Diagnostik, Therapie, 115–261. Georg Thieme Verlag, Stuttgart, New York 1990.

[6] Riccardi, G., A. A. Rivellese: Effects of dietary fiber and carbohydrate on glucose and lipoprotein metabolism in diabetic patients. Diabetes Care *14* (1991) 1115–1125.

[7] Scheppach, W.: Bedeutung von Ballaststoffen für die Entstehung und Therapie gastroenterologischer Erkrankungen. Akt. Ernährungsmedizin *16* (1991) 143–145.

7.6 Insulin therapy

J. Schulze, H. Rietzsch

7.6.1 *Introduction*

The problem of the therapy of NIDDM lies in its heterogeneity and in the stage by stage course of the disease, which by definition is "insulin independent". The degree of insulin resistance and its compensation by endogenous hyper-, normo- or hypoinsulin secretion are responsible for its sequential pattern of pathogenesis and the clinical picture of genetically programmed type II diabetes mellitus [2].

A further particularity is represented by environmental factors which favor manifestation (overeating or malnutrition, physical inactivity, stress, concomitant illness, surgery, pregnancy, diabetogenic medication, etc.), factors of considerable importance for the fate of type II diabetic patients (metabolic syndrome). A therapeutic concept which does not take this cluster of risk factors into consideration, but concentrates only on disturbed carbohydrate tolerance, remains nothing other than unsatisfactory blood glucose cosmetics. Associated risk factors can be therapeutically influenced in the long-term by consistent diabetic basic therapy and phase-adapted oral hypoglycemics, lipid-lowering drugs and anti-hypertensives.

Despite this approach, about 5 – 10% of all patients per year suffer a secondary failure of conventional anti-diabetic therapy. The European Consensus Conference recommends that insulin be administered "not too early and not too late" to avoid hyperglycemic-related symptoms and so-called late complications which are caused by chronic metabolic imbalances of the carbohydrate, lipid and protein metabolisms (Euro-Norm).

7.6.2 *Indications for insulin therapy in type II diabetes*

Long-term insulin therapy is indicated in:

1. Type II diabetics with primary or secondary sulfonyl urea failure
2. Severe diabetic late complications: high grade retinopathy, pronounced polyneuropathy, advanced nephropathy

Temporary insulin therapy is indicated in:

1. Major surgery
2. Severe infections
3. Corticosteroid treatment and intercurrent illness

4. Absorption disorders from oral hypoglycemics
5. Pregnancy (oral diabetics contraindicated)

Long-term metabolic decompensations are accompanied clinically by typical symptoms, for instance muscular weakness, loss of weight, fatigue, lack of drive and depressive mood. Such symptoms as well as previously detected diabetic complications in younger type IIa diabetics justify the immediate commencement of insulin therapy! Hyperosmolar coma in the typical type II diabetic requires a relatively frugal use of insulin in comparison to the ketoacidotic imbalance.

For the majority of type II diabetics, the decision to move to insulin, a constraining measure, will require a precise individual risk-benefit analysis based on age, life expectancy, accompanying risk factors and late complications which have already been detected.

The C-peptide measurement before and 6 minutes after glucagon stimulation has proven itself to be helpful in the decision for or against insulin. With the help of the test results it is possible to draw conclusions about endogenous insulin secretion as an indication for or against the need for insulin [4].

▶ *Aids in determining the indication for insulin therapy in type II diabetes*
- Proof of ketoacidosis
- Blood glucose imbalance with weight loss
- Typical diabetes symptoms in secondary sulfonyl urea failure

In cases of doubt:

Proof of reduced insulin secretion by the B-cells by means of glucagon stimulation:

Cave: The glucagon test should not be performed with decompensated carbohydrate metabolism, because high blood glucose has an additional toxic effect on the B-cells. This can result in a falsified reduction of the secretion response after glucagon stimulation. A temporary insulin therapy for recompensation of a metabolic imbalance does not generally disturb the C-peptide assay.

Performing the glucagon test: The C-peptide level in serum is determined before and 6 minutes after i.v. injection of 1 mg glucagon. The serum samples must be kept refrigerated until they are analysed. The test should be conducted in the fasting state. Blood pressure must be monitored.

Assessment of the glucagon test: After stimulation C-peptide should not exceed 1.1 nmol/l, if a reduced insulin secretion capacity is to be assumed. A fasting C-peptide of over 0.6 nmol/l indicates that there is sufficient endogenous insulin.

The glucagon test does not allow for conclusions to be drawn about the degree of insulin resistance. This means that despite evidence of sufficient endogenous insulin production, exogenous insulin may in fact be necessary.

Contraindications to the glucagon test: Pheochromocytoma, severe hypertension.

7.6.3 *Strategies of insulin therapy in type II diabetes*

A number of general procedures have been introduced for the application of insulin which could also be used for type II diabetes. There are, however, certain particulars for their use. Before insulin therapy can commence, an intensive repetitive training is necessary to familiarize the patient with the intended insulin regime, the corresponding eating habits and the necessity of blood glucose self-monitoring. Recently there have been new indications for the combined first line use of acarbose or biguanides with insulin (see section 7.7). New adjustments should be made with human insulin. On the other hand there are no indications for changing well-adjusted patients from a highly-purified animal insulin.

7.6.3.1 *Combination therapy insulin plus acarbose*

Data available on the effect of alpha disaccharidase inhibitors show acarbose to be a new, potent antidiabetic agent which contributes to the reduction of postprandial glucose peaks and thereby the improvement of the dietetic metabolic state by means of competitive inhibition of intestinal alpha glucosidase. Acarbose acts antihyperglycemic by "smoothing" postabsorptive glucose levels. The substance is effective in type II as well as in instable type I diabetes. These then represent favorable additive effects with an insulin therapy beside the combination possibilities with diet and oral anti-diabetics (see section 7.5). According to studies on the artificial pancreas (biostator) and our own clinical experiences, there was an insulin saving effect (20 – 30%) and smoothing of postabsorptive blood sugar peaks in insulin independent type II diabetics. The lowering of fasting blood sugar values occurs only after 6 – 8 weeks after administering acarbose; the same holds true for HbA_1 and triglycerides.

7.6.3.2 *Combination therapy insulin plus sulfonyl urea*

With continued residual secretion, normal body weight and advanced age combination therapy offers the advantage of a simple and safe therapy regimen for many patients with sulfonyl urea failure. It has been possible to prove that equivalent metabolic control can be obtained with less insulin and fewer injections per day in comparison to insulin monotherapy [1]. The application of the insulin can be made as desired. The morning injection in combination with sulfonyl urea before breakfast and the latter alone in the evening has proven itself effective (fig. 1). By the same token, the single evening injection has been shown to lower

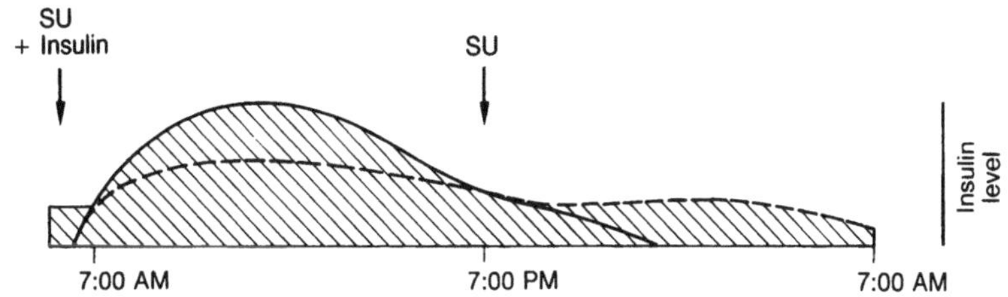

Fig. 1: Example of combined treatment with sulfonyl urea plus delayed-effect insulin (insulin administration in the morning).

the nocturnal blood sugar value. The insulin dosage increase should take place very slowly, so as to not suppress the endogenous insulin production. Generally intermediate or basal insulin are used. If more than 24 IU insulin or several injections should be necessary, the treatment form should be discontinued and insulin monotherapy pursued.

7.6.3.3 *Conventional insulin therapy*

For all type II diabetics below the age of 60, in whom diabetes-specific complications should be expected because of their life expectancy, normoglycemic adjustment is required. Clinical experience has shown that after long-term, "insufficient" sulfonyl urea therapy with a poor metabolic state, often also with secondary hyperlipoproteinemia, insulin therapy does not immediately lead to the desired success. Despite the administration of higher insulin doses, sometimes up to 80 – 120 IU, hyperglycemia and hyperlipoproteinemia remain for long periods (resistance, receptor down regulation, glucotoxicity). Aside from these complicated special situations, which often require longer periods of hospitalization for clarification and treatment, type II diabetics without obesity with an unsatisfactory metabolic state, can generally be adjusted with two administrations of insulin. Generally insulin preparations with set portions of NPH and regular insulin are used. Industry offers this insulin in various preparations (tab. 1). The composition consists of about one-third regular and two-thirds delayed insulin. The insulin is generally injected at breakfast and before dinner. In rare cases *one* insulin injection leads to a satisfactory optimization of the metabolism (fig. 2).

7.6.3.4 *Intensive insulin therapy*

Viewed critically, only about 10 – 20% of the patients attain a normalization of the blood glucose, according to the requirements of the NIDDM Policy Group, with the conventional insulin therapy [3]. In the other patients, who must fear late complications, regular insulin administration at meals and possibly even a late evening injection of basal insulin should be recommended. This procedure can, with the help of modern injection aids and training for self-monitoring, and

Tab. 1: Common human insulin

Preparation[1]	IU/ml	depot principle	Effect after s. c. injection (hours)[3]		
			Begin	Maximum	Duration
Short-acting insulins					
H-Insulin Hoechst	40	–	0.5	1 – 2	5 – 8
H-Insulin 100 Hoechst for OptiPen	100	–	0.5	1 – 2	5 – 8
H-Tronin 40	40	–	0.5	1 – 2	5 – 8
H-Tronin 100 (for H-Tron Pumpe)	100	–	0.5	1 – 2	5 – 8
Huminsulin Normal 40	40	–	0.5	1 – 4	6 – 8
Huminsulin Normal 100	100	–	0.5	1 – 4	6 – 8
Huminsulin Normal Lilly for Pen	100	–	0.5	1 – 4	6 – 8
Insulin Velasulin Human	40	–	0.5	1 – 3	5 – 8
Insulin Velasulin Human (PP) (for Nordisk Infusor/Insuject)	100	–	0.5	1 – 3	5 – 8
Insulin Actrapid HM	40	–	0.5	2 – 5	6 – 8
Insulin Actrapid HM Penfill (for NovoPen)	100	–	0.5	2 – 5	6 – 8
Actrapid HM NovoLet	100	–	0.5	2 – 5	6 – 8
Intermediate-acting insulins					
Basal-H-Insulin Hoechst	40	NPH[2]	0.5 – 1	4 – 6	11 – 20
Basal-H-Insulin 100 Hoechst for OptiPen	100	NPH	0.5 – 1	4 – 6	11 – 20
Huminsulin Basal (NPH) 40	40	NPH	0.5 – 1	2 – 10	18 – 20
Huminsulin Basal (NPH) 100	100	NPH	0.5 – 1	2 – 10	18 – 20
Huminsulin Basal (NPH) Lilly for Pen	100	NPH	0.5 – 1	2 – 10	18 – 20
Insulin Insulatard Human	40	NPH	1 – 1.5	4 – 12	16 – 24
Insulin Insulatard Human-X[4]	100	NPH	1 – 1.5	4 – 12	16 – 24
Insulin Protaphan HM 40	40	NPH	1 – 1.5	4 – 12	16 – 24
Insulin Protaphan HM Penfill	100	NPH	1 – 1.5	4 – 12	16 – 24
Protaphan HM NovoLet	100	NPH	1 – 1.5	4 – 12	16 – 24
Mixed insulins					
Depot-H15-Insulin Hoechst	40	15% H-Insulin +	0.5 – 1	1 – 6	11 – 20
Depot-H15-Insulin Hoechst for OptiPen	100	85% Basal-H-Insulin			
Depot-H-Insulin Hoechst	40	25%-H-Insulin +	0.5 – 1	3 – 6	12 – 18
Depo-H-Insulin 100 Hoechst for OptiPen	100	75% Basal-H-Insulin +			

Komb-H-Insulin Hoechst	40	50% H-Insulin +	0.5	1 – 4	10 – 16
Komb-H-Insulin 100 Hoechst for OptiPen	100	50% Basal-H-Insulin			
Huminsulin Profil I	40	10% Huminsulin Normal +	0.5	2 – 9	12 – 18
Huminsulin Profil I for Pen	100	90% Huminsulin Basal			
Huminsulin Profil II	40	20% Huminsulin Normal +	0.5	1 – 8	12 – 16
Huminsulin Profil II for Pen	100	80% Huminsulfin Basal			
Huminsulin Profil III	40	30% Huminsulin Normal +	0.5	1 – 8	12 – 15
Huminsulin Profil III for Pen	100	70% Huminsulin Basal			
Huminsulin Profil IV	40	40% Huminsulin Normal +	0.5	1 – 8	10 – 15
Huminsulin Profil IV for Pen	100	60% Huminsulin Basal			
Insulin Mixtard 15/85 Human-X[4]	100	15% Velasulin Human +	0.5 – 1	1 – 6	12 – 24
		85% Insulatard Human			
Insulin Mixtard 30/70 Human	40	30% Velasulin Human +	0.5	1 – 12	14 – 24
Insulin Mixtard 30/70 Human-X[4]	100	70% Insulatard Human			
Insulin Mixtard 50/50 Human	40	50% Velasulin Human +	0.5	4 – 8	12 – 24
Insulin Mixtard 50/50 Human-X[4]	100	50% Insulatard Human			
Insulin Actraphane HM 10/90 Penfill	100	10% Actrapid HM +	0.5	2 – 8	14 – 24
		90% Protaphan HM			
Insulin Actraphane HM 20/80 Penfill	100	20% Actrapid HM +	0.5	2 – 8	14 – 24
		80% Protaphan HM			
Insulin Actraphane HM 30/70	40	30% Actrapid HM +	0.5	2 – 8	14 – 24
Insulin Actraphane HM 30/70 Penfill	100	70% Protaphan HM			
Insulin Actraphane HM 30/70 NovoLet	100				
Insulin Actraphane HM 40/60 Penfill	100	40% Actrapid HM +	0.5	2 – 8	14 – 24
		60% Protaphan HM			
Insulin Actraphane HM 50/50 Penfill	100	50% Actrapid HM +	0.5	2 – 8	14 – 24
		50% Protaphan HM			
Insulin Monotard HM	40	30% amorph, MC-Insulin,	2 – 2.5	6 – 16	18 – 24
		70% kristallin, MC-Insulin			
Long-acting insulins					
Insulin Ultratard HM 40	40	100% kristallin, Zink	3 – 4	8 – 24	24 – 28

[1] All preparations patented tradenames; [2] NPH = Neutral Protamin Hagedorn; [3] This is an approximation; [4] for Insuject-X

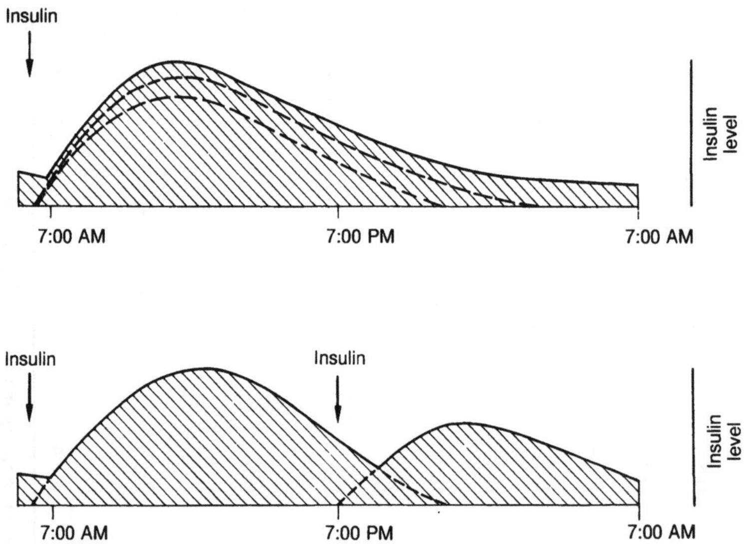

Fig. 2: Schematic of conventional insulin therapy (top = single administration, bottom = double administration of a mixed insulin).

flexible metabolic control, become as well-accepted as the treatment of type I diabetes (fig. 3).

An alternative for younger type II diabetics with residual secretion is the functional insulin substitution using the basis-bolus concept. This procedure differs only slightly from the above mentioned variations. The only change is the addition of the morning basal insulin injection (fig. 4).

7.6.3.5 *Insulin pump treatment*

In rare cases insulin pump treatment may be required for type II diabetes. This is true for patients with significant insulin resistance, in whom an improvement of the blood glucose control has not been managed. The reduction of the insulin required by pump therapy from 150 IU to 80 IU per day is an example of this. Usually it is possible to get by with temporary subcutaneous pump treatment. With higher hepatic insulin resistance there is the possibility of intraperitoneal application of the insulin via a port system. This method is presently in the clinical trial stage. In association with the insulin pump treatment one should consider temporary intravenous insulin infusion which is used for breaking insulin resistance, for instance, in severe infections or emergency situations.

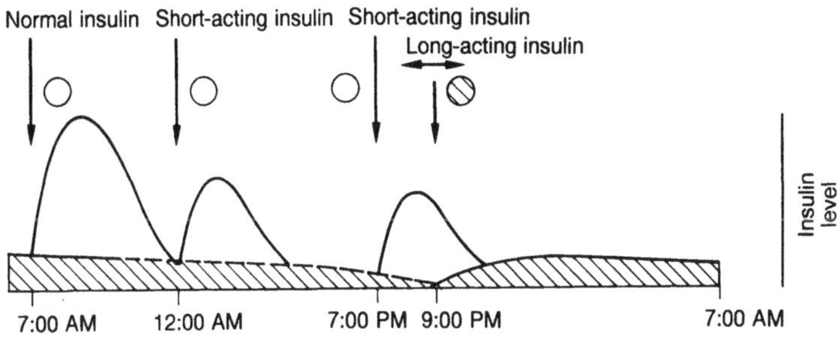

Fig. 3: Schematic of intensified insulin therapy according to the basis-bolus concept (short-acting insulin administration at the main meal times and long-acting insulin at night)

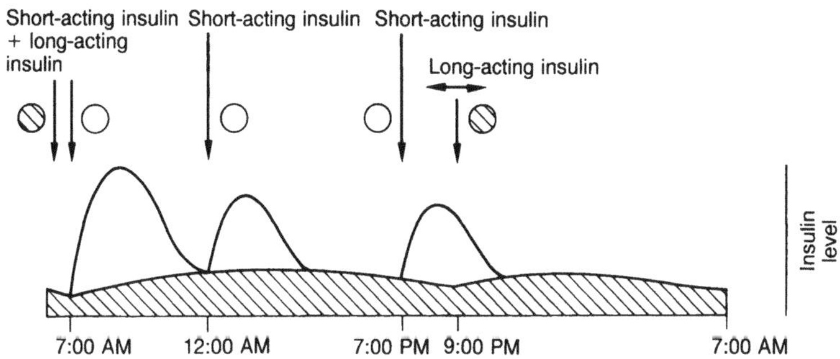

Fig. 4: Schematic of intensified conventional insulin therapy (ICT) according to the basis-bolus principle.

7.6.4 Supplementary measures in insulin therapy

Without thorough training in the metabolic control and handling of injection aids, the use of blood and urinary glucose test strips as well as instruction of the patients and family members about possible related complications, insulin therapy remains a method which is fear-ridden. The injection technique has improved dramatically in the last few years. The bothersome task of disinfecting materials has become a thing of the past. Single use, disposable syringes represent a universal injection medium which should be a part of every diabetic's repertoire. These syringes are available for the common U 40 insulin. They are also available for U 100 insulin which is used in other EU countries and pens and pumps. Various pens are popular. The following aspects should be taken into consideration when using such injection aids:

1. Type of insulin and the availability in the corresponding pen ampule
2. Handiness of the pen and the "patient's technical abilities"; the patients should be allowed to select the type of insulin which they wish from amongst those appropriate.

3. Individual instruction in using the pen is mandatory. A demonstration ampule is available for this purpose.
4. For hesitant patients, the Novolet system is a welcome method for overcoming the difficulties involved in learning how to give injections. The system also contains a touch system for those with impaired vision.

Thorough training and instructions, also for elderly patients and their family, allow for precise metabolic regulation, avoidance of hyperglycemia or comata by self-monitoring of estimates of the course and therapy consistency. This brings us closer to the basic principle so important for the type II diabetic – lowest insulin dosage possible and dosage adjustment, so as to avoid overinsulination which can lead to adverse lipogenesis with increasing obesity and hyperlipoproteinemia. Beyond that, this procedure reduces threatening hypoglycemia.

7.6.5 *Summary*

Heterogeneity and the progressive course of NIDDM make an individual medical therapy mandatory, which should be oriented on the current pathophysiological situation. Important predicators for the therapeutic success are the remaining insulin secretion capacity, measured with the C-peptide, and concomitant diseases of the metabolic syndrome, which according to the current state of knowledge represent the cause and consequence of insulin resistance. Before the decision is made to use a differentiated insulin therapy, the possible combinations with acarbose, metformin and/or sulfonyl ureas should be exhausted. Should the control parameters (glycemia, lipids) remain above the therapeutic goal despite these measures, and the patient is either within or below normal weight range with diabetes of longer duration and diabetes-specific complications, insulin treatment is absolutely mandatory. The patient then enters into a new quality of therapy. This should be accompanied by intensive training with intensive self-monitoring.

References

[1] Bachmann, W.: Kombinationstherapie mit Sulfonylharnstoffen. Dtsch. Med. Wschr. *113* (1988) 652–654.

[2] DeFronzo, R. A.: The triumvirate beta cell, muscle, liver: A collusion responsible for NIDDM. Diabetes *37* (1988) 667.

[3] European NIDDM Policy Group: A Desktop Guide for the Management of Non-insulin-dependent Diabetes mellitus (NIDDM). IDF Bulletin *35* (1990) 1–11.

[4] Faber, O. K., C. Binder: C-peptide response to glucagon: a test for the residual B-cell function in diabetes mellitus. Diabetes *26* (1977) 605–610.

[5] Hanefeld, M., J. Schulze: Medikamentöse Differentialtherapie des Typ-2-Diabetes, Ärzteblatt Sachsen 7 (1992) 744–752.

7.7 Differential therapy with antidiabetics

M. Hanefeld

7.7.1 A manual for differential therapy

The options described in the previous chapters, and their combinations, are essentially those which are available for drug differential therapy (tab. 1). There are still no medications which directly overcome insulin resistance in that

Tab. 1: Medications for the treatment of type II diabetes

Inhibitors of the intestinal glucose release (alpha glucosidase inhibitors, guar)
Anorectics – D-fenfluramine
Biguanides (metformin)
Sulfonyl ureas
Insulin

they intracellularly potentiate the insulin effect. Therefore, antihyperglycemic medications, which impede the blood glucose increase, are first indicated for the early phases of the diabetes and possibly for high-risk patients with IGT or pre-stages of diabetes. There seems to be an advantage to simultaneously reducing the basal and/or glucose-stimulated hyperinsulinemia. From this it is possible to deduce that for the early phases of NIDDM acarbose, metformin and – to some extent – D-fenfluramine (fig. 1) are first on the list. The Dresden school thereby

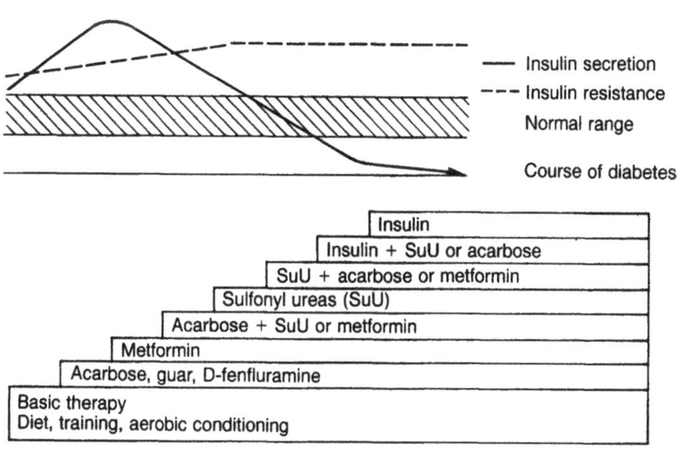

Fig. 1: Stages in the therapy of NIDDM.

finds itself for the most part in agreement with the concept implied by Mehnert and Standl [5]. This makes insulin resistance and the remaining insulin secretion capacity decisive criteria for the selection of the first-line drug. Both of these parameters are difficult to measure in practice. In addition, there is the fact that not every NIDDM exhibits a primary insulin resistance. The physician depends for the most part on clinical data and laboratory values which are quickly available to reach his/her decision (tab. 2). Excess weight and constant weight are a sign of sufficient insulin secretion reserve, according to the rule of thumb, "If you're fat, you've got insulin." If they are available, basal and one- and two-hour insulin values after 75g glucose are a significant help in estimating the B-cell capacity still remaining.

Tab. 2: Clinical and paraclinical indicators for the insulin secretion capacity in NIDDM

	Residual insulin secretion	
	sufficient	exhausted
History	Duration of diabetes < 5 yrs. Weight = ↑ No diabetes symptons (thirst, etc.)	Duration of diabetes > 5 yrs. Weight ↓ Increasing symptoms
Status	No or only mild diabetes-specific complications	Neuropathy Albuminuria (proteinuria) Proliferative retinopathy
Laboratory	Base- excess, lactate = C-peptide > 1.1 nmol/l after stimulation serum insulin > 1s range (basal and stimulated)	Acidosis, lactate ↑ C-peptide < 1.1 nmol/l after stimulation serum insulin ↓, diminished and delayed postprand. rise

This is more easily done using the C-peptide assay in the glucagon test. A C-peptide value > 1.1 nmol/l six minutes after i.v. glucagon stimulation and an increase of 2 to 3-fold over the basal value indicate a sufficient remaining secretion. The same is true if the insulin value is over the 95 percentile or the 1s range of the specific insulin reference value. Of course, the absolute insulin and C-peptide concentrations are to a large extent dependent on the current blood glucose situation. Nevertheless, they can be used as an important aid in deciding.

If the clinical and laboratory data indicate there is sufficient remaining secretion capacity, acarbose and metformin should be seen as the treatment of choice. As there are no comparative long-term studies of these medications, the decision must be made on the basis of the mode of action, the contraindications and the side effects.

7.7.1.1 *When acarbose, when metformin?*

Acarbose is, on the basis of its profile of action, advantageous in patients with NIDDM whose blood sugar increases in the course of the day, especially postprandially. Due to the fact that less than 1% of acarbose is absorbed in the small intestine and that the breakdown products which are taken up in the colon are excreted quickly and completely into the kidneys and respirations, an accumulation should not be expected, even with impaired liver and renal function. For that reason, acarbose has the advantage of greater safety over metformin in elderly, often multimorbid patients. This is also true for the combination therapy with sulfonyl ureas. Metformin is particularly effective in patients whose increased nocturnal hepatic gluconeogenesis leads to high fasting blood glucose concentrations. Metformin's domain is the middle-aged obese diabetic with elevated blood lipids, because here the complex actions on the excess weight, the insulin resistance of the liver and the hyperlipidemia are particularly beneficial (tab. 3) [2, 5]. Its use in sulfonyl urea failure should be limited to this circle of patients. The reverse approach would appear more reasonable, i. e. the addition of sulfonyl ureas in NIDDM with insufficient or decreasing metformin effect [5] (fig. 1).

Tab. 3: Differential therapy with oral anti-diabetics as first line drug in NIDDM

	Acarbose	Metformin	SU
Elderly	+ + +	– –	–
Multimorbidity	+	– – –	+
FBG↑↑	+	+ +	+
postprandial BG↑↑	+ +	+	+
Hyperinsulinemia	+ +	+ +	–
Beg. insulin deficiency	–	–	+ + +
Obesity	+	+	– –
Hypertriglyceridemia	+	+	–
Hypertension	+	+	–

7.7.1.2 *Sulfonyl urea – when, how, which?*

As already explained, sulfonyl ureas belong to the phase of the beginning relative lack of insulin. This is often found in type IIa diabetes or is announced by the HbA_{1c} increase or weight loss under the previous monotherapy. In elderly patients or those with liver and/or kidney disease, "soft" sulfonyl ureas with lower retention and hypoglycemic shock danger, such as tolbutamide, are preferable. Glibenclamide, the most effective and best investigated second generation sulfonyl urea derivate, is especially indicated for those younger than 70 [1].

Glipizide is advantageous in impaired renal function, because its active components are hardly retained. Only second generation sulfonyl ureas, glibenclamide and glipicide, should be considered in combination with insulin.

7.7.1.3 *Insulin use – as early as necessary, as late as possible*

There can be no doubt that the use of insulin at the proper time is the most reliable method of primary and secondary prevention of late complications in NIDDM. Nevertheless, on the basis of consistent epidemiological data [3, 4], the premature use of insulin should be avoided, because body weight and other risk factors are increased with its use. Last but not least, despite all the modern aids, there are a number of social problems connected with the use of insulin in elderly patients.

Therefore, the therapeutic goals and the risk-benefit ratio should be weighed carefully when deciding for one of the options or their combination (tabs. 4, 5). The combination treatment of insulin with sulfonyl ureas represents, where it is sufficient, a reasonable compromise. However, this treatment is only wise when the metabolic control is managed with one injection which contains the maximum 24 units of a basal, intermediary or combination insulin. If this is not possible, regular insulinization with several injections is preferable.

Tab. 4: Therapeutic effects of various monotherapies on the metabolic syndrome in type II diabetes

	Insulin	Sulf. urea	Metformin	Acarbose
Obesity	↑ ↑	↑	↓	=
Hyperglycemia	↓ ↓	↓	↓	↓
Insulin resistance	↑ =	↑ =	↓	↓ ?
Hyperinsulinemia	↑	↑	↓	↓
Triglycerides	↓ ↑	=	↓	↓ =
Cholesterol	=↓	=	↓	=↓
HDL-C	↑	=	=↑	=
Hypertension	=↑	=	=	=
Atherosclerosis	↑ ?	↑ ?	↓ ?	↓ ?

Tab. 5: Side effects of various monotherapies in type II diabetes

	Insulin	Sulf. urea	Metformin	Acarbose
Hypoglycemia	+ +	+	–	–
Gastrointestinal disorders	–	–	+	+ +
Blood count	–	(+)	(–)	–
Lactic acidosis	–	–	+	–
Fatal complications	(+)	+	+	–

7.7.2 *Summary*

The selection of an oral hypoglycemic is for the most part determined by the remaining insulin secretory capacity, patient age and concomitant illnesses. With hyperinsulinemia, i. e. with increasing plateau of the Starling curve of the insulin secretion, acarbose and metformin are the first line drugs. With increasing relative insulin deficit sulfonyl ureas and insulin are required. Acarbose has advantages for elderly patients and those with dominating postprandial hyperglycemia. Metformin is indicated in younger NIDDM patients with high fasting blood glucose values.

The combinations acarbose plus metformin, acarbose plus sulfonyl urea and sulfonyl urea plus acarbose should be considered as intermediary steps. The combination sulfonyl urea plus insulin reduces the insulin required and allows for a single daily injection in appropriate cases.

References

[1] Gerich, J. E.: Oral hypoglycemic agents. New Engl. J. Med. *321* (1989) 1231–1245.

[2] Hermann, L. S.: Biguanides and Sulfonylureas as combination therapy in NIDDM. Diabetes Care *13* (Suppl. 3) (1990) 37–42.

[3] Janka, H. U., A. G. Ziegler, E. Standl et al.: Daily insulin dose as a predictor of macrovascular complications in diabetes mellitus. Diab. Metab. *13* (1987) 359–364.

[4] Knatterud, G., C. Klimt, M. Goldner et al.: Effects of hypoglycemic agents on vascular complications in patients with adult onset diabetes. VIII Evaluation of insulin therapy. Final report *31* (Suppl. 5) (1982) 1–26.

[5] Mehnert, H.: Diabetes mellitus. In: H. Mehnert (Hrsg.): Stoffwechselkrankheiten, 115–258. Thieme Verlag, Stuttgart 1990.

[6] Schernthaner, G.: Kritische Analyse der antidiabetischen Therapie mit Metformin: Stoffwechselwirkungen, antiatherogene Effekte und Kontraindikationen. Akt. Endokr. Stoffw. *13* (1992) 44–50.

8 Special therapeutic aspects

8.1 Treatment of hypertension

J. Schulze, Silke Meisel, M. Hanefeld

Treatment of hypertension in type II diabetes mellitus is more than just reducing the blood pressure.

The primary goal of the treatment is, beside the classical ones – the prevention of atherosclerotic vascular diseases, particularly stroke, coronary and nephrosclerosis, as well as left ventricular hypertrophy and cardiac insufficiency, such as has been formulated in the consensus paper of the German Hypertension League [2] – the prevention of microangiopathy, especially concerning the kidneys.

8.1.1 Basic therapy

Basic therapy aims at a complex improvement in the cluster of atherogenic factors. It focuses on the optimization of insulin effect on the musculature, liver and fat tissue through weight normalization and an increase in physical activity.

The basic therapy is founded on 5 pillars of non-drug intervention:

1. Basic diet (tab. 1) [5]
2. Correction of obesity, especially in android obesity [7] (partial fasting)
3. Physical conditioning (aerobic endurance training), which, along with weight reduction, is associated with an increase in insulin sensitivity [8].
4. Exclusion of accompanying risk factors (alcohol, nicotine, stress, NaCl abuse; normalization of glycemia and lipids)
5. Education/self-monitoring (individual and group counseling according to a strict instructional program [13]) and blood pressure measurement courses for physicians' assistants and support personnel [3].

Successful treatment of hypertension is only achievable through patient education, self-monitoring and flexible adaptation of the treatment measures. Also helpful for a tailored therapy are blood pressure profiles, drawn from self measurement or through an objective 24-hour monitoring.

8.1.2 Anti-hypertensives – benefits and risks

Only after the exhaustion of these basal therapeutic measures, which show equally beneficial effects on blood pressure, weight, diabetes and lipid metabolism, should the application of drug therapy no longer be delayed. With values at or above

Tab. 1: Non-drug basic therapy of hypertension in metabolic diseases [5]

Health education

- Alcohol abstinence
- Quitting smoking
- Endurance training (jogging, cross-country skiing, rowing, bicycling, touristic hiking)
- Sufficient rest phases

Diet

- Fat reduction to 30% of energy intake
  10% saturated fatty acids
  10% monosaturated fatty acids
  10% polyunsaturated fatty acids
  Plenty of fresh water fish
- Salt reduction to below 8 g/day
- Carbohydrates
  large amounts of unprocessed fruits and vegetables, few refined carbohydrates
- Proteins
  high percentage of plant proteins (esp. soy beans, beans, millet)

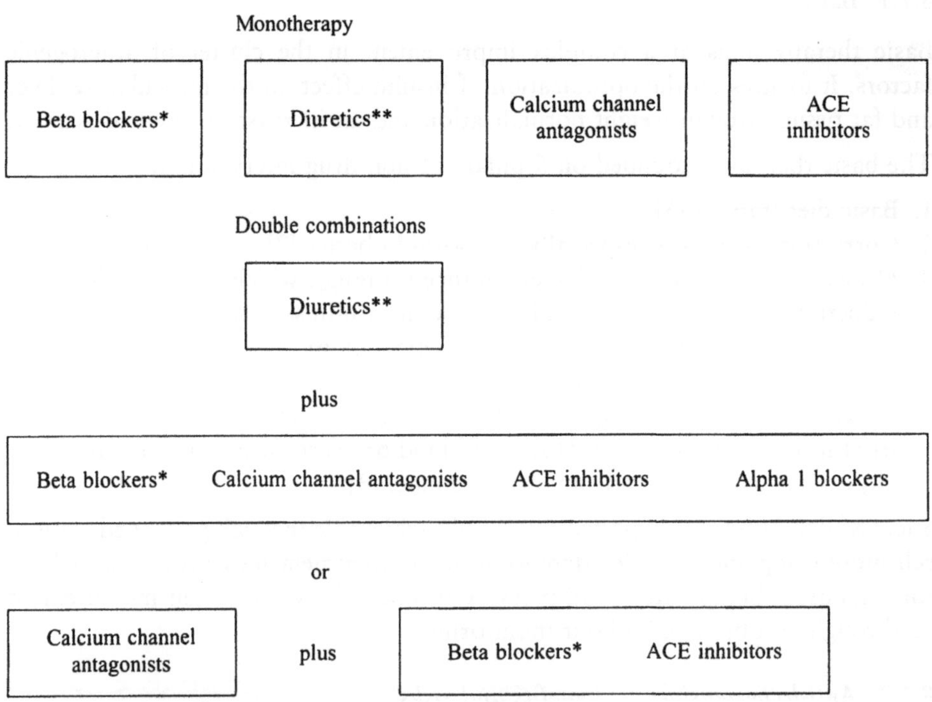

* Beta 1 selective blockers preferred
** Triamterene, aldosterone antagonists preferred, not in nephrophathy

Fig. 1: Therapy suggestions of the German Hypertension League [2].

140/90 mmHg and with multiple risks, the indication for "metabolically neutral" and progression-preventing anti-hypertensive drugs is given. This also applies to isolated systolic hypertension (fig. 1) [2]. The first choice of medicines are calcium channel antagonists, ACE inhibitors and alpha 1 blockers. The second choice for consideration are selective beta blockers, potassium sparing diuretics (triamterene or aldosterone antagonists), vasodilators and sympatholytics. Due to diabetogenic and undesirable effects on the lipid and purine metabolisms, thiazide diuretics and non-selective beta blockers should no longer be used in patients with pre-manifest or manifest diabetes or dyslipoproteinemia with hypertension [1, 15]. The newer antihypertensive medicines are not only effective and largely metabolism-neutral, they also have beneficial effects on further associated risk factors (tab. 2) [6, 16].

According to current knowledge, alpha 1 blockers, ACE inhibitors, some calcium channel antagonists, and some beta 1 blockers should be favored due to a demonstrable reversal potential for left-ventricular hypertrophy. In addition, for both ACE inhibitors and alpha 1 blockers, an improved insulin sensitivity could be demonstrated with the use of the glucose clamp technique [12].

Also, in regard to accompanying lipid disorders, calcium channel antagonists and ACE inhibitors behave neutrally. The long-term use of peripheral alpha 1 blockers of the doxazosine variety leads to a HDL-cholesterol rise through an increase in the lipoprotein catabolism [9]. Loop diuretics, e.g. furosemide, with monitoring of electrolytes are indicated for patients showing a tendency towards edema, whereby small doses of diuretics in combination with an ACE inhibitor have been shown to be very effective.

The currently used anti-hypertensives and their clinical value for hypertension, with respect to the metabolic syndrome, will be briefly summarized (tab. 3) [5].

Diuretics: Hydrochlorothiazide preparations can increase the triglyceride level up to 25% and the LDL cholesterol around 6% [11]. The insulin sensitivity is lowered and the HbA_1 and blood glucose rise. These medications should, therefore, be given in NIDDM – when necessary – only as a combination with ACE inhibitors and in low dosages. The same is true for furosemide. The danger of diabetes manifestation is increased in patients with lipid metabolism disorders. Potassium-retaining diuretics (triameterene) are less effective and are accompanied by the danger of potassium retention in diabetics with kidney damage.

Beta blockers: Non-selective beta blockers are obsolete for use in diabetes and lipid disorders due to their negative metabolic effects. Beta 1 selective blockers (atenolol, metoprolol) also reduce insulin sensitivity significantly, raising thereby the serum insulin level and the HbA_{1c}. In addition, triglycerides increased by about 20% and the HDL cholesterol fell significantly in controlled studies with selective blockers. Diuretics and beta blockers both share a reduction of libido and potency – already a problem for most people with metabolic diseases.

Tab. 2: Side effects and advantages of various classes of antihypertensives in diabetes [6].

	Diuretics	Non-cardio-selective beta blockers	Cardioselective beta blockers	Angiotensin-converting enzyme inhibitors	Calcium channel antagonists
Worsening of glucose tolerance	+	(+)	(+)	–	–
Reduced awareness of hypoglycemia	–	+ + (in those requiring insulin)	+ (seldom)	–	–
Poor lipid profile	+	+	?	–	–
Other common side effects	Hypokalemia, volume depletion, impotence	Lowered physical performance ability, impotence		Dry cough	Leg edema occasional flush
Beneficial effects	Decreased edema		Cardioprotective and anti-arrhythmic effect Reversal of left hypertrophy	Improved Na-excretion, possibly reno-protective improved reversal of LVH	Anti-arrhythmic effect (in special forms of arrhythmia) Reversal of LVH

LVH: left ventricular hypertrophy

Tab. 3: Blood pressure reducing medications in diabetes and lipid metabolism disorders [5].

	Important representatives	Relative indications	Relative contraindications	Remarks
Diuretics	Hydrochlorothiazide Furosemide Triamterene	Coronary insufficiency Kidney insufficiency	Dehydration Gout Impotence	Combination treatment with ACE inhibitors, control electrolytes, triamterenes only in combination
Beta blockers (cardio-selective)	Atenolol Metoprolol Talinolol	Angina pectoris Secondary prevention after infarction Rhythm disorders	Coronary insufficiency Bradycardia PAD, Asthma	Masks warning symptoms of hypoglycemia
ACE inhibitors	Captopril Enalapril Ramipril	Coronary insufficiency Albuminuria	Kidney artery stenosis Single kidney	Monitor for hyperkalemia
Calcium blockers	Nifedipine Diltiazem Isradipine Felodipine	Angina pectoris Peripheral arterial circulatory disorders	Treatment with digoxin + beta blockers	
Alpha 1 blockers	Doxasosine Urapidil	Coronary insufficiency	Coronary insufficiency with aortic or mitral stenosis Pregnancy Orthostatic dysregulation (esp. Prazosin)	

PAD: peripheral arterial disease

Calcium channel antagonists: The representatives of the vasodilators currently available on the market have no significant effect on diabetes and lipid metabolism. Their anti-anginal and hypoxia tolerance improving properties are of additional benefit in diabetics with atherosclerosis.

ACE inhibitors: They have no negative effects on metabolism. An improved insulin effect after ingestion of ACE inhibitors has even been described. They take on particular importance in the treatment of early stages of diabetic nephropathy. By lowering the intraglomerular hypertension they have been able to reduce micro-albuminuria. The early stages of nephropathy were reversible with the administration of ACE inhibitors and the progression of advanced stages could be delayed.

Alpha 1 blockers: The positive effects of prazosine on the blood lipids and glucose tolerance were first proven by Leren [10]. However, due to tachycardia and an increased tendency towards orthostatic dysregulaton and sodium retention, their use has remained limited. With doxazosine, a post-synaptic alpha 1 blocker, the tendency towards tachycardia has been essentially eliminated. Atherogenic lipids have been lowered and the vaso-protective HDL raised under this medication. Insulin sensitivity and diabetes control were significantly improved as well.

8.1.3 Summary

In addition to lowering elevated blood pressure and HbA_1, the therapy of hypertension in type II diabetes must also be directed at the total complex of disturbed metabolic functions. This so-called basic therapy aims at a complex improvement in the cluster of atherogenic factors through a health-promoting lifestyle, weight reduction, physical activity, education and self-monitoring. Only after the exhaustion of non-drug measures for treating diabetics with hypertension, is the application of metabolically-neutral, antihypertensive medication indicated. Calcium antagonists, alpha 1 or beta 1 blockers with ISA and ACE inhibitors should be favored because of their beneficial metabolic effects and reversal of dangerous left-ventricular hypertrophy. Blood pressure profiles, drawn from self measurement or 24-hour monitoring, are helpful for a successful therapeutic control.

References

[1] Bengtssun, C., G. Blohme et al.: Do antihypertensive drugs precipitate diabetes? Brit. Med. J. *289* (1984) 1495–1497.

[2] Deutsche Liga zur Bekämpfung des hohen Blutdrucks e. V. Empfehlungen für die Behandlung des Hochdruckes bei Diabetes, Heidelberg 1989.

[3] Gleichmann, S., U. Gleichmann: Patientenedukation bei Hypertonie – Welche Methoden sind praxisgerecht? Internist *32* (1991) 119–126.

[4] Hachamovitch, R., E. M. Sonnenblick et al.: Left ventricular hypertrophy in hypertension and the effects of antihypertensive drug therapy. Curr. Prob. Cardiol. *13* (1988) 369–421.

[5] Hanefeld, M.: Hochdrucktherapie bei Diabetes und Fettstoffwechselstörungen. Medicamentum *33* (1992) 64–68.
[6] Hasslacher, C., E. Ritz: Hypertonie und Diabetes mellitus. Internist *31* (1990) 180–190.
[7] Kaplan, N. M.: Das tödliche Quartett: Zentrale Adipositas, Glukosetoleranz, Hypertriglyzeridämie und Hypertonie. In: Neue Perspektiven im Umgang mit kardiovaskulären Risikofaktoren, 25–41. Beilage zu The Lancet, April 1991, Deutsche Ausgabe.
[8] Krotkiewski, M., K. Mandroukas, L. Sjöström et al.: Effects of long-term physical training on body fat, metabolism, and blood pressure in obesity. Metabolism *28* (1979) 650–658.
[9] Landinoss, C. K., S. L. Neuman: The effects of antihypertension agents on serum lipids and lipoproteins. Arch. Intern. Med. *148* (1988) 1280–1288.
[10] Leren, P.: Am. J. Med. *82* (suppl.1 A) (1987) 31–35.
[11] Lithell, H.: Effect of antihypertensive drugs on insulin, glucose and lipid metabolism. Diabetes care *14* (1991) 203–209.
[12] Messerli, F. H.: Clinical determinants and consequences of left ventricular hypertrophy. Am J. Med. *75* (1983) 51–56.
[13] Mühlhauser, I. et al.: Die Bedeutung der Patientenschulung in der Behandlung chronischer Krankheiten: Diabetes mellitus, Hypertonie, Asthma bronchiale. Die Internistische Welt *8* (1987) 1–14.
[14] Pollare, T., H. Lithell et al.: Application of prazosin is associated with an increase of insulin sensitivity in obese patients with hypertension. Diabetologia *31* (1988) 415–420.
[15] Poulter, N.: Thiazide und Betablocker bei Hypertonie: Es ist Zeit zur Neuorientierung. The Pharmaceutical Journal *224* (1990) 626–627.
[16] Weinberger, M. H.: Optimierung der Senkung kardiovaskulärer Risiken unter einer antihypertensiven Therapie. In: Neue Perspektiven im Umgang mit kardiovaskulären Risikofaktoren, 43–59. Beilage zu The Lancet, April 1991, Deutsche Ausgabe.
[17] Williams, G.: Hypertension in diabetes mellitus. In: J. C. Pickup, G. Williams (eds.): Textbook of Diabetes, 719–735. Blackwell scientific publications, Oxford 1991.

8.2 Treatment of dyslipoproteinemia

M. Hanefeld

8.2.1 *Introduction*

In the evaluation of dyslipoproteinemia, we must assume that persons with NIDDM represents a high risk group for atherosclerosis. In this, dyslipoproteinemia plays a decisive role. This is based, firstly, on the fact that NIDDM and the disorders associated with it as well as the disappearance of the relative atherosclerosis protection in women eo ipso stipulate the classification in the category of EAS* "lipid metabolism disorders and two additional risk factors". Another reason is the atherogenic potency of a dyslipoproteinemia due to the diabetes-specific modifications of the lipoproteins and the thereby related disorders in the breakdown and cholesterol reverse transport described in section 5.2. Thirdly, it must be taken into account that at the time of NIDDM diagnosis, atherosclerotic lesions are already present in a high percentage of cases, so that for the most part we must establish action limits for secondary prevention.

Action limits: The target values for the most important lipid fractions shown in tab. 1 were drawn from the criteria of the NIDDM Policy Group [4] and the EAS [1]. At present, there is no substantiated understanding of the treatment of further lipid anomalies like hyperapobeta-lipoproteinemia and Lp(a) increase, although there is no doubt as to their importance as substantial individual risk factors.

Tab. 1: Target values for ideal blood lipids in NIDDM

	(mmol/l)	(mg/dl)
Total cholesterol	<5.2	< 200
Triglycerides	<1.7	<150
HDL cholesterol	M >0.9	>35
	F >1.1	>42
LDL cholesterol	<3.5	<135
Total cholesterol /HDL cholesterol	<5	

8.2.2 *Basic therapy*

8.2.2.1 *Excluding secondary factors for disorders in lipoprotein metabolism*

In multi-morbid type II diabetics there are a variety of secondary diseases and complications, which can be a cause of secondary hyperlipoproteinemias or exacerbate primary diseases (tab. 2). It should therefore be clarified by means of

* EAS*: European Atherosclerosis Society

Tab. 2: Causes of secondary dyslipoproteinemia in NIDDM

Causes	Proof
Metabolism	
– Imbalanced diabetes	HbA_{1C} ↑ Fructosamine ↑
– Secondary hyperinsulinism (exogenous insulin, SuU)	Insulin ↑ Insulin-resistence during clamp
– Android obesity	WHR M >1.0 F >0.85
– Alcoholism	Gamma GT ↑ Upper abdominal sonography
Medications	
– Beta blockers	History
– Thiazide diuretics	
– Estrogen-rich contraceptives, adrenal cortical steroids, anabolics	
Hormonal	
– Estrogen deficiency	Gonadotropin ↑ Estrogen ↓
– Hypothyroidism	TSH ↑, T_4 ↓
Diseases	
– Chronic kidney diseases	
– Cholestasis	
– Bulimia	

a detailed history and diagnosis, whether the factors named here play a role. In cases where beta blockers and thiazide diuretics are used, a switch should be made to alpha blockers, ACE inhibitors and calcium channel antagonists which are metabolism neutral and/or have positive effects on diabetes and lipid metabolism (see section 9.1). Whether the modern ovulation inhibitors with low estrogen doses still have negative effects on lipid metabolism is questionable and must be tested on an individual basis through follow-up controls of the lipids. Much more common in women with NIDDM are estrogen deficiency syndromes occurring already in their early 40's and requiring supplementation. These deficiencies are also responsible for the higher risk of osteoporosis in this patient group. A rise in the triglycerides and drop in HDL cholesterol should always be viewed in relation to the diabetes control. With HbA_{1c} values over 7.5% despite maximum oral therapy, the question is definitely raised as to whether insulinization is necessary. This should be clarified by a glucagon test. C-peptide values < 1.1 nmol/l after i.v. glucagon stimulation indicate an insulin insufficiency [2]. Vice versa, with a therapy-refractory hypertriglyceridemia in NIDDM, which is only poorly controlled at a high dose of insulin, one must consider the possibility of excessive triglyceride synthesis as a result of iatrogenous peripheral hyperinsulinemia. With C-peptide values > 1.1 nmol/l, an attempt at insulin discontinuation in association with a reduction to ideal weight and physical conditioning is indicated for breaking the insulin resistance.[15].

8.2.2.2 Selection of an appropriate oral anti-diabetic

Sulfonyl ureas, metformin and alpha glucosidase inhibitors also vary regarding their effects on the lipoprotein spectrum. While sulfonyl ureas do not significantly influence triglycerides and HDL cholesterol, a lowering of the triglycerides has been repeatedly described for metformin and acarbose [6, 9]. Therefore, these medications should be given preference, in obese cases of NIDDM and hypertriglyceridemia with sufficient insulin reserves.

8.2.2.3 Diet

A diet according to the recommendations of the Diabetes and Nutrition Group of the EASD, as presented in section 8.3, thoroughly meets the EAS guidelines for a lipid-lowering, atherosclerosis-preventing diet [1] (tab. 3).
Due to the restrictions on refined carbohydrates, however, diets with less than 35% fat are difficult to attain in middle and northern Europe. Therefore, a strict fat-restricted diet must be maintained as a goal when dealing with a dyslipoproteinemia linked to NIDDM. Recent studies have shown that 3 factors are most decisive for the effect on the lipoprotein profile: 1. the fiber content and the avoidance of refined carbohydrates; 2. the fatty acid pattern; 3. a high percentage of plant proteins. The resulting recommendations for diabetics with lipid metabolism disorders are shown in tab. 3.

Commercially available fish oils in dosages of 8 – 16 g do have an excellent triglyceride-reducing effect [11], however, they can lead to a worsening of the diabetic metabolic condition. Guar lowers cholesterol to a slight degree. A slight triglyceride reduction was observed for pectin. These adjuvant substances have the advantage of being natural ballast which supplant the energy concentration of food and raise intestinal motility. The diet presents a special problem in the case of the infrequent chylomicron syndrome. In this case, a drastic reduction of fat intake is unavoidable. Beyond an exclusion of fat, the tolerated amount of fat is attained with an initial 10 g fat per day and stepwise increase of the fat supply.

8.2.2.4 Physical conditioning

Adequate conditioning should be an integral part of the therapy of NIDDM up to old age. The basic rules for this were presented in section 8.4. It can be safely assumed today that aerobic conditioning in the form of endurance training not

Tab. 3: Lipid-reducing diet for NIDDM with dyslipoproteinemia

	Amount	Food type
Fats	<30%	No butter, hardened margarine, whipped cream, whole milk
– saturated fats	7 – 10%	No fatty cheeses, fatty cold cuts or sausage, meat and sauces, palm oil, coconut oil
– monounsaturated	10%	Olive oil, safflower oil
– polyunsaturated	10%	Sunflower, soy and flax oil
Cholesterol	<300 mg	2 eggs/wk allowed, no egg yolks
Low fat animal and plant proteins	12 – 15%	Fish, poultry, beef, veal, game, lamb, soy and algae products
Carbohydrates	>45%	No sugar, white bread or fine
– mono and disaccharides	<10%	baked goods
– complex carbohydrates, raw fiber and ballast materials	>40%	All fruits and vegetables, beans, peas, spaghetti, whole grain bread, oat products, müsli

only lowers the triglycerides, but also raises the vasoprotective HDL cholesterol, especially the HDL_2 fraction. Regular training is particularly effective in patients with hypertriglyceridemia and hyperinsulinemia [7, 8]. The complex effect on the various forms of HLP are presented in fig. 1. While the effect on triglycerides already takes place 2 – 3 weeks after the start of training, HDL cholesterol first begins to rise after 2 – 3 months. The LDL cholesterol concentrations are not significantly influenced.

8.2.3 Drug therapy

If the Euro-Norms for "good" lipid control have not been reached after the exhaustion of non-drug therapy possibilities and the optimization of the diabetes control, the indication for the use of lipid-lowering drugs should be generously applied, as long as the preconditions named in tab. 4 have been met. Because diabetics constitute a group with additional risk factors, a target value of 3.5 mmol/l for LDL cholesterol should be aimed for. This is particularly true concerning the secondary prevention of previously existent atherosclerotic vessel complications. The same indications as those for non-diabetics hold true for the differential drug therapy of lipid metabolism disorders (tab. 5) [3, 11, 13]. Fibrates (bezafibrate, fenofibrate, gemfibrozil) are the first drugs of choice for hypertriglyceridemia and low HDL cholesterol. They are more likely to have positive effects on the carbohydrate metabolism and insulin resistance. After the intake of the conventional nicotinic acid preparations (nicotinic acids, betapyridyl carbinol, xanthinol nicotinate) an acute worsening of diabetes and the IGT was

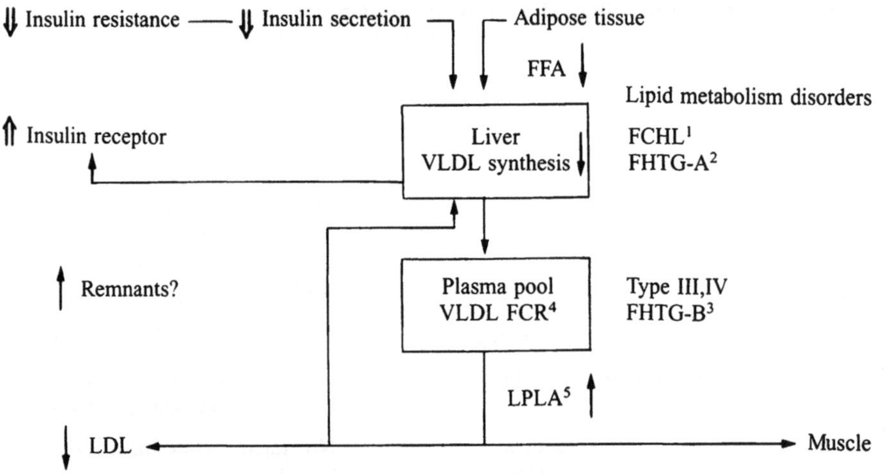

[1] Familiar combined hyperlipoproteinemia
[2] Familiar hypertriglyceridemia-A with pronounced increase in the VLDL synthesis
[3] Familiar hypertriglyceridemia-B with defective VLDL break-down
[4] FCR: fractional catabolic break-down rate
[5] Lipoprotein lipase activity

Fig. 1: The effect of physical conditioning on the lipoprotein metabolism in hyperlipidemias [8].

Tab. 4: Requirements for the use of lipid-lowering drugs in NIDDM

- Two pathological values are present, which were obtained under standard conditions.
- The possibilities of correction of a secondary dyslipoproteinemia have been exhausted (diabetes optimization)
- The dyslipoproteinemia presents a risk from the point of view of the overall situation.
- No general or diabetes specific contraindications are present.
- Compliance is given.

repeatedly observed, such that these drugs could only be used in NIDDM being treated with insulin. Acipimox, a new nicotinic acid derivative, leads to a long-lasting drop in the fatty acids and, at least in the mid-term, improves glucose control as pertains to the regulation of the Randle glucose fatty acid cycle [14].

Anion exchange resins (cholestyramine, colestipol) are still the first choice in treating polygenous hypercholesterolemia. One cholestyramine pectin combination (Vasosan P®) was able to significantly reduce side effects [10]. The cholesterol synthesis enzyme (CSE) inhibitors surpass all previous cholesterol-reducing drugs regarding effectiveness and compliance. Compared to the anion exchange resins, they have the advantage that they also lower triglycerides and the VLDL and

Tab. 5: Medications for the treatment of lipid metabolism disorders in diabetes

Lipid metabolism disorder	First choice medications	Additional
Hypertriglyceridemia	Bezafibrate, fenofibrate, gembrozil, acipimox, fish oils	Acarbose, metformin, nicotinic acid
Combined hyperlipidemia	Fibrates, CSE inhibitors (lovastatin, simvastatin pravastatin, acipimox)	Nicotinic acids, anion exchangers
Hypercholesterolemia	CSE inhibitors, anion exchangers	Guar, fibrates
Chylomicron syndrome	Fish oils, acipimox, gembrozil	Other nicotinic acid derivatives and fibrates

chylomicron remnants, which play an important role in the dyslipoproteinemia of diabetics [5]. The combination of lovastatin and gemfibrozil was shown to be an effective and safe therapy of mixed HLP in NIDDM with intact liver and kidney function.

The combination of acipimox plus fibrate is effective for treating therapy-refractory hypertriglyceridemia. In the case of severe hypercholesterolemia, the combinations of anion exchange resins plus CSE inhibitors, anion exchange resins plus fibrate or, in the case of anion exchange resin intolerance, CSE inhibitors plus fibrate have all proven to be effective. With the presence of intact kidney and liver function and excluding an accompanying medication with immune suppressors, no objections exist to this last combination. As has already been discussed, in the use of lipid-lowering drugs, a number of side effects must be monitored which can have a stronger effect under the special conditions of NIDDM (tab. 6).

Tab. 6: Diabetes-typical side effects of commonly used lipid-lowering drugs

Fibrates:	Lithogenic bile, impotence Monitor kidney performance! Increase in the effect of sulfonyl ureas
Nicotinic acid derivatives: (except acipimox)	Worsening of the carbohydrate tolerance, hyperuricemia
CSE inhibitors:	Not known
Anion exchangers:	Not known
Fish oils:	Worsening of the carbohydrate tolerance

8.2.4 Summary

In the indication evaluation for a lipid-lowering therapy, the realization that NIDDM represents a high risk group is of fundamental importance. Secondary dyslipoproteinemias are common. Therefore primary importance should be placed on optimizing glucose control, eliminating excess weight, improving diet and physical conditioning, and discontinuing the use of lipid-raising and/or HDL cholesterol-lowering medications. Only after these measures have been exhausted over 6 – 8 months is a lipid-lowering drug indicated. Here, several diabetes-specific aspects must be considered.

References

[1] Assmann, G. (Hrsg.): Fettstoffwechselstörungen und koronare Herzkrankheit. Primärprävention, Diagnostik und Therapie. MMW Medizin Verlag, München 1988.

[2] Binder, C.: C-Peptide und B-cell function in diabetes mellitus. In: J. Pickup, G. Williams (eds.): Textbook of diabetes, 348 – 356. Blackwell scientific publications, Oxford 1991.

[3] Dunn, F. L.: Treatment of lipid disorders in diabetes mellitus. Med. Clin. N. Am. *72* (6) (1988) 1379 – 1398.

[4] European NIDDM Policy Group. A desktop guide for the management of non-insulin-dependent diabetes mellitus (NIDDM). IDF Bulletin (suppl.), April 1990.

[5] Garg, A., S. M. Grundy: Lovastatin for lowering cholesterol levels in non-insulin-dependent-diabetes mellitus. N. Engl. J. Med. *318* (1988) 81 – 85.

[6] Gerich, J. E.: Oral hypoglycemic agents. New. Engl. J. Med. *321* (1989) 1231 – 1245.

[7] Hanefeld, M., J. Huttunen: Exercise. In: A. G. Olsson (ed.): Atherosclerosis. Biology and clinical science, 481 – 486. Churchill Livingstone, Edinburgh 1987.

[8] Hanefeld, M., S. Fischer, U. Julius et al.: More exercise for hyperlipidemic patients. Ann. Clin. Res. *20* (1988) 77 – 83.

[9] Hanefeld, M., S. Fischer, J. Schulze et al.: Therapeutic potentials of acarbose as first-line-drug in NIDDM insufficiently treated with diet alone. Diabetes Care *14* (8) (1991) 732 – 737.

[10] Hanefeld, M., W. Leonhardt, L. Schmidt et al.: Vasosan® – eine Cholestyramin-Pektin-Wirkstoff-Kombination mit höherer Wirksamkeit und weniger Nebenwirkungen. Medicamentum *28* (8) (1987) 170 – 172.

[11] Jensen, T.: Fisch oil administration in diabetes. In: C. E. Mogensen, E. Standl (eds.): Pharmacology of diabetes, 153 – 162. De Gruyter, Berlin 1991.

[12] Lopes-Virella, M. F., J. A. Coldwell: Pharmacological treatment of lipid disorders in diabetes mellitus. Diab. Metab. Rev. *3* (1987) 691 – 722.

[13] Schernthaner, G.: Kritische Analyse der antidiabetischen Therapie mit Metformin: Stoffwechselwirkungen, antiatherogene Effekte und Kontraindikationen. Akt. Endokr. Stoffw. *13* (1992) 44 – 50.

[14] Sirtori, C. R., G. Gianfranceschi, M. Sirtori et al.: Reduced triglyceridemia and increased high density lipoprotein cholesterol levels after treatment with acipimox, a new inhibitor of lipolysis. Atherosclerosis *38* (1981) 267 – 271.

[15] Weck, M., M. Hanefeld, S. Gehrisch et al.: Insulinbehandlung bei adipösen Typ-II-Diabetikern als Teilursache für exzessive Hyperlipidämie und Insulinresistenz oder Probleme in der Glukosekontrolle – Ein circulus vitiosus? Z. Klin. Med. *4* (1987) 853 – 856.

8.3 The treatment of hyperuricemia

H.-E. Schröder

8.3.1 *Basic therapy for the reduction of medication use*

In any case of hyperuricemia, one should first thoroughly exhaust the non-drug therapy possibilities. Basal treatment, based on a re-orientation of eating habits, weight reduction and physical conditioning, fully meets the basic principles for treatment of type II diabetes (see sections 7.1 to 7.4). For the diet consultation for patients with hyperuricemia, we focus on the recommendations of the German Nutrition Society, according to which the portion of carbohydrates should contribute up to 60%, the fat content up to 30% and the protein content over 10%. Milk proteins are to be preferred among proteins, because they are purine-free. The permitted weekly purine intake, expressed in terms of the urea content, is pegged at 2–3 g [1]. Variations of these recommendations are necessary to account for further metabolic imbalances (see section 7.3).

The size of the portion usually consumed is decisive for the estimation of the purine intake. Purine-rich foods (tabs. 1 and 2) probably play no significant role when they are only enjoyed in small portions. In contrast, purine-poor foods can constitute a significant purine load when they are consumed in large amounts to cover calorie needs [1]. Uric acid values can be decreased by 120 μmol/l as a result of a consistent basic therapy, so that low-grade hyperuricemia can be corrected already with these measures [3].

8.3.2 *Choosing a uric acid reducer*

There are two drug classes with varying sites of action available for the drug therapy of hyperuricemia [3]. The *uricostatic agents* suppress exogenous and endogenous uric acid formation and thereby ease the renal excretion capacity. The most important representative of this group is allopurinol, an isomer of hypoxanthine. Due to the long half-life of the main metabolite, oxipurinol, the dose can be administered once daily. In contrast, the *uricosuric agents* increase renal uric acid excretion and thereby lower the serum uric acid level. They do not influence uric acid formation. The danger of uricosuric agents is in their mechanism of action. If the initial dose is too high, the massive rise in renal uric acid excretion can lead to the crystallization of uric acid in the renal tubules or kidney parenchyma. The consequences are kidney stone formation and in extreme cases renal failure. Dehydration with acidification of the urine promotes this process. For this reason, it is necessary to prescribe uricosuric agents in gradually

Tab. 1: Important purine-rich foods

Food	mg uric acids per 100 g	Portion size	
		Portion	in (g)
– Meat, game, poultry: beef filet, cutlet, stewing meat, mutton, rabbit, venison	70 – 130	35 – 195	50 – 150
– Fish: Sole, halibut, oysters	90 – 127	36 – 190	40 – 150
– Mushrooms: Boletus, chanterelles	25 – 50	38 – 75	150
– Vegetables: Spinach, asparagus, beans (green), green cabbage, carrots, red cabbage, cauliflower	25 – 70	38 – 105	150 – 250
– Beer	16	80	0.5 l

Tab. 2: Important foods very rich in purine

Food	mg uric acids per 100 g	Portion size	
		Portion	in (g)
– Offal: Thymus, liver, heart, kidneys	240 – 1030	300 – 1030	100 – 125
– Meat: veal filet, pork, rabbit, mutton	145 – 190	220 – 280	150
– Game and poultry: Goose, duck, chicken, turkey	110 – 240	165 – 300	150
– Fish: Herring, smoked herring, sardines in oil, smoked sprats, salmon, shellfish, carp, pike, cod	140 – 560	210 – 525	50 – 150
– Legumes: Peas (green and yellow), white beans, lentils	130 – 185	51 – 220	25 – 150

increasing doses with urinary pH values controlled at 6.2 to 6.8 and the assurance of a fluid intake of 2.0 to 2.5 l over the course of the day. The most important example of this group is benzbromaron, which shows the strongest effectiveness with good tolerability. The long half-life of its metabolites enables the preparation to be prescribed once a day.

Due to their mechanism of action, the uricostatic agents are recommended for all forms of over-production, the uricosuric agents, in contrast, for renal excretion disorders [2]. A test of renal uric acid excretion is, however, necessary to differentiate therapy. The method of urine collection required is not practical for everyday office use.

8.3.3 Recommendations for the practice

We recommend an initial basal treatment with allopurinol in an increasing dosage with monitoring of the serum uric acid level for 1 – 3 months. If the uric acid level has not yet normalized at an allopurinol dose of 300mg, treatment is to be continued with a combination of allopurinol and benzbromaron, in free or defined combination, for which the maximal doses given in tab. 3 are generally not necessary. If a hyperuricemia is not correctable with the therapeutic doses given in tab. 3, the patient should be transferred to a specialized out-patient clinic for individual diagnosis and therapy planning.

Tab. 3: Dosage schema of the most important uric acid reducers

Preparation	Starting dosis	Therapeutic dosis*
Allopurinol	100 mg	100 – 300 mg
Benzybromaron	25 – 50 mg	50 – 100 mg
Standard combination (Allopurinol/benzbromaron)	100/200	100/20 – 300/60 mg

* These high dosages are rarely needed with the patient-specific application of the uric acid reducers

Is it necessary to treat every hyperuricemic? A drug-induced uric acid reduction is only necessary, when the following symptoms are present:

- Serum uric acid level constantly above 480 μmol/l
- Less than 60 years old
- Development of gout (kidney, skeletal)
- Urolithiasis
- Hypertension
- Poorly-controlled type II diabetes
- Pronounced dys- or hyper-lipoproteinemia, as well as
- Reduced kidney function.

Uric acid reducers and renal insufficiency: The dosage of the preparations must be adjusted to the remaining kidney function. Allopurinol should be limited to 200 mg at serum creatinine values of 180 μmol/l, and to 100 mg at serum creatinine values of 350 μmol/l. Of the uricosuric agents, only benzbromaron may be used, and in a reduced dosage (25 - 50 mg) up to a serum creatinine level of 350 mmol/l.

Uric acid reducers and important interactions: Along with a worsening of the glucose tolerance, thiazides and furosemides can induce hyperuricemia. If these preparations must be further prescribed, uric acid reducers are necessary for long-term application. Cytostatics of the 6-mercaptopurine variety must be reduced to 25% of the normal dosage to prevent toxic side effects in simultaneous allopurinol therapy. Glibenclamide and insulin do not influence the serum uric acid level. Tolbutamide and metformin can possibly lead to a worsening of hyperuricemia through a reduction in renal uric acid excretion.

8.3.4 Summary

The basis of therapy for hyperuricemia should in all cases be a reduction in dietary purine intake . Mild hyperuricemia can be thus corrected. The uricostatic agent, allopurinol, in a dose of up to 300 mg is well suited to serve as a basic therapy for the drug-induced reduction of the uric acid level. Pronounced renal uric acid excretion disorders can often be better improved with a uricosuric agent. For a combined application, commercial preparations with 100 mg allopurinol and 20 mg benzbromaron are available. Based on the severity of the purine metabolic disorder, it must be decided, whether a short trial of drug therapy or a long-term therapy is necessary.

References

[1] Schröder, H.-E.: Stufendiagnostikprogramm und Differentialdiagnose der Störungen des Purinstoffwechsels und begleitender Krankheiten. In: P. Thiele, G. Heidelmann, H.-E. Schröder (Hrsg.): Hyperurikämie und Gicht. 81 – 115. Fischer, Jena 1986.

[2] Schröder, H.-E.: Pharmaka zur Behandlung der Hyperurikämie und Gicht. In: P. Thiele, G. Heidelmann, H.-E. Schröder: Hyperurikämie und Gicht. 131 – 149. Fischer, Jena 1986.

[3] Spann, W., S. Wolfram: Diät. In: N. Zöllner (Hrsg.): Hyperurikämie, Gicht und andere Störungen des Purinhaushalts. 260 – 299. 2. Aufl. Springer, Berlin, Heidelberg, New York 1990.

8.4 Treatment of coagulation disorders and blood flow disorders

U. Julius

8.4.1 *The therapy of thrombophilia*

8.4.1.1 *Introduction*

The connections between metabolic parameters and disorders in coagulation and in the rheologic blood properties (see section 5.5) suggest that an *eumetabolization* could contribute significantly to the reduction of thrombophilia in diabetics.

Pertaining to this, it is important that
- patients not smoke,
- patients are physically active
- blood pressure is well controlled
- excess weight is reduced
- plant oils (also fish oils) are consumed in the diet
- venous stasis is avoided
- diseases, which could lead to polyglobulism, are sufficiently treated.

The same indications and contraindications are applicable to diabetics and non-diabetics in the use of pharmaceutics which influence coagulation.

Differences exist between:

1. Primary prevention
An acute vascular event (e.g., a myocardial infarction) has not yet occurred. Due to "thrombophilia" in (older) type II diabetics, it is desirable that the opportunities for the primary prevention be actively used (e.g., acetylsalicylic acid for the prevention of arterial occlusions).

2. Secondary prevention
An event or a particular condition has already occurred or emerged. It is important to prevent a relapse or a threatening complication. The available study results are primarily focussed on this sort of therapy and have been able to show impressive effects. This is particularly true for interventional-radiologic interventions in the arterial system.

8.4.1.2 *Acetylsalicylic acid*

Acetylsalicylic acid possesses important anti-aggregational effects. In various studies, the following effects of this substance could be documented:

- Protection from stroke and reduction in the frequency of fatal outcomes patients with transient ischemic attacks or minor strokes

- Decreased mortality and/or development of myocardial infarction in cases of unstable angina
- Decreased re-occlusion rate after percutaneous transluminal angioplasty of major arteries and in the coronary arteries
- Prevention of a recurrent vascular occlusion after a disobliterative endarterectomy or after the performance of an aorto-coronary bypass
- Secondary prevention after a myocardial infarction.

The prescription of acetylsalicylic acid can already be introduced in low doses in the presence of a peripheral arterial disease in stages I or II (according to Lafontaine).

The daily dose should lie between 100 and 300 mg. Two recent studies have also demonstrated the clinical efficacy of smaller doses (30 mg/day) [1, 7] for secondary prevention after transient ischemic attacks or minor strokes. The smaller doses are associated with fewer side effects. The optimal dosage for diabetics has until now still not been definitively defined.

Laboratory investigations are not necessary for the monitoring of this therapy. Long-term therapy is possible and it is advisable, given the presence of an atherosclerotic vascular disease. Doses higher than those discussed are only necessary where the antiinflammatory effect of the substance is desired.

8.4.1.3 Anticoagulants

The use of anticoagulants of the coumarin type leads to the reduction in the coagulation capability of the blood by influencing the coagulation system in plasma. One should differentiate between absolute and relative indications:

1. Absolute indications
- Subsequent to deep vein thrombosis (over 3 – 6 months) and pulmonary embolism (6 – 12 months); after recurrent thromboembolism potentially lifelong
- Atrial fibrillation with arterial embolism
- Artificial heart valves, chronic heart wall aneurysms, cardiomyopathy
- Anti-thrombin III deficiency

2. Relative indications
- Chronic arterial occlusive disease (contraindications often disallow this)
  Differences
  arterial thrombosis → acetylsalicylic acid recommended
  embolic occlusion → anticoagulants recommended
- After arterial bypass operation.

The measurement of the thromboplastin time serves to monitor this therapy form, the partial value should lie between 15 and 25%. Hemorrhages are to be expect in 3 – 5% of the anticoagulated patients. For this reason, the use of these substances is often problematic in older type II diabetics.

The considerations regarding "low-dose anticoagulation" (partial value between 30 and 50%) for the prevention of stroke in patients with atrial fibrillation are interesting. In this case, the danger of hemorrhage is lower.

8.4.1.4 Heparin

Heparin accelerates the inactivation of thrombin and other coagulative factors via anti-thrombin III. One differentiates between prophylactic and therapeutic use.

1. Prophylactic use (2 – 3 x 5000 U/day)
Increased thrombosis risk in the venous system, e.g.,
- Post-operative
- With immobilization
- With extended bed rest
- With intensive diuretic treatment
- During risky fasting treatments.

The application of low-molecular weight heparin preparations allows for a single daily injection with a relatively comparable effecicacy. Studies regarding this are underway, which will be significant for future preparation choices.

2. Therapeutic use (initial bolus: 10,000 – 15,000 U; continuous infusion 20,000 – 40,000 U per day)
- Deep venous thrombosis
- Standard after fibrinolysis or a thrombectomy
- Pulmonary embolism
- Arterial occlusion
- Disseminated intravascular coagulation
- Procedures involving extracorporal circulation (dialysis, lipid apheresis, heart surgery)

8.4.1.5 Fibrinolytic agents

The procedures of *fibrinolysis* (with streptokinase or urokinase or tissue plasminogen activator) have become well established in the therapy of acute myocardial infarction, lung embolism, arterial occlusion, the occlusion of bypasses or shunts or life-threatening vein thromboses in hospital.

The lowering of a mild hyperfibrinogenemia with the consequence of an improved myocardial microcirculation could be demonstrated for *fibrate therapy*.

8.4.2 Rheologically oriented therapy

The therapy of a deficient peripheral and central circulation and thereby a deficient nutrient supply of tissue should take into account three biological functional units [3]:

1. *Circulatory properties of the blood*
- Maintenance of microcirculation
- Hemolysis-protection and membrane flexibility
- Prevention of erythrocyte aggregation
- Suppression of thrombocyte aggregation
- Increase in the blood circulation speed and prevention of low-flow conditions.

2. *Immediate effects on the vessel endothelium*
- Influencing the arterial and venous tone
- Regulation of a disturbed thromboxane-prostacycline balance (biosynthesis)
- Improvement in the vessel wall permeability in capillaries (filtration) and venules (resorption).

3. *Effects in the perivascular tissues (interstitium)*
- Suppression of an ischaemia-related cytotoxic edema
- Stimulation of oxygen and glucose uptake and utilization
- Increase in tissue tolerance of hypoxia
- Prevention of pathological lipid oxidation through neutralization of toxic oxygen radicals.

This list demonstrates that numerous pharmaceuticals already introduced into practice take aim at rheological phenomena (e.g., acetylsalicylic acids, Ca-antagonists, blood pressure regulating drugs, vitamin E). The plasma viscosity is optimized through a lowering of the raised fibrinogen level. It is to be expected that new compounds will open further possibilities in the future.

Three therapeutic procedures should here be mentioned, which can be applied for *an improvement of the circulatory properties of the blood.*

If the blood circulatory properties are impaired with a hematocrit > 45% and if an ischaemia is present, an isovolemic hemodilution should be considered: blood letting (400–500 ml), simultaneous infusion of rheomacrodex, hydroxyethyl starch or autologous plasma. The hematocrit is thereby lowered to 35 – 38%. An acute myocardial infarction presents a contraindication. The polymorbidity of older type II diabetics often does not allow this therapy.

Pentoxifyllin is a methylanthine derivative. It increases the erythrocyte flexibility and suppresses the thrombocyte aggregation. Its main area of use is in chronic cerebral and peripheral circulatory problems. 800–1200 mg/day in 2–3 single doses (long-acting preparation) is prescribed. An infusion therapy is also possible.

Extracts of ginkgo biloba reduce erythrocyte stiffness and tendency to erythrocyte aggregation. Its indications for use are peripheral artery diseases with intermittent claudication as well as brain performance disorders. The clinical importance of this extract must still be placed in relationship to changes observed in the microcirculation.

8.4.3 Summary

The eumetabolization and exclusion of factors with negative influence on coagulation and rheology are important above all for younger diabetics, even when micro or macro-angiopathy have still not been observed.

For older type II diabetics, eumetabolization is generally not the greatest desired therapeutic goal. In these patients, acetylsalicylic acids should be used for prevention of a vascular occlusion in known atherosclerotic vascular diseases. The indications for the prophylactic application of heparin are to be observed. Acetylsalicylic acid and heparin have proven themselves in the area of secondary prevention. Anticoagulants are occasionally used in secondary prevention, and the absolute indications for long-term use are relatively few. A good willingness to cooperate on the part of the patient, is an essential precondition for this therapy.

In each case, the application of the treatment therapies which are offered under "rheologically oriented therapy", must be decided upon by the physician.

References

[1] Dutch TIA Trial Study Group: A comparison of two doses of aspirin (30 mg vs. 283 mg a day) in patients after a transient ischemic attack or minor ischemic stroke. N. Engl. J. Med. *325* (1991) 1261–1266.

[2] Ebenezer, Chr.: Behandlung rheologisch bedingter Störungen der Mikrozirkulation. Rationale hämorheologische Therapie mit Rökan. Mainzer Verlagsanstalt und Druckerei, Will und Rothe, Mainz 1990.

[3] Ernst, F.-D.: Mikrozirkulation und Hämorheologie. Münch. med. Wschr. *130* (1988) 863–866.

[4] Gerok, W., F. Hartmann, M. Pfreundschuh et al.: Klinik der Gegenwart. Urban & Schwarzenberg, München, Wien, Baltimore 1991.

[5] Oehler, G., B. Kemkes-Matthes: Blutgerinnung und Thrombose. Thrombose-Schriftenreihe. Sandoz AG, Nürnberg 1991.

[6] Rustige, J., J. Senges, W. Schöps et al.: Zu wenige Patienten mit akutem Herzinfarkt erhalten eine Thrombolyse. Deutsches Ärzteblatt *88* (1991) D-4790-D – D-4792.

[7] SALT Collaborative Group: Swedish Aspirin Low-dose Trial (SALT) of 75 mg aspirin as secondary prophylaxis after cerebrovascular ischaemic events. Lancet *338* (1991) 1345–1349.

9 Late complications of diabetes

9.1 The diabetic foot

9.1.1 *The ischemic diabetic foot*

Sabine Fischer, H. Rietzsch

9.1.1.1 *Epidemiology*

Arterial circulatory disorders of the extremities are 5 times more frequent in diabetics than in non-diabetics, the risk of gangrene of the foot 20 times more frequent. According to findings of the Schwabing Study, evidence of peripheral arterial circulatory disorders in diabetics is an unfavorable prognostic finding. Arterial occlusive disease, for the most part in stage I, was present at the first examination in 67.4% of those diabetics who died of cardiovascular illness within 5 years of diagnosis, compared to 12.7% of those who were still living. Characteristic for diabetics is the fact that women are affected by macroangiopathy as often or even more often than men [9, 16].

9.1.1.2 *Pathological anatomy and pathophysiology*

Besides the macroangiopathy, microangiopathy is also typical for the diabetic. Circulatory disorders of the legs often appear very peripherally in diabetics, in 2/3 of the cases in the calf and foot [19], only 1/4 of the occlusions are found in the thigh vessels. The macroangiopathy of the diabetic does not generally differ from that of the non-diabetic. It is however, usually more pronounced than with the non-diabetic, is more diffuse and progresses more quickly. Often a number of vascular regions are affected, which is then a factor in the prognosis. In all probability the macrovascular complications begin to form increasingly during the pre-diabetic phase.

The so-called Mönckeberg mediosclerosis is viewed as typical for the diabetic. This is a tubular calcification of the tunica media of the arterial wall in mid-sized arteries of the muscular type, whereby the intima remains intact, i. e. there is no restriction in the vascular volume (fig. 1). It is suspected of being dependent on the duration of the diabetes [19] and most common in the arteries of the lower extremities. Wall thickening with cellular proliferation and fibrous network formation on the smallest arterioles and capillaries as well as thickening occurs in the capillary basement membrane. These vascular changes occur in all vascular domains. The diabetes as such is important for the formation of macrovascular

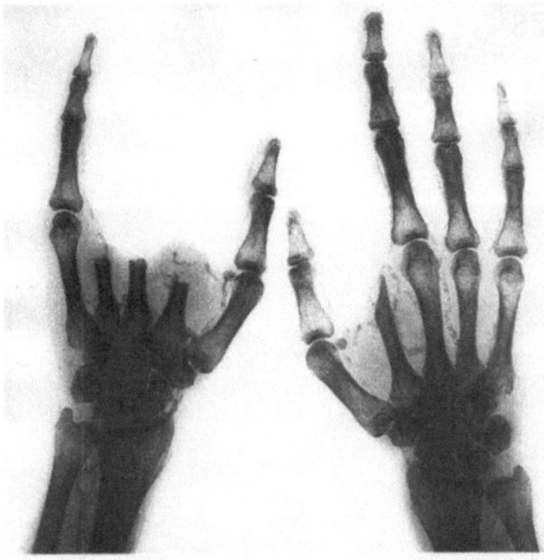

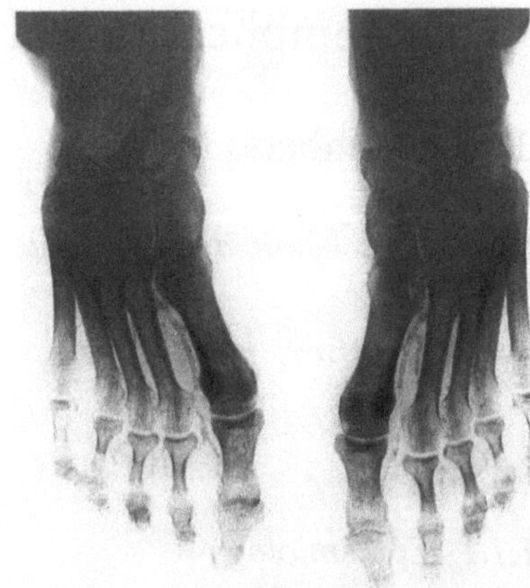

Fig. 1a: Pictures of a Mönckeberg mediosclerosis: the hands of a 40-year old female diabetic with 30 years of living with diabetes (condition after finger amputations due to acral necroses, severe post-operative wound healing disturbances).

Fig. 1b: Feet of a 60-year old male diabetic with pronounced diabetic late complications (retinopathy, nephropathy (peritoneal dialysis) and ulcers between the toes).

changes, but risk factors such as hypertension, hypertriglyceridemia, hyperinsulinemia and pathological coagulation [9, 16] which occur more frequently in diabetics than in the normal population are important as well. Breddin was able to show an elevated thrombocyte aggregation for diabetic men [5]. From the San Antonio Heart Study it is possible to conclude that the atherosclerotic changes are also in part caused by hyperinsulinemia and obesity [8]. As the macroangiopathy begins to take form prior to onset of the clinical manifestation of diabetes, there can be little association with the duration of the diabetes.

The atherosclerotic changes occur as a result of anomalies of the flow dynamics and mechanical peculiarities, especially at vessel branches and places where the mechanical demands are greater. Beside the hypertension, the metabolic disorder per se, and especially the hyperglycemia, are pathogenetically instrumental in the development of the microangiopathy. This leads to enzymatic and non-enzymatic glycosylation of proteins and corresponding functional anomalies which induce the changes in the basal membrane, the changes in the blood flow properties and the disturbed oxygen transport. The diabetic microangiopathy is therefore influenced by the duration of the diabetes and the quality of the metabolic control [15].

9.1.1.3 Clinical picture

When taking the patient history it is necessary to inquire about intermittent claudication symptoms, which can also occur in the foot as a result of the frequent peripheral localization, along with other risk factors of atherosclerosis and smoking. With a concomitant diabetic neuropathy, typical pain may not occur or only be perceived to a limited extent, so that clinical misdiagnosis is possible. Quickly fatigued legs, sensation of cold or paresthesia, may occur in the early stages of the disease. Rest pain indicates an advanced stage of vascular disease (Fontaine stage III, see below); it occurs most frequently when the leg is elevated or in cold weather. If the leg is lowered or the surrounding temperature increased, the pain subsides. Nocturnal leg cramps are not generally a sign of peripheral circulatory disorders, but are often considered as such by patients. Diseases of veins or complaints of the joints or spinal column must be excluded by means of differential diagnosis.

If there are peripheral vascular changes and possibly an accompanying neuropathy, minor injuries can lead to severe healing disorders with the formation of ulcers or necrosis, if treatment is not begun promptly and followed consistently.

When examining the patient it is necessary to perform a subtle examination of the heart and bilateral blood pressure, of the total vascular status with bilateral palpitation of the A. carotis, A. subclavia, A. radialis, A. femoralis, A poplitea (often difficult to palpitate), A. tibialis posterior and A. dorsalis pedis, as well as bilateral auscultation of the A. carotis and A. femoralis. As a result of the peripheral attack, it is frequently possible to still detect the foot pulse although necroses and ulcers already exist. Both legs must be carefully examined, especially with respect to skin color, wounds, injuries and fungus mycoses. Skin temperature should be taken, comparison of the legs made, edema, vein diseases and changes in joints examined. It is also important that the spaces between the toes be examined so that small necroses or interdigital mycoses are not overlooked. If there are manifest circulatory disorders, the skin is usually pale and cool, frequently slightly cyanotic, especially when the leg is elevated. As other vascular provinces are generally affected, renal function (serum creatinine, microalbumin test, protein excretion in 24-hr. urine, urine culture) should be examined, a resting ECG, echocardiography, duplex sonography of the carotids and an ophthalmologic examination should be performed. Blood tests serve to detect coagulation disorders, hyperlipoproteinemia, changes in the electrolytes, renal function disorders, anemia, etc.

The intermittent claudication distance (walking speed 120 steps per minute, difficult if concomitant heart failure, severe CHD, arthroses, diseases of the spinal column or diabetic neuropathy are present) must be determined in the course of further examinations. This is important if the complaints are present only under stress.

Treadmill ergometry (better standardization of the intermittent claudication distance) and occlusion plethysmography should be mentioned in the framework of the apparative diagnosis. Nowadays, oscillography has faded into the background somewhat. Ultrasound examinations are used to localize stenoses or occlusions and to determine their extent and severity. The cruro-brachial index is also determined by means of Doppler ultrasound, i. e. the quotient from systolic malleolar arterial pressure and systolic upper arm pressure. The systolic malleolar arterial pressure is normally greater than that of the systolic upper arm pressure so that the cruro-brachial index is usually between 1.0 – 1.2, values below 1 being pathologic. This ratio should not, however, be used with pronounced Mönckeberg mediosclerosis or edema. Because the absolute pressure in the leg is decisive for the circulation of the leg, some investigators determine only the malleolar pressure (valid only with normal BP) (tab. 1).

Tab. 1: Malleolar arterial pressure and cruro-brachial index in Fontaine stages II and III

Stages	Malleolar arterial pressure	CBI
Compensated occlusion		
(IIa)	>80 mmHg	0.7 – 0.9
(IIb)	60 – 80 mmHg	0.5 – 0.7
Decompensated occlusion		
(III)	<60 mmHg	<0.5

Duplex sonography can be used for evaluation of the vessel wall or suspicion of aneurysms. It can also serve to assess the success of vascular surgery. If, on the basis of the history, clinical examination and non-invasive investigative methods, there is the suspicion of severe arterial circulatory disorders with possible need of an operation, a percutaneous transluminal angioplasty (PTA) or a lysis therapy, angiography then is indicated and necessary. Angiography is always indicated in stage III and IV and with acute deterioration of a previously existent claudication, even in stage IIb. The need for angiography in stage IIa is a personal decision, for example with young patients or to fill a social need (e.g. the patient has to walk longer distances at work). The decision to perform angiography should be more aggressively pursued the more proximal the occlusion or stenosis is and the shorter the history of illness. The danger of the development of an acute renal insufficiency or worsening of existing renal insufficiency as a consequence of contrast medium should be kept in mind with diabetics. It is possible to determine the location and the extent of the stenosis or occlusion and assess the collateral supply with angiography. The indication for angiography must be viewed very narrowly and focus itself on the therapeutic consequences. A stenosis of > 60% causes ischemia.

To functionally determine the circulatory disorder, the Fontaine stage assessment is equally suitable for non-diabetics as well as diabetics:

Stage	I:	Asymptomatic, possibly atypical discomfort on the foot or leg in certain positions, frequently incidental findings
	II:	Intermittent claudication: After a certain distance, cramp-like pain as a result of stress-related muscle ischemia; patient is forced to rest, after a certain period of rest the pain subsides, the patient can walk again until the pain returns.
	IIa:	Intermittent claudication distance 1 – 2 km to 200 m
	IIb:	Intermittent claudication distance < 200 m
	III:	Rest pain, partially beginning trophic disorders, complaints when extremities are raised or horizontal, when lowered the complaints often subside as a result of the increased perfusion pressure.
	IV:	Necrosis, ulcers, gangrene; poorly healing tissue lesions in the region of the foot
	IVa:	Stationary necrosis
	IVb:	Advancing gangrene: It should be noted that not every poorly healing wound is necessarily stage IV; it is possible that it is a stage IIb with stable intermittent claudication distance and a malleolar pressure of 80 mmHg without rest ischemia.

Depending on the location of the occlusion there is the aortic type, the pelvic type, the thigh and the peripheral occlusive location. Multiple stenoses or occlusions of various locations are also not rare (two- and multi-staged occlusions). The prognosis for these is worse and therapy complicated (fig. 2):

Aortic type:	Total occlusion of the aorta abdomalis or the aortic bifurcation → Leriche syndrome
Pelvic type:	Occlusion of the pelvic axis, usually the A. iliaca comm. and externa; no pulse distally below the groin
Thigh type:	A. femoralis superfic. especially in the adductor channel and below the ramification of the A. profunda femoris or affliction of the entire length; if the A. profunda femoris remains permeable → good prerequisite for the formation of a collateral circulation; lack of pulse distal from the A. poplitea on.
Peripheral:	Occlusion or stenosis in the region of the calf or foot vessels; pain frequently in the arch of the foot! Most frequent type of occlusion in diabetic! (In contrast, non-diabetics exhibit proximal stenoses or occlusions more frequently).

9.1.1.4 Therapy

Prophylactic measures are of considerable importance for avoiding or stopping the progress of atherosclerotic vascular complications. Among these is not-smoking, detection and regulation of hypertension (BP < = 140/90) and hyper-

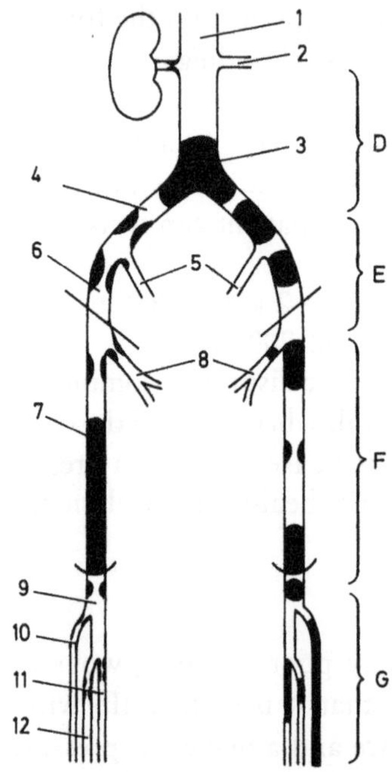

Fig. 2: The most important stenosis and occlusion localizations in the lower body half, generally found in patients with peripheral circulation disorders: (1) aorta abdominalis, (2) a. renalis, (3) aorta bifurcation, (4) a. iliaca comm., (5) a. iliaca int., (6) a. iliaca ext., (7) a. femoralis superfic., (8) a. profunda femoris, (9) a. poplitea, (10) a. tibialis ant., (11) a. tibialis post., (12) a. peronea. Localization types (see text): taken in a modified form from: Kappert [10].

lipoproteinemia (see section 8.2). Furthermore, combating obesity with the aim of at least reducing insulin resistance and hyperinsulinemia and thereby attaining a euglycemic blood sugar from the beginning of the disease. The aim of the therapy, which is often more difficult and longer-term than with non-diabetics, due to the complexity of the situation, is to slow the progression of the vascular disease (secondary prevention), extension of the pain-free walking distance, regression of an extremity-threatening ischemia, i. e. a stage III or stage IV to a stage II and certainly to avoid amputation (amputation of toes in advanced stages of gangrene is however, often unavoidable to save the leg).

Diet, risk factors, general therapy

Beside the specific therapeutic aspects, the basic therapeutic measures are also very important. Among these is the fat-modified diabetic diet (see sections 7.2 and 8.2).

If there are already cardiovascular disorders, the necessity of optimum diabetic control is even greater, and, for the most part, normoglycemia should be the goal. If the condition has already reached stage IV, the blood glucose values in the daily profile should be between 6 and 7 mmol/l. This requires tight blood glucose, fructosamine and HbA_1 or HbA_{1c} monitoring, self-monitoring of the blood glucose is absolutely essential. Insulin therapy is almost always unavoidable with peripheral arterial disease in stage IV. Only in exceptional cases, when the blood glucose and HbA_{1c} values are optimal, for instance with lower dosages of a glibenclamide therapy, can this be continued.

Smoking is absolutely prohibited with manifest atherosclerotic diseases and the consistent treatment of other risk factors such as a hypertension or hyperlipoproteinemia is of the utmost importance. Frequently a coronary heart disease is also present. This must be carefully regulated. Coronary insufficiency, which may be present, must be treated. Edema is to be eliminated, anemia or electrolyte disturbances are to be balanced. Mycoses are to be properly treated. Progression to stage IV is to be avoided by prophylactic means (avoid tight or poor footwear, proper foot care, no hot foot baths, etc.). Analgesics are often required in stages III and IV. Drug treatment must be reviewed with respect to possible side effects on the peripheral arterial disease (e.g. non-selective beta-blockers and thiazide diuretics should be replaced by other suitable medication).

Angiographic measures

The diabetic must, at an early date, receive clear guidelines to avoid and recognize peripheral arterial occlusive disorders. Complex training of the diabetic is very important in this respect. In this manner it is possible to avoid long and expensive hospitalization.

The ultimate goal is to absolutely avoid an amputation. If one leg is already amputated the prognosis for the second leg is worse. The principle therapeutic objective with macroangiopathy is the correction of the stenosis or ischemia, i. e. the operative vascular reconstruction or the reopening of stenosis or occlusions or, in case this is not possible, the formation of a good collateral circulation. In this respect the possibility of a vascular operation or a percutaneous transluminal angioplasty (PTA) or a local lysis therapy should be considered at an early date in the stages IIb, III, and IV, which are defined by the critical circulation of the extremity. Only by restoration of the atherosclerotically altered vascular system can the perfusion pressure be increased which might make it possible to overcome more peripheral stenoses and supply more peripheral vascular regions. If an opening of the lumen in these stages is not possible, drug therapy has to be the treatment of choice.

An operation is indicated in longer stenoses or occlusions in the pelvic or thigh region and older occlusions (older than 3 months), if the vessel has a peripheral

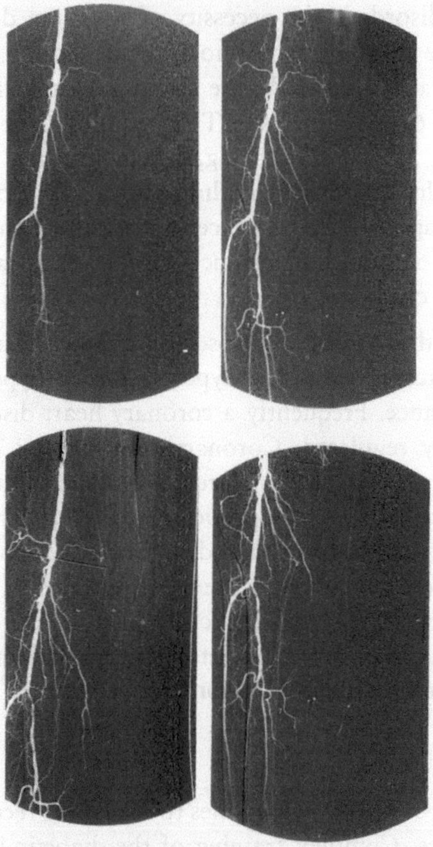

Fig. 3a: Arteria femoralis superficialis right: before (upper images) and after (lower images) a PTA (66-year old patient with Diab. mellitus Type II, HLP and hypertension). Several stenoses in the thigh region. Clinical claudicatio intermittens; walking range before the PTA 400 m, after the PTA 1000 m, in addition, atherosclerotic changes in the lower leg arteries are present.

connection. Especially in the case of multi-stage occlusions the possibility of an operation on proximally located stenoses should be considered at an early date. Anticoagulants should be used post-operatively, particularly in bypass operations that extend beyond joints. Heparin can be injected by the patient for up to six months, maximum one year in cases of coumarin necroses.

PTA is used in diagnosing significant stenoses of the aortoiliacal and femoropopliteal axis (stenosis of the A. femoralis superific. the middle and distal A. iliaca comm. and ext. occlusion up to 5 – 10 cm long) (fig. 3). Platelet aggregation inhibitors or anticoagulants are then indicated to avoid the danger of a reocclusion [10].

Lysis therapy is indicated in thromboembolic occlusions or embolic occlusions with ongoing ischemia, especially with acute worsening and development of a

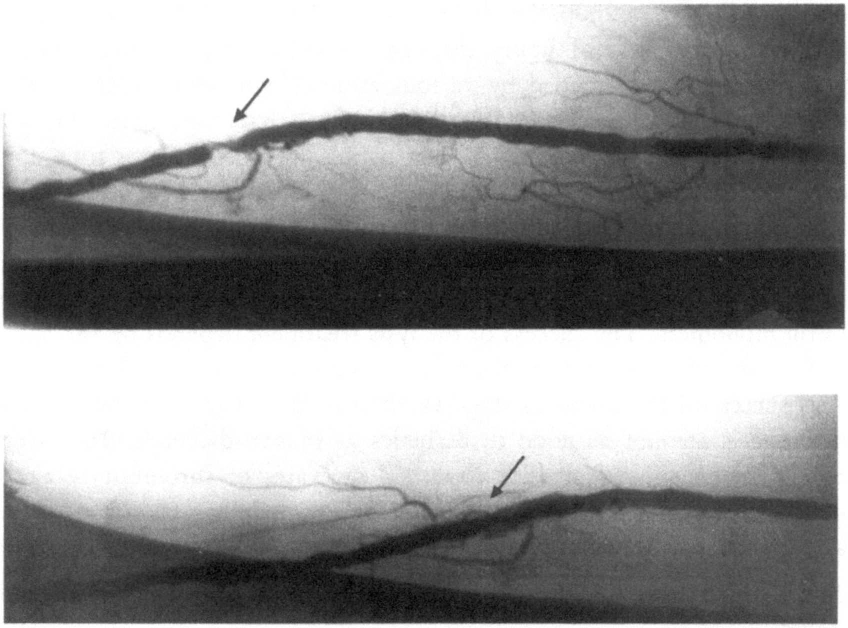

Fig. 3b: 85-year old female long-term diabetic (type II diabetes), acral necroses on several toes of the left foot with the additional presence of neuropathy. The high degree stenosis of the arteria femoralis superficialis before the PTA (upper image), after PTA border amputation and healing of the lesions (lower image).

stage IIb, III (or IV). The age of the occlusion should be less than three months. The more distal the occlusion, the lower the age of the occlusion should be, if the lysis is to be successful. Local lysis is preferable to a systemic lysis because of its lower rate of complications (local lysis: normal reptilasis time, normal fibrinogen). Streptokinase and urokinase or rtPA (recombinant tissue plasminogen activator) are used as thrombolytics, whereby the trend is to the latter two forms of medication as a result of the short lysis times and lower frequency of complications. Streptokinase and urokinase are injected directly into the thrombus via an intraarterial catheter using x-ray monitoring (small amounts of the fibrinolytic in minute-long intervals while inserting the catheter centimeter for centimeter), so that the lysable material is removed. The end of the catheter must be located in the region of the stenosis or occlusion so that the substance is delivered to the diseased area and does not flow off through collaterals. The high complication rate should be kept in mind with a combination of lysis with PTA (total dosage 30,000 – 50,000 IU streptokinase or 100,000 – 150,000 IU urokinase [14]). Contraindications for local lysis are active gastrointestinal ulcers, malignant hypertension, manifest hemorrhaging diathesis, polytrauma, vascular aneurysms as cause of the vascular occlusion [14], vitreous hemorrhage, recent operation, active retinopathy diabetic stage II to III. A local lysis can also be performed over several hours through an indwelling catheter. Different approaches are recommended by various authors, whereby the trend is towards shorter lysis times (e.g. 30,000 IU streptokinase/h, lysis time up to 3 hr, or 100,000 IU urokinase/hr, lysis time up to 3 hr or 2.5 mg rtPA/hr, lysis time up to 3 hr or 5,000 – 10,000 IU streptokinase/hr, lysis time up to 72 hr or 20,000 – 50,000 IU urokinase/hr or 1 – 2 mg rtPA/hr, lysis time up to 48 hr, heparin must always be applied parallel to urokinase or rtPA: 500 – 1000 IU heparin/hr). The efficiency of the local lysis can be monitored on the basis of the increase in D-dimers or fibrin monomers. The success of the lysis treatment depends on the age, length, and genesis of the occlusion, the peripheral effluent system and the clinical stage (less successful treatment in stage IV than in II or III). Lysis results in arterial thrombosis are not as good in diabetics as in non-diabetics. To maintain the patent lumen, treatment with coumarin derivates or thrombocyte aggregation inhibitors should follow. Marcumar is supposed to be superior to treatment with acetylsalicylic acid in the first year after PTA.

The following describes the most important therapeutic measures in the individual stages.

Stage II

Active vascular exercise using the interval principle, with the objective of promoting collateral formation by means of reactive hyperemia is most recommended in stage II. Examples are walking or tiptoe or rolling exercises. If for example walking is chosen, the patient walks 2/3 of the pain-free distance, pauses briefly and repeats this several times. This exercise is then performed several times a day and the distance slowly increased. This then improves the circulation in the muscles; the efficacy of the exercise is better in the proximal vascular processes than in the distal vascular constrictions. Influences on the possible success of the walking are shown in tab. 2. The effect of the exercise (increase in distance of 80 – 150%) is supposed to be about the same as that with vasoactive substances (increase of the distance 50 – 200%) [3]. Walking is therefore the therapy of choice for improving walking distance [3].

The so-called vasodilators are no longer as important because of their tendency to lead to the so-called "steal effect". By means of dilatation of healthy arteries blood is taken from the atherosclerotically changed vascular sections. This leads to an increase in the skin circulation (good effect on "cold feet"), but the muscle flow is lowered or remains unchanged. The objective of vasodilators is the stimulation of the formation of collaterals and their extension. Primary coronary insufficiency must be excluded, because an increase in heart minute volume is necessary to supply the collaterals. In cases of severe circulatory disorders,

Tab. 2: Prognostic factors in the framework of walking exercise (Bollinger) [14]

Favorable	Unfavorable
– Short history (< 1 year)	– Long history
– One-sided occlusion	– Double occlusions
– Femoral occlusion	– Pelvis and multi-stage occlusions
– Good hemodynamic parameters (stage II)	– Poor hemodynamic parameters (late stage II, stage III)
– Intact locomotor system	– Diseased locomotor system (spinal disease, arthritis)
– Normal cardiac and pulmonary function	– Cardiopulmonary insufficiency
– Positive motivation	– Lack of motivation

however, the capillaries in the periphery are already extended, and vasodilators do not have any effect in this stage.

A positive effect in circulatory disorders in stage II (significant increase of the pain-free distance with pentoxiphyllin vs. placebo) could be shown for pentoxiphyllin (intravenous and oral application) [17]. With this medication there is general improvement of the circulation of the extremities. The circulation of the previously poorly supplied extremities increases, because pentoxiphyllin is suspected to have hemorheologic effects and only acts as a weak vasodilator (improvement of the erythrocyte and leucocyte flexibility [14]). A corresponding increase of the pain-free distance has also been obtained with naftidrofuryl [12] and buflomedil (compared to placebo, i.v. and oral) [2]. Naftidrofuryl has a blood viscosity reducing effect by means of maintaining the flexibility of the individual erythrocytes. Other authors have reported a reduction of the oxygen consumption under stress by means of optimization of the cell metabolism by naftidrofuryl and buflomedil [14] (see tab. 3 for an overview of the preparations).

Better results were attained in a double-blind study with the combination of exercise treatment and pentoxiphyllin than with walking alone [11]. The use of vasoactive substances alone is indicated if exercise treatment is not possible due to concomitant illness (e.g. severe arthritis) [3]. In a comparison of the efficacy of a five-week hemodilution versus pentoxiphyllin treatment in 20 patients with arterial peripheral disease, the maximum distance improved significantly more following hemodilution. The pre- and post-stenotic blood flow rate increased significantly only in the hemodilution group, whereby the decrease in the hematocrit is viewed as the decisive hemorheologic change [21].

In general one is reserved about vascular-reconstructive measures in stage II. If a PTA is possible, this should be performed at the proper time. Only in the case of very difficult to treat disease, of short duration, should the surgical option be considered.

Tab. 3: Overview of vasoactive medications (Müller-Bühl, Diehm) selection [14]

Substance oral	Tradename	Average daily dosage
Pentoxifyllin		600 – 1200 mg
100/400/600 mg	Trental	
400 mg	Claudicat ret.	
Naftidrofuryl		300 mg
100 mg	Dusodril	
Buflomedil		450 – 600 mg
150 mg	Bufedil	
300 mg	– forte	
600 mg	– long	
150/300 mg	Defluina peri 150/300 mg	

For intravenous administration

Pentoxifyllin Amp.	Trental	1 amp. 100 mg 1 inf. amp. 300 mg
	Rentylin	1 amp. 100/300 mg
	Claudicat	1 amp. 100/300 mg
Naftidrofuryl	Dusodril	1 amp. 40 mg
	– Pi (infusion)	1 amp. 200 mg
Buflomedil	Bufedil	1 amp. 50 mg
	Defluina peri injection solution	1 amp. 50 mg

Acetylsalicylic acid is said to significantly slow the progression of atherosclerosis in the femoropopliteal region [10], which is interesting in view of the findings of Breddin et. al, that in diabetic men the thrombocyte aggregation is spontaneously increased [5]. Acetylsalicylic acid is therefore indicated in the course of secondary prevention of atherosclerosis in stage II (dosage 30 – 300 mg/die) [3]. If there are multiple peripheral occlusions or stenoses at strategically important places, or longer, diffuse stenoses, which can not be corrected with an operation or PTA, this is a relative indication for anticoagulation [10]. Anticoagulants are also indicated by the presence of a dilated angiopathy with emboli sources which can not be removed. Thrombocyte aggregation inhibitors act in particular, on those processes on the arterial wall (plaque formation), anticoagulants on thrombosis complications in the area of the stenosis or aneurysm [3].

Stage III

Exercise treatment is contraindicated in stage III [10, 14], because the circulation is already critically low at rest. Patients must be immobilized until the circulatory situation has improved, legs should be slightly lowered, kept warm by means of loose cotton bandages and protected from pressure necroses. The possibilities of an operative vascular reconstruction or PTA or local or systemic lysis therapy should be considered first. If an operation, PTA or lysis therapy is not possible or the patient refuses to undergo these procedures, treatment with prostaglandin E1 (prostavasin) can be initiated. Prostaglandin E1 is licensed in Germany for the treatment of peripheral arterial disease in stage III and IV [3, 10]. Its efficacy has been proven in studies of both intraarterial and intravenous administration [1, 13] and is supposed to be equally good for diabetics as non-diabetics [1]. Possible side effects are nausea, malaise, headache, decreased blood pressure, tachycardia, angina, confused state, seizures, allergic reactions, and isolated cases of pulmonary edema or congestive heart failure. Pain, reddening, swelling and sensation of warmth may occur in the extremity infused following intraarterial administration. Coronary insufficiency, cardiac arrhythmia, IHD, myocardial infarction within the last 6 months, pneumonia, severe obstructive pulmonary disorders, hemorrhaging, and severe hepatic diseases are contraindications.

Prostaglandins are supposed to have a potent vasodilatory effect on the vascular musculature. In patients with critical extremity ischemia there is extreme dilatation of the collateral arteries [18]. Furthermore, they inhibit thrombocyte and erythrocyte aggregation and improve the rheological properties of the blood [13]. The walking distance can be significantly improved and rest pain significantly influenced by prostavasin in patients with intermittent claudication and very limited walking distances [6]. In addition, acral lesions heal better and the analgesic needs are reduced [14, 13]. However, new recommendations from the Drug Commission of the German Federal Health Authorities have been made on the basis of reports about the severe side effects in those with previous myocardial damage or elderly patients, especially following intravenous application, for the inclusion of these recommendations in the contraindications for prostavasin. Prostavasin should, according to these recommendations, only be administered by a physician experienced in angiography and under constant cardiovascular monitoring. If there is a tendency towards heart failure, or IHD is present, the treatment should only be performed under hospitalized conditions. The indication for prostavasin therapy should be subjected to a very strict risk-benefit analysis.

A comparison of prostaglandin and adenosine triphosphate in stage III and IV (1 x daily i. a. application over 3–4 weeks) demonstrates significantly better results with respect to reduction of rest pain, decrease of analgesic use, ulcer healing, and amputation rate for prostavasin [4, 22].

Other therapeutic measures aim to improve the blood flow properties, e.g. by increasing the erythrocyte flexibility (pentoxiphyllin oral or as infusion). In a study, in which diabetics were also included, in patients in whom an operation was not indicated or the previous therapy was insufficient, an improved healing of ulcers, an easing of pain, an increase in the pain-free walking distance and thereby the regression of the clinical stages III and IV before therapy was shown with pentoxiphyllin; only the blood viscosity was not significantly improved [20]. Following i.v. administration of prostavasin or pentoxiphyllin in a multi-center study (hospital treatment of patients in stage IV for 4 weeks), better results were observed following prostavasin with respect to healing of necrosis, analgesia consumption and long-term results [23]. It is also possible to use naftidrofuryl in the treatment of severe forms of ischemia [7]. Pure vasodilators are contraindicated in these stages.

Another therapeutic approach consists of the reduction of the whole blood viscosity (isovolemic hemodilution with low-molecular dextrans, e.g. phlebotomy and simultaneous administration of hydroxyethyl starch with the objective of reducing the hematocrit value < 0.40, with IHD to 0.40 – 0.42) [10]. A hemodilution treatment is effective in patients with initial hematocrit values > 40% (contraindications: coronary insufficiency, renal insufficiency, anemia). The increase of thrombocytes following phlebotomy is compensated by the administration of thrombocyte aggregation inhibitors. Hemodilution treatment is indicated in stage III and IV, and in patients in stage II with short walking distance and inoperability. A hypervolemic hemodilution, i. e. only infusion of low molecular dextrans without preceding phlebotomy, is difficult due to the cardiovascular strain, but should possibly be considered with hematocrits < 40%.

The administration of acetylsalicylic acid or anticoagulants is also necessary in these stages.

Acupuncture treatment of the extremity, intraarterial oxygen insufflation and subcutaneous oxygen injection are obsolete measures, which could cause worsening of arterial circulatory disorders or even amputation of the extremity.

The primary objective remains avoiding amputation, which is only indicated with the danger of a toxic circulatory failure or uncontrollable sepsis in stage IV.

In general it should be noted that drug therapy only has limited efficacy in regions where the circulation is severely disturbed. This is due to the fact that the possibilities for compensation have, for the most part, been exhausted and the capillaries in the disturbed skin regions to some extent are no longer supplied with blood.

Laser angioplasty and rotation angioplasty are new developments in the field of vascular reconstruction in the treatment of peripheral circulatory disorders. There are, however, no studies available on the superiority of these methods to PTA.

Stage IV

If all of the prophylactic and therapeutic measures for the previous stages fail, the occurrence of gangrene is always associated with acute danger for the extremity. This deleterious complication can develop from any ischaemic disease of the lower extremities. The angiopathic diabetic foot always presents a diverse clinical dilemma. Because of the combined peripheral and sensory deficits of diabetic polyneuropathy, the symptoms of pain associated with necrosis, or the earlier signs of intermittent claudication may be lacking. There are also forms of diabetic angiopathies both without and with only slight inhibition of the sense of pain.

There are therefore two forms of angiopathic diabetic foot (for differential diagnosis see sec. 9.1.2).

1. *Ischaemic gangrenous foot without neuropathy*: The presence of this is determined by the decrease of the perfusion pressure in the arteria tibialis posterior. Pressures below 50 mmHg lead to such trophic disorders that necrosis or wounds from operations cannot heal.
2. *The ischaemic gangrenous foot with peripheral diabetic polyneuropathy* shows a pronounced weakening of the resistance to infection, which is connected with a particularly high risk of amputation.

Compared to the purely neuropathic foot, the existence of acral necrosis in the angiopathic foot is the result of circulation-based trophic disorders. In general these are then cause of a reduced load capacity in the foot. The necrosis of tissue can follow a number of paths:

1. The acute ischaemic foot with occlusion of the arteries (obliteration, embolism, thrombosis) is represented in only a relatively small percentage of the disease.
2. Advanced necroses may result from a trophic skin damage and develop through many different kinds of microinjuries (rhagades, improper foot care, injuries of any kind).
3. All forms of mycosis pedis are frequently entry points of infection in diabetics.
4. The degree of the circulatory disorder dictates the outcome, i. e. if and how quickly the body's own defenses can stop the process. The progression of the necrosis is determined by the degree of the inflammation. Microthrombi in the region of the small vessels fuel or promote this vicious circle.
5. The existence of such a gangrene is possible in every stage of the arterial occlusive disease (I-III) depending on the extent of the injury and the current accompanying circumstances (permanent stress, bacterial flora).

Frequent locations of gangrene:

- individual toes
- metatarsophalangeal joint of the first and fifth toe. Here there is a slight soft-tissue cover. The process quickly reaches the synovium and the bradytrophic

connective tissue. From here, the infection spreads distally and into the middle foot region.
- Calluses and fissures on the heel
- Mycotic nail beds and mycosis in the regions between the toes.

The ischaemic gangrenous diabetic foot is an instance of *acute emergency* and requires an interdisciplinary, therapeutic approach. Every necrosis and inflammation in the foot should be cause to immediately consult an experienced diabetologist. The therapeutic efforts are, in the end, determined by the vascular situation. It is not possible to obtain the same convincing therapeutic successes as is the case with the purely neuropathic foot. In addition, the affected patients frequently have severe vascular changes, with the corresponding clinical symptoms, in other regions of the body (heart, brain). A clearly increased frequency of amputation with greater post-operative risk can be observed in these polymorbid patients.

Therapeutic measures

Hospitalization of the patient in an internal medicine ward, specializing in diabetes, that has angiologic, angiographic, interventional-radiology, surgical and vascular-surgery capacities.

General measures for stabilization of the local findings: In many cases systemically applied antibiotics help to hinder the toxic spread of infection and therefore the number of emergency operations. Further drug measures are: total heparinization, hemodilution (target: hematocrit < 0.42), treatment of lipid metabolism imbalances and above all, an optimal control of diabetes with insulin.

Initial local treatment: dry gangrene: no manipulation, wait for clear demarcation, only with suspicion of blocked secretion is incision indicated, absolute immobilization is not necessary. Slightly hanging position of the leg is advantageous.

Moist gangrene: irigate, debride, release pus, elevate extremity slightly. Absolute immobilization required.

Immediate clarification of the vascular situation with all available means (clinical examination, sonography, angiography, DSA) so as to determine the possibilities for reperfusion (fibrinolysis, embolectomy, PTA and related methods, vascular-surgical reconstruction, bypass). The vascular reconstruction is the causal therapy, only thereafter are more advanced steps indicated.

Conservative treatment: If there is no possibility of vascular reconstruction, the initial treatment may be continued in an attempt to stop the necrotic process and heal the wound. While it is not very promising, this procedure has indeed helped some diabetics to retain their leg. Although their efficacy is a subject of some controversy, vasoactive substances may be used.

Local wound treatment: Wounds which are to be principally viewed as infected, require intensive treatment. Systemic antibiotic treatment must be adapted to the findings of the wound smear. Surface necrosis must be carefully removed. If possible the complete demarcation of the necrosis should first be clarified. It is not unusual that the necrotic process is forced deeper as a result of manipulation in the diseased tissue.

Basic principle: Dry treatment of dry wounds – moist treatment of moist wounds.

Irrigation with isotonic sodium chloride solution is applicable as long as there is a florid inflammation. Only in exceptional cases should these have antiseptic or antibiotic additives. The irrigation of the deeper regions of the wound should be conducted with the aid of catheters. The use of 3% hydrogen peroxide can be recommended for the general antisepsis and cleansing of the wound surface. A final rinse with isotonic sodium chloride solution is, however, necessary in such procedures. We have had good experiences with the use of cellulose containing powders (for instance Deshisan®) for drying the floor of the wound. The wounds, which generally heal relatively slowly, are to be regularly debrided. Proteolytic salves should only be used when it can be assured that deeper connective tissue will not be partly digested by them. The edges of the wounds should be regularly freshened, fibrin coating should be removed. The granulation tissue should be protected from drying out with grease tulle (Oleotüll®), excessive granulation etched away with a silver nitrate stick. The vulnerable edges of wounds should be covered with zinc oil (with nystatin additive, where necessary). The use of silver nitrate represents a possibility for long-term antisepsis of the granulation zones. Exposed bone areas are to be removed to below the level of the wound. Skin transplantation should be viewed critically, because, particularly in the plantar region the secondary scar tissue is generally better able to bear weight than the transplanted material. The treatment of acral lesions always includes the prophylactic treatment of both feet (mycosis, callous removal, bone oil). Physiotherapeutic treatment such as galvanic current, physical exercise and, depending on the local findings, walking, support the treatment.

Amputation: If the demarcation includes bone and tendon, an amputation must be performed. Following successful vascular reconstruction, a border zone amputation is generally sufficient. Bone, and above all tendon, are to be cut back to the depth of the wound. The question of closing the wound is to be decided critically. Primary sutures should be avoided in cases where there is still minimum circulation, because the perfusion pressure is not usually sufficient to ensure the circulation in the adaptation area. A secondary healing of the wound, although longer in duration, appears to be the more reasonable alternative. In addition, this method allows for a more simplified removal of demarcated diseased tissue which was left at the amputation.

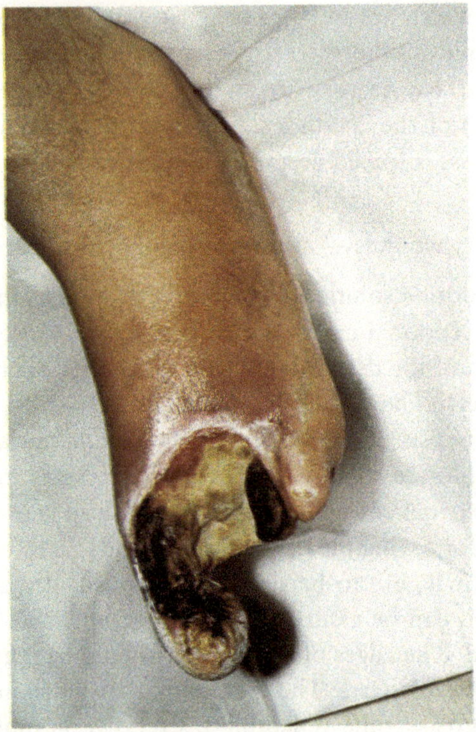

Fig. 4: Condition on admittance after the removal of the 2nd to 4th toes due to arterial occlusive disease of the thigh type in the a. femoralis superficialis. The necrosis is advanced.

Aids in determining the height of the amputation:

- *Spontaneous amputations* are generally possible. They are, however, more a thing of the past.
- *Border zone amputations* are indicated in all biologically younger patients following improvement of the circulation.
- *Transmetatarsal forefoot amputation* does not generally allow for primary wound closure and is generally only indicated when circulatory conditions are still satisfactory.
- *Operations in the region of the tarsal bones or amputation to the height of the lower ankle* (amputation according to Syme) are rare procedures. Stable scarring can be attained if open, non-functional surfaces of the joint are scraped back to the spongiosa.
- *Lower leg amputations are always better than amputations above the knee,* because the prosthetic care for them is better. The formation of longer back flaps of skin and a good primary wound closing are important for lower leg amputations. Here, too, the knowledge of the circulatory conditions below

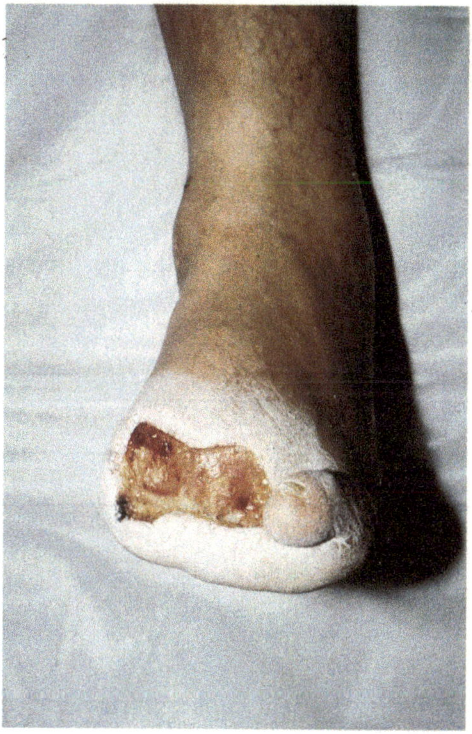

Fig. 5: Condition after border zone amputation after previous performance of a femoro-popliteal vessel bypass. In their further development, the results could be brought to full healing.

the knee are very important for the surgeon. Tight sutures should not be used with poor circulation.

- A higher amputation is always preferable in *elderly patients*, provided the circulation is good, because rehabilitation is quicker. Along with the lower leg and above the knee amputation the Baumgartner intraarticular amputation in the knee may also be practiced.

Prostheses: After lesions in the foot have healed, it is necessary to fit the patient with orthopedic shoes. The scarred area should be relieved of pressure and the foot given a soft bed. Of the more extensive operations the transmetatarsal forefoot operation causes the least amount of difficulty as far as shoes are concerned. The artificial foot, necessary following amputation in the ankle region, is difficult to fit. This calls for a relatively heavy load for the splints. Well-formed, developed and strong stockings are a prerequisite for complication-free prothesis following lower leg or above the knee amputations.

Secondary prevention: At this point it appears extremely important to point out measures which combat a renewed deterioration of the circulation:

- optimal diabetic control
- treatment of a possible lipid metabolic disorder
- use of platelet aggregation inhibitors, depending on the degree of retinopathy coumarin derivates
- no smoking
- vascular exercise
- consultation of specialists, even better a specialized team.

Table 4 gives an overview of the therapeutic principles in the specific stages of Fontaine.

Tab. 4: Overview of the most important therapeutic principles in the various Fontaine stages

Basic therapy					Revascularization			
Fontaine stage	1	2	3	4	5	6	7	8
I	××	(×)	–	–	–	–	–	–
IIa	×	(×)	(×)	×	(×)	–	–	–
IIb	×	××	××	××	××	×	(×)	×
III	(×)	×	××	–	×	××	×	×
IVa	(×)	×	×	–	×	×	××	×
IVb	(×)	(×)	×	–	(×)	–	××	–

1 Combat risk factors
2 Antithrombotic therapy
3 Vasoactive medication
4 Ergotherapy
5 Non-surgical therapy: PTA
6 Non-surgical therapy: lysis therapy
7 Surgical therapy
8 Other (hemodilution)

Expression of thanks

We would like to thank Prof. Dr. K. Köhler, Director of the Radiologic Clinic of the Dresden Medical Academy for the x-rays.

9.1.1.5 *Summary*

Atherosclerotic vascular diseases are the most frequent and important complications for the type II diabetic. Beside the macroangiopathy, the microangiopathy is specific for the diabetic. Peripheral arterial occlusive disease in the diabetic does not principally differ from that of the non-diabetic. It does however, occur more diffusely in the diabetic, is often more pronounced and tends to progress more quickly. As a result of the possible additional neuropathy, the clinical complaints may be reduced.

Diagnostically, the detailed clinical examination yielded by Doppler sonography and the anticipated consequences of angiography stand out in the foreground. Basic therapeutic principles are the best for possible normoglycemic metabolic control and the treatment of other existing risk factors. Active vascular exercise is emphasized in Fontaine stage II, accompanied by particularly rheologically-effective substances such as pentoxiphyllin or naftidrofuryl. Shorter walking distance should be considered an indication for surgery or PTA. If stage III is already present immobilization of the extremity is required to inhibit necrosis. The possibilities of operative vascular reconstruction or a PTA or lysis therapy should be exhausted. If these types of treatment are not possible, prostaglandins can be used. In such cases the indication should be defined quite narrowly due to the potential severity of the side effects. Acetylsalicylic acid is indicated in both stages II and III or anticoagulants in the presence of multiple stenoses or occlusions or lesions at strategically important places. The principle therapeutic goal is regression from stage III to stage II or extension of the walking distance in intermittent claudication. The ultimate goal is to hinder necrosis or gangrene.

In stage IV, the treatment should always be initially performed in hospitals by an experienced team of physicians. The goal is, by means of the most conservative amputation possible and directed use of aid, to maintain the functional ability of the leg. Polypharmacy can not always be avoided in such cases. The five mainstays of therapy in this final stage are, to the extent possible, improvement in hemoperfusion by means of PTA or vascular reconstruction, improvement in perfusion through medication and optimization of the hematocrit, combat infection, optimize the metabolic state with insulin and debridement.

References

[1] Balzer, K., W. Rogatti, K. Rüttgerodt: Therapeutische Wirksamkeit von Prostaglandin E1 – intraarterielle und intravenöse PG E1 – Therapie bei AVK im Stadium III/IV. Therapiewoche *39* (1989) 2736–2742.

[2] Bisler, H.: Klinische Erfolge der Buflomediltherapie bei arterieller Verschlußkrankheit. Therapiewoche *33* (1983) 2204–2210.

[3] Bollinger, A.: Medikamentöse Therapie bei peripherer arterieller Verschlußkrankheit. Schweizer Med. Wochenschrift *118* (1988) 1283–1289.

[4] Böhme, H., M. Brülisaner, U. Härtel et al.: Periphere arterielle Verschlußkrankheit im Stadium III und IV – Kontrollierte Zwei-Zentren-Studie zur Wirksamkeit von intraarterieller Prostaglandin E1-Infusion. Med. Welt *40* (1989) 1501–1503.

[5] Breddin, H. K., H. J. Krzywanek, P. Althoff et al.: PARD: Platelet aggregation as a risk factor in diabetics; results of a prospective study. Horm. Metabol. Res. (suppl. 15) (1985) 63–68.

[6] Diehm, C.: Intravenöse Prostaglandin E1-Therapie bei Patienten mit peripherer arterieller Verschlußkrankheit (AVK) im Stadium III – eine doppelblinde placebokontrollierte Studie. In: H. Heidrich, H. Böhme, W. Rogatti (Hrsg.): Prostaglandin E1-Wirkungen und therapeutische Wirksamkeit, 133–143. Springer Verlag, Berlin 1988.

[7] Greenhalgh, R. M.: Naftidrofuryl for ischemic rest pain: A controlled trial. Brit. J. Surg. *68* (1981) 265–266.

[8] Haffner, S. M.: Prediction of NIDDM by body fat distribution and hyperinsulinemia. In: E. Standl (ed.): Perspectives of the Hyperinsulinemia/Insulin Resistance Syndrome in NIDDM, MMV Medizin Verlag, München 1990.

[9] Janka, H. U., P. Grünwald, G. Waldmann et al.: Karotisstenosen, Kardiovaskuläres Risikoprofil und assoziierte Makroangiopathie bei ambulanten Diabetikern: Die Schwabinger Studie zur Makroangiopathie bei Diabetikern. Vasa *11* (1982) 111–116.

[10] Kappert, A.: Lehrbuch und Atlas der Angiologie. Verlag Hans Huber. Bern, Stuttgart, Toronto 1989.

[11] Kiesewetter, H., J. Blume, F. Jung et al.: Gehtraining und medikamentöse Therapie bei der peripheren arteriellen Verschlußkrankheit. Dtsch. Med. Wschr. *112* (1987) 873–878.

[12] Maass, U., H. G. Amberger, H. Böhme et al.: Naftidrofuryl bei arterieller Verschlußkrankheit. Kontrollierte mutizentrische Doppelblindstudie mit oraler Applikation. Deutsch. Med. Wschr. *109* (1984) 745–750.

[13] Mörl, H., E. Rogge, E. Schollmayer: Die Bedeutung von Prostaglandin E21 in der Behandlung der AVK. Herz und Gefäße *12* (1992) 71–79.

[14] Müller-Bühl, U., C. Diehm: Angiologie. Verlag W. Kohlhammer, Stuttgart, Berlin, Köln 1991.

[15] Pirart, J.: Diabète et complications dégénératives. Presentation d'une étude prospective portant sur 4400 cas observés entre 1947–1973. Diabete Metab. *3* (1977) 97–107.

[16] Prevalence of small vessel and large vessel disease in diabetic patients from 14 centers. The World Health Organisation Multinational Study of Vascular Disease in Diabetics. Diabetologia *28* (Suppl. 1) (1985) 615–640.

[17] Rudofsky, G., K. F. Haussler, H. P. Küntal et al.: Zur intravenösen Pentoxifyllin-Behandlung der chronischen peripheren arteriellen Verschlußkrankheit. Med. Welt *39* (1988) 1136–1140.

[18] Scheffler, P., D. de la Hamette, G. Leipnitz: Therapeutic efficacy of intravenously applied prostaglandin E1. Vasa *28* (Suppl.) (1989) 19–25.

[19] Standl, E., H. U. Janka: Der diabetische Fuß. In: H. Mehnert, K. Schöffling (Hrsg.): Diabetologie in Klinik und Praxis, 2. Aufl., 513–528. Thieme, Stuttgart 1984.

[20] Sternitzky, R., K. Seige: Clinical investigation of the effects of pentoxifylline in patients with severe peripheral occlusive vascular disease Curr Med Res Opin 1985 9 (9) 602–610.

[21] Triebe, G., U. Münnich, F. Liebold: Therapievergleich zwischen Hämodilution und Pentoxiphyllin bei arterieller Verschlußkrankheit. Dtsch. Med. Wschr. *117* (1992) 523–530.

[22] Trübestein, G., M. Ludwig, C. Diehm et al.: Prostaglandin E1 bei arterieller Verschlußkrankheit im Stadium III und IV – Ergebnisse einer multizentrischen Studie. Dtsch. Med. Wschr. *112* (1987) 955–959.

[23] Trübestein, G., S. von Bary, K. Breddin et al.: Intravenous prostaglandin E1 versus pentoxiphylline therapy in chronic arterial occlusive disease – a controlled randomised multicenter study. Vasa *28* (Suppl.) (1989) 44–49.

9.1.2 *The neuropathic diabetic foot*

H. Rietzsch

9.1.2.1 *Epidemiology*

Diabetic foot complications can be of fatal importance for the patient. Beside the consequences of arterial occlusive disease, at least two-thirds of the cases are the result of neuropathy [1] or at least to a considerable degree. The neuropathic diabetic foot is characterized by the innervation disturbance of the skin, integumentary appendage, vascular and skeletal musculature, as well as impairment of the sensory nerve functions. An infection through a skin lesion can lead to an explosive exacerbation of the disease with organ-threatening necrosis [7]. The number of amputations in diabetic patients is therefore considerably higher than that of the overall population [4].

Tab. 1: Amputations of the lower extremities (toes, feet, lower leg, above the knee) per 10,000 persons in the USA between 1976 and 1978 [1]

Age (years)	Patients with Diabetes mellitus	Patients without Diabetes mellitus
0–44	14.1	0.5
45–64	45.0	1.9
>64	101.4	9.9
Total	59.7	2.0

The patient population with diabetic foot complications is often equated with those with circulatory leg complications and an amputation is performed too quickly and too extensively. In the Declaration of Saint Vincent, a reduction of the amputation rate of 50% was set as the goal. This goal aims on the one hand at the proper indication of this form of therapy and on the other hand a more exhaustive use of prophylactic therapy. The diabetic foot, as a frequent and serious complication of diabetes mellitus, causes at least 20% of the overall treatment costs of the already expensive therapy of this chronic disease. It is not unusual that symptoms of a diabetic foot complication lead to the diagnosis of a type II Diabetes mellitus which has remained unknown and uncompensated for a long time. Beside the neuropathy, there are frequently also diabetes-related changes in the cardiovascular system, in type II diabetics less frequently in the eyes and kidneys. At this point it should be mentioned that the current state of care for diabetics, with respect to foot complications, is very much in need of improvement in all of Germany. Hardly more than 10% of diabetics have their feet examined on a regular basis, let alone are given a reasonable prophylactic treatment. The training of the diabetic and the physician are an important part of overcoming this problem.

9.1.2.2 *Pathological anatomy and pathophysiology*

Long before necroses develop, pathological changes begin to take place on the diabetic-neuropathic foot. The trophic foot edema can be viewed as a consequence of the autonomous innervation disorder with impairment of the microcirculation. A hyperfusion can be observed. The discrepancy of good circulation of the neuropathic foot to the trophic disorders has to be seen in the increased shunt blood with reduced exploitation of oxygen. This condition takes on particular importance in the nutritive supply of the bone. The occurrence of osteolysis is often followed by osteomyelitis with extensive abscesses of soft tissue and sepsis. The mechanical load capacity of the skeleton of the foot is considerably reduced by the changes in the bones, there are foot deformities, pathological fractures, collapse of the plantar arch in the sense of a Charcotic foot. It is noticeable in clinical practice that especially those patients are affected by these complications, in whom the diabetic-neuropathic genesis indicates a possible alcohol-related damage to the nervous system (Bureau-Barrière Syndrome I). The innervation of the sweat and sebaceous glands of the skin of the feet is relatively disturbed. This results in a reduced load capacity for the sin. The skin is noticeably dryer and broken, with a tendency to hyperkeratosis. These changes form the basis for the occurrence of calluses and fissures, a possible site of entry for infection. It is not unusual that hyperkeratosis take on extreme dimensions, so that they act like a foreign body and lead to pressure necrosis on the sections of tissue below them. The consequences are hematoma, which ulcerate outwards and become infected. This can lead to a classical neurotrophic ulcer. This occurs in the main weight bearing areas of the foot – the heads of metatarsals I and V and the heel. Foreign bodies and irregularities in shoes or tight shoes (fashionable shoes) have a comparable pathogenetic effect. Injuries which occur as a result of improper foot care can also result in the formation of an ulcer. The peripheral, sensory symmetric polyneuropathy, which blocks pain transmission and the biologically reasonable reaction to inflammatory pain, is the basis for the appearance and chronicity of the ulcer. This can be the only explanation as to why patients with greasy and wet foot ulcers go on for years after quickly having lost interest in treatment, which of course only supports the lack of interest in foot complications in diabetes mellitus.

Other localizations of pressure ulcers are to be expected in the presence of a motor and sensory, peripheral symmetric diabetic polyneuropathy. The motor components of the neuropathy lead to muscle atrophy and the preferred impairment of the adductors. As a result, calluses due to pressure and rubbing ulcers can be found on the dorsal skin areas of joints.

Diabetic gangrene is not a nosological unit. Chantelau [1] makes a very practice-related distinction:

1. Neuropathically infected foot
2. Ischaemic-gangrenous foot with peripheral, arterial occlusive disease
3. Foot with peripheral neuropathy and arterial occlusive disease.

9.1.2.3 Clinical findings and diagnosis

The diagnostic objectives in diabetic foot syndrome are:

Early detection of predisposing foot symptoms

- Inspection of the foot
  Skin condition, edemas, swellings, erythema, mycotic infections, condition of toenails, horny skin, corns, decubitus ulcers
  Inspection of the shoes is mandatory!
- Neurological examination
  Tuning fork test, warmth discrimination, reflexes, motor and sensory velocity of nerve conduction
- Architecture of the foot
  Rigidity of the basic joint of the big toe, arch of the foot, if necessary, additional orthopedic consultation
- X-ray diagnosis
  Early detection of osteolysis, changes in joints, manifestation of gout
- Angiological examination
  Doppler sonography, vein occlusion plethysmography, cruro-brachial index, angiography
- Pedography
  Pressure distribution and uptake in the sole of the foot [3, 4]
- Gait pattern
- Bone scintigram
  Proof that bone is affected with ambiguous x-ray findings, for purposes of follow up

Examinations in cases of necrosis, ulcer, general signs of infection

- Inspection
  Spread of necrosis (skin, connective tissue, tendons, bones)
- Microbiological diagnosis
  Wound smear, blood culture
- Neurological and angiological examination

- X-ray diagnosis
- Bone scintigram
  Proof that bone is affected with ambiguous x-ray findings, for purposes of follow up

A precise classification of the foot lesions is absolutely necessary to plan the therapy. Table 2 shows the differential diagnosis procedure.

Tab. 2: Differential diagnosis in the diabetic foot

	Neuropathy	Angiopathy
History:	Long-term diabetes mellitus + nephropathy + retinopathy + indication for decompensation HbA_{1c} ↑↑	Additional risk factors + disorder of lipid metabolism + chronic ischaemic heart disease + nicotine abuse + intermittent claudication
Location:	Plantar rarely dorsal, decubitus necrosis and calluses	Acral toe, foot
Sensitivity: (Tuning fork test)	Reduced, often lacking	
Pain:	Little to none	Present
Inspection:	Foot warm, pink, dry, smooth contours, voluminous foot	Foot cold, pale, atrophic dermis and subdermis
Foot pulses:	Present (sometimes difficult to detect with edema)	Lacking
X-ray:	Early osteolysis	Unremarkable bone structure often even in necrotic area

Symptoms of both kinds can be found in feet with peripheral neuropathy and arterial occlusive disease. The classic neuropathic ulcer (fig 1.) is characterized by the following findings in typical locations:

- Hyperkeratotic edge
- Torpid ulcer floor, sometimes deep, smeary
- Necrosis limited to area of ulcer
- Stationary findings often for longer periods of time
- Do not tend to heal with continued use of foot
- Uncomplicated bacterial flora and blastomyces

The complications connected with such findings (figs. 2 and 3) are:

- Connective tissue and plantar aponeurosis affected with pronounced phlegmon and quickly spreading necrosis
- Spread to articular capsules

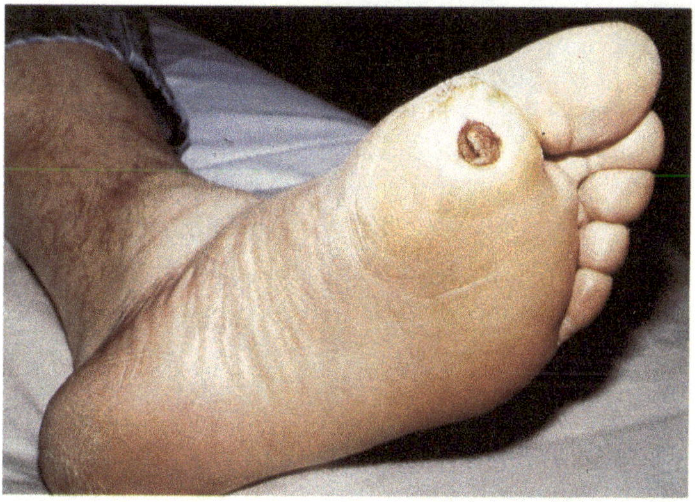

Fig. 1: Neurotrophic ulcer at a typical location. The patient has been a diabetic for 13 years. The local findings have existed for over one year. The involvement of the joint cavity is well-recognizable. Osteolysis could not be proven. The condition healed within 6 weeks.

- Osteomyelitis with sequestering, most often in the region of the toes and the middle foot (not a necessity)
- Infection rises along synovial sheath
- Fever, sepsis
- Problem bacteria: staphylococcus, pseudomonas aeruginosa, proteus mirabilis, klebsiella, e. coli, enterococcus. *Gaseous gangrene* should be considered in any case.
- Check *tetanus* immunization and update, if necessary.

9.1.2.4 Therapy

Prevention is, of course, the best medicine here, too. The diabetic, as a chronic patient, requires intensive care with the aim of optimal metabolic control. This means that all of the instructions which are appropriate for the treatment of diabetic polyneuropathy also hold true. Because diabetic polyneuropathy in advanced stages exhibits irreversible late complications, the treatment of the foot must be directed against the appearance of necroses or the beginning of such relapses. The following should be emphasized in this respect:

Education of the patients

During each diabetic training program the problem of foot complications should be given the greatest attention:

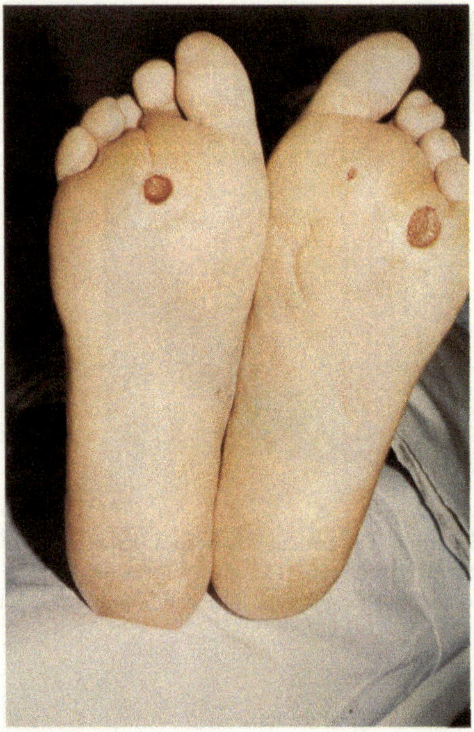

Fig. 2: Local findings of a patient with severe destructive osteomyelitis on both feet. They present the classic picture of malum perforans. The remaining medial ulcer on the left leg quickly healed after the resection of the metatarsophalangeal joints according to Cleyton. The poorly-healing lateral ulcer lies in the region of an unfavorable plantar OP scar.

- Daily inspection of the foot
- Nail care, if necessary with support from the physician
- Calluses
  - Remove cause (shoes, pressure sores)
  - Removal with pumice following footbath possible
- No cutting instruments for foot care
- Lukewarm footbaths only, use thermometer
- Grease skin after footbath
- Cotton socks without folds or darns
- Beware of mycotic infections, treatment mandatory, careful in pools!
- No bare feet, even at home
- No local, additional warmth
- Special foot exercises and sufficient movement is very important.

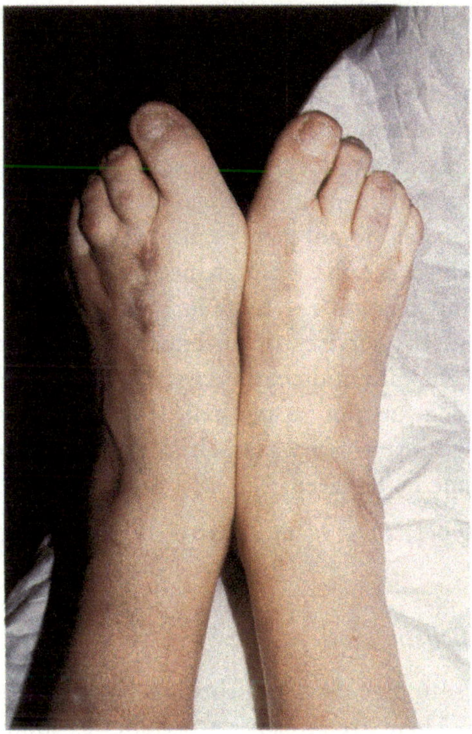

Fig. 3: View of the same patient. The beginning foot deformation (Charcot) is clearly recognizable. As a rule, dorsal incisions heal without complications.

Shoes

Orthopedic shoes are not generally necessary for minimal changes. The patient should wear soft shoes, which are not tight, do not rub or put pressure on the feet. These shoes may also be combined with a soft insert.

Principle: The shoe must be fitted to the foot, not the other way around!

Unfortunately, many patients still wear completely inappropriate shoes, even with severe foot complications. Holes in the sole, sometimes hard, poorly fitting inserts, which have been passed from shoe to shoe can be found. Occasionally, foreign bodies which have fallen into the shoe or nails sticking up out of the sole have to be removed. Such conditions can be responsible for more or less sudden appearance of necrosis.

In any case, the decision to prescribe orthopedic shoes must be made on a case-to-case basis. Transferring the patient to a specialist may be helpful. Some institutions use pedographs which graphically illustrate the distribution of pressure on the sole of the foot. Pressure of more than 50 N/cm^2 is considered to be a threat for decubitus ulcers. Orthopedic shoes are indicated in such situations. This is of course also true for patients in whom necroses have healed or where amputations have been performed.

The orthopedic shoe for the diabetic foot must be suited to the specific situation, which is particularly important in the case of local findings, so as to prevent the recurrence of lesions. The first commandment in footwear is to avoid pressure sores. This means that shoes for diabetics do not have to meet the usual demands placed on orthopedic footwear, which are the maintenance and restoration of the functional units and the natural shape of the foot. In order to form a soft and pressure-free bed for the foot, the services of an experienced orthopedic shoemaker should be sought, as is the case in diabetic centers. These shoes have a consistently hard sole and a rolling function at the ball of the foot to relieve the metatarsophalangeal joints. The insert is always soft. It is subject to wear and tear and must from time to time be replaced.

Ulcers can seldom be cured by shoes, to prevent relapses they are absolutely essential.

Specialized outpatient clinics for diabetic foot

It would be preferable if patients with diabetic foot problems could visit special outpatient clinics for consultation. There are already such clinics at some treatment centers. Studies by Hanfland and Paetow [2, 3, 5] have confirmed the effectiveness of such institutions. Care in the areas surrounding a special outpatient clinic resulted in a conservative, organ-maintenance treatment for 68% of the patient population admitted to hospitals, while the usual care of another hospital investigated resulted of a 49% amputation rate. In addition, there was a particularly high post-operative mortality rate and a very high percentage of above-the-knee amputations. In the treatment of the complicated diabetic foot, the experience of the personnel in the specialized care provided was important. An integrated, inpatient and outpatient treatment of the diabetic foot complications must be viewed as particularly favorable [3]. Particularities in the course of treatment and rehabilitation of each patient can be of interest for the stabilization and maintenance of the treatment success. Where specialized outpatient care is possible, the often long-term hospitalization can be shortened and therefore the overall costs of the treatment reduced. The high potential for relapse following the healing of skin lesions must be given particular attention. The treatment team of diabetologists and experienced orthopeds and orthopedic shoemakers allows for the uncomplicated continuous adaptation of the footwear in accordance with the not infrequent changes of the load capacity of the foot. The fact that the patient and general practitioner have the permanent possibility to obtain the specialized care necessary, without delay, is especially important. This allows severe deterioration and readmittance to the hospital to be reduced considerably, as has been demonstrated in our "Outpatient Clinic for the Diabetic Foot" which is associated with our diabetes ward.

Treatment of the neuropathic infected foot

1. Hospitalization is generally necessary. The patient should be admitted to a specialized clinic where the diabetologist and the orthopedic surgeons are accustomed to working together. The patient should be primarily admitted to a medical ward with an experienced diabetologist. The affected foot must be *completely immobilized*. Even a light load (as a compromise) before the wound is healed extends the course of the disease. Visits to the toilet should be included in such considerations.
2. Normoglycemic metabolic control with insulin:
   This generally requires an intensive conventional insulin therapy (ICT). Insulin pump treatment (CSII) may be necessary and helpful. The supportive neuropathy treatment with alpha-liponic acid has proven itself clinically. Other neuropathy-inducing habits such as alcohol consumption should be avoided.
3. Daily local treatment:
   - Antiseptic footbath
   - Debridement
   - Removal of calluses
   - Rinsing of wounds with NaCl 0.9%, hydrogen peroxide 3% only on the surface
   - Moisturizing of the wound with continuous rinsing or tulle gras, depending on the local findings
   - Bandages must be changed several times per day when necessary
4. Antibiotic therapy
   - Systemic antibiotics following the antibiogram (wound smear from the deeper region of the wound) penicillin/cephalosporin + clindamycin + aminoglycoside
   - Long-term treatment with clindamycin with bone lesion (x-ray/scintigram) for several months. If clindamycin is not tolerated gastrointestinally, other antibiotics effective on gram-positive bacteria (lincomycin, teicoplanin) can be considered as alternatives
   - Local antibiotics are to some extent controversial. Gentamycin chains (Septopal®) and antiseptic gauze (Sofratüll®) generally offer good results
5. Antimycotic therapy:
   Sol. Castellani SR is convincing for the treatment of skin mycoses. Beyond that nystatin zinc oil can be used. Nail mycoses should also be treated. The use of ungt. Kal. iodati 35% SR has proven effective.

6. Skin transplantation is generally not required.
7. Amputation and sequester removal:
   Amputation should be conducted as sparingly as possible. The neuropathic foot, with its intact blood supply has considerably better chances of healing than does the angiopathic foot. If an operation is necessary, it should be planned at the borderline after sufficient antibiotic treatment and demarcation. A severe, uncontrollable sepsis in the neurotrophic diabetic foot represents a rare exception, which can be seen as an indication for a more extensive amputation.
8. Skin care:
   Prevention and removal of horny skin, nail care and greasing of the skin with ol. ped. tauri are indicated.
9. Orthopedic footwear after healing of wound [6]:
   Provisional footwear can only serve as a compromise solution for long-term courses. The so-called "heel shoe" allows early mobilization and better treatment of the patient in cases of ulcers in the frontal region of the foot. Patients should not continue to wear the shoes that they have been wearing. If necessary a second pair of shoes or slippers should be worn.
10. General drug therapy (heparin, acetylsalicylic acid for prevention of thrombosis).

9.1.2.5 *Summary*

Besides retinopathy and nephropathy, the "diabetic foot" represents a severe late complication of diabetes. Unfortunately, this condition is far too often underestimated in clinical practice, as demonstrated by the large number of patients who are still not being treated appropriately. On the one hand, there is far too often the admission for surgery with the result being a hasty operation and amputations which are too extensive. On the other hand, there are the patients whose neuropathic ulcers are "treated" with salves and such for long periods of time without any healing.

The prevention of the diabetic foot syndrome is most important in acting against the early symptoms. Education and motivation of the patient are the main objectives in this regard. Specialized care of patients with diabetic feet in clinics can contribute greatly to managing the goal of the Declaration of Saint Vincent to reduce the amputation rate by 50%.

References

[1] Chantelau, E., M. Spraul, M. Schmid: Das Syndrom des diabetischen Fußes. Dtsch. med. Wschr. *114* (1989) 1034–1039.

[2] Hanfland, J.: Welchen Beitrag leistet eine Spezialambulanz bei der Behandlung von Patienten mit „diabetischem Fuß"? Med. Welt *38* (1987) 1405–1409.

[3] Kardorff, B.: Ergebnisse einer integrierten ambulanten und stationären internistischen Behandlung des „diabetischen Fußes“. Präv.-Rehab. 4 (1992) 1 – 8.
[4] Most, R., P. Sinnock: The epidemiology of lower extremity amputations in diabetic individuals. Diab. Care 6 (1983) 87.
[5] Paetow, P.: Operative und konservative Therapie des „diabetischen Fußes“ in einem Krankenhaus der Grundversorgung. Präv.-Rehab. *3* (1991) 112 – 118.
[6] Schaff, P. S., W. E. Siebert: Ulcusprophylaxe am diabetischen Fuß. Orthopädie-Schuhtechnik 6 (1988) 16 – 23.
[7] Standl, E., H. U. Janka: Der diabetische Fuß. In: H. Mehnert, K. Schöffling (Hrsg.): Diabetologie in Klinik und Praxis, 2. Aufl., 513 – 528. Thieme Verlag, Stuttgart, New York.

9.2 Diabetic polyneuropathy

H. Rietzsch

9.2.1 Introduction

Around 200 years ago, Rollo described diabetic polyneuropathy as a form of diabetes mellitus manifestation. Representing 30% of all polyneuropathies, it is today, along with alcohol-induced polyneuropathy, a very significant subgroup of this disease. There remains no doubt that the possibly life-threatening metabolic imbalances form the grounds for therapeutic measures in the treatment of diabetes mellitus. The consequences of a form of therapy, which only causes the disappearance of the immediate dangers of diabetes mellitus, seem, however, to decidedly favor diabetes-related nerve damage. In the daily clinical practice, neuropathy symptoms are often underestimated, diagnosed too late and can then only be unsatisfactorily therapeutically influenced. The enormous growth in understanding, especially in the past two decades, has enabled this long underestimated diabetes complication to move increasingly into the center of consideration. Through investigations of the morphology, metabolism and function of the affected nerves, it quickly became apparent that the classical, clinically-defined conception of polyneuropathy was no longer sufficient for the description of the disease picture. Thus, the lack of evidence of nerve lesions, for example as the result of measurements of the velocity of nerve conduction, does not exclude the possibility of a diabetic polyneuropathy. The understanding of the disease is being improved at this time, especially through new knowledge regarding "autonomic diabetic neuropathy". Disorders and symptoms which appear in relation to this are still often observed and investigated isolated from each other. Increasingly, however, the awareness has grown that the autonomic polyneuropathy precedes the peripheral and that, therefore, the development of irreversible damages ("the point of no return") can be prognosticated earlier. Taking these new data into account, the term "diabetic polyneuropathy" is a preferred term for describing diabetic nerve damage. The diagnosis of this diabetes complication thereby becomes more comprehensive. It presents a therapy-accompanying and therapy-determining factor in diabetes treatment. Recent investigations have given rise to the hypothesis that diabetic polyneuropathy may play a key role in the syndrome of diabetic late complications. It is to be expected that, in the future, sensitive methods for the early measurement of such disorders could serve in the evaluation of a successful diabetes treatment. The nerve metabolism disturbed by hyperglycemia is seen as the main cause of diabetic polyneuropathy. From this position emerges the therapy target of the achievement of normal glycemia for the prevention of diabetic late complications.

One must continually provide maximal attention to a patient with diabetic polyneuropathy. Subtle clinical investigation results and also discrete indications from the disease picture should always be interpreted from the standpoint that the patient is robbed of a large part of his/her self-awareness through the disease. The heart attack which occurs painlessly and is treated too late or the long-dismissed severe foot complication can all too often become serious blows in the course of the disease and in the life of the diabetic.

9.2.2 *Epidemiology and pathogenesis*

Diabetic polyneuropathy is categorized as a diabetic late complication. This statement gives the deceptive impression that an assumed latency of the clinical symptoms might justify a delay of systematic therapeutic intervention. Pirart [9] has shown that clinical symptoms of diabetic polyneuropathy could already be found at the time of diagnosis in 7.5% of the diabetics. The prevalence of polyneuropathy increased to 40% at 20 years and 50% at 25 years of living with diabetes. These figures substantiate that diabetic polyneuropathy already begins to develop at the onset of the diabetic disorder. According to Vinik (Ann Arbor 1987), the occurrence of a diabetic polyneuropathy can be reckoned with in 90% of all diabetics. The figures found in the literature vary between 10 and 100% [7]. The frequency of diabetic polyneuropathy is about equal in both IDDM and NIDDM. In type I diabetes, the first clinical symptoms of polyneuropathy become detectable at the earliest after one year, such as, for example, diminished sensitivity to vibration in the feet. [12]. This is different in type II diabetes, where metabolic disorders precede the clinical diagnosis by years and the symptoms of polyneuropathy are not infrequently apparent at the first examination, and where it is possible that the diabetes mellitus is discovered, for example, through a foot complication. Neuropathy occurs more frequently in elderly diabetics.

9.2.3 *Pathological anatomy*

Histological investigations of the nerves have shown segmented zones of the Schwann cells with de- and re-myelinization regions, finally with axon degenerations. In the case of neuropathological pain, the selective attack on the thin nerve fibers could be detected [2]. A reduction in the number of capillaries has been found to positively correlate with the severity of the neuropathy. In cases of local neuropathy, an atrophy of the muscle fibers can be detected, such as in "diabetic amyopathy". Pathological anatomical changes have been found in the nerve fibers of the autonomous nervous system up to the ganglia.

9.2.4 *Pathophysiology*

Several hypotheses are being discussed regarding the pathophysiology of the nerve damage, though none has yet been supported with final proof.

1. An increase in the breakdown of glucose to sorbitol by aldose reductase leads to a decrease in the concentration of free myoinositol, a 6-valent alcohol, upon which a disorder of the phospolipid-coat membrane and the Na-K-ATPase occurs. An energetic desufficiency in the nerve fibers is a consequence.
2. Much discussed is the hypoxia hypothesis, according to which a micro-angioorganopathy of the vasa nervorum results in an insufficient supply to the nerves. This idea would also coincide with the myoinositol metabolism hypothesis. The selective attack on the thin nerve fibers could be thus explained. In addition, the flow properties of the blood worsen with an unfavorable glycemic condition.
3. The disturbed axonal transport of neurotransmitters has been investigated.
4. The special significance of the non-enzymatic glycosylation of the nerve proteins is still not clear. It has been proven that poor glycemic control is an essential factor in the development of diabetic polyneuropathy. In untreated type II diabetes there is a correlation between the disturbance of the velocity of nerve conduction and the HbA_1 level [10]. Nocturnal neuropathy pains can be successfully treated through the normalization of the blood glucose by means of an insulin pump. As well, the manifestation of the autonomic diabetic polyneuropathy is equally frequent in type I and type II diabetics, which is also seen as a proof of the causal significance of hyperglycemia [8].

9.2.5 *Classification and clinical symptoms of the forms of diabetic neuropathy*

The different clinical pictures have led to a classification of diabetic polyneuropathy in which both clinical and sub-clinical criteria exhibit influence. From the practical point of view, divisions according to clinical picture are advantageous:

1. Autonomic diabetic polyneuropathy
2. Distal, symmetric, sensorimotor polyneuropathy
3. Focal neuropathy.

These differentiations include the possibility that the forms may be combined with one another.

9.2.5.1 *The autonomic vegetative polyneuropathy*

Due to its great importance from a pathophysiological point of view, this neuropathy form should be given significant attention. Irreversible damage to the autonomous nervous system have frequently occurred before symptoms of the peripheral neuropathy appear and are detected. Particularly alarming is the evidence of an extremely elevated mortality in diabetics with autonomic polyneuropathy. For example, Ewing [4] found a 50% mortality 2 years after a diagnosis of an autonomic neuropathy. Hasslacher [5] also found a one to threefold increased mortality for diabetics with autonomic neuropathy compared to those without. Important connections obviously exist for autonomic neuropathy to the other so-called late complications of diabetes mellitus. The question arises regarding the causal relationship of neuropathy, nephropathy and retinopathy. The influence of the nerve disorder on the microcirculation of the affected organs must be viewed as a possible progression factor [6].

The vegetative nervous system, with its omnipresent distribution in the organism, makes its presence known through a large number of possible deficiency symptoms in the various organ systems. For practical purposes, these can be divided into visceral and peripheral disorders.

Polyneuropathy-related disorders of the cardiovascular system

Clinical

Orthostatic dysregulation with an, in part, significant drop in blood pressure level is an expression of a disorder of the sympathetic nervous system. Through the variations in blood pressure, especially through the orthostatic effect, hypertension can possibly be overlooked. In diabetics with autonomic vegetative neuropathy, the physiological nocturnal drop in blood pressure is often lacking, which results in an elevated average daily pressure. This symptom is now accessible due to the capability for 24-hour blood pressure measurement with pulse control. A resting tachycardia with a heart rate of up to 90/min is already an obvious sign of a cardiac, parasympathetic related neuropathy. In differential diagnosis, a tachycardia must be considered as a possible consequence of a comedication with nifedipine, prazosin or other pharmaceuticals. This disorder can be verified by the subsequent rigidity of the heart rate, e.g., the lack of the respiratory variability present in healthy individuals.

Special diagnostics

In principle, orienting parameters can be achieved through simple investigations. The respiratory-related heart rate variability can be documented with deep in- and exhalation in five second intervals with a simultaneous ECG monitoring. A heart rate change of less than 10/minute leads to suspicion of a cardiac autonomic neuropathy. In combination with the Valsalva Pressure Test (the mercury column of the blood pressure meter is pressed to 40 mm Hg for five seconds via a mouthpiece) the diagnosis of damage to the parasympathetic nervous system can be established though proof of the lack of a heart rate decrease. The evaluation of the ECG graphs taken can be performed according to the following schematic:

Quotient	$\frac{\text{shortest R-R interval in the ECG}}{\text{longest R-R interval in the ECG}}$
Normal range	over 1.21
Borderline range	1.11 – 1.20
Pathological	under 1.10

This is supplemented by the measurement of the QT interval in the ECG. In cases of an autonomic cardiac neuropathy, it is lengthened, which can explain the increased risk of sudden cardiac death. Here, the significance of the damages to the cardiac, visceral pain sensation should be pointed out. Low-pain or painless heart attacks are the consequence. The orthostatic reaction can be measured with the commonly-used Schellong test.

With computer-aided investigation methods for measuring heart rate changes during rest, with forced breathing, during the Valsalva Pressure Test and with the Ewing test, the symptoms can be very well-documented, such as are illustrated by the examination results put together with the "ProSciCard" system (figs. 1 and 2).

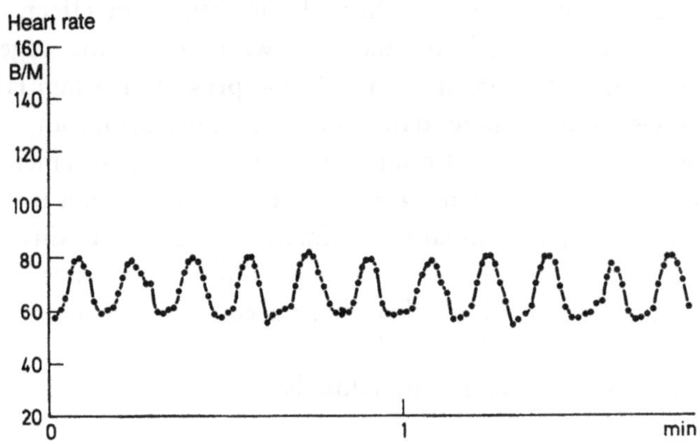

Fig. 1: Heart rate variation during forced breathing in a patient without parasympathetic nervous system damage, normal findings, R-R variation coefficient of 12.4%; 55-year old type II male diabetic, HbA_{1C} 7.1%, (ProSciCard, original).

Along with hypertension manifestation, the 24-hour blood pressure and pulse measurement can be used to clearly identify noctural hypertension, such as illustrated by the examination examples produced with the "SpaceLabs"system (figs. 3 and 4). In the future, such specialized examinations will also be very helpful in tracing this neuropathy form in the daily practice.

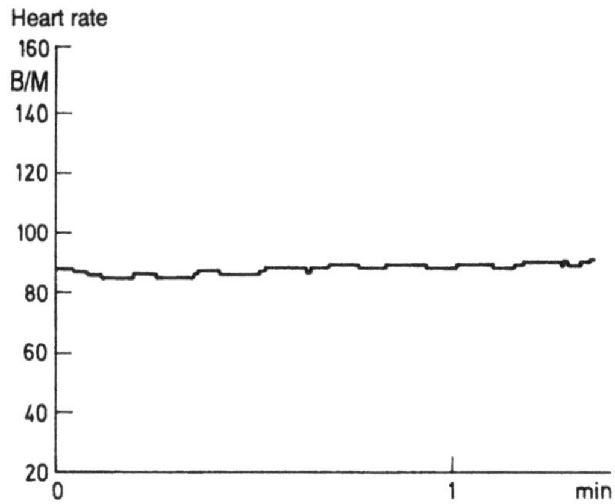

Fig. 2: Heart rate rigidity during forced breathing in a patient with a pronounced cardia autonomic neuropathy, R-R variation coefficient of 1.66%; 43-year old type II male diabetic, HbA_{1C} 9.5% (ProSciCard, original).

Polyneuropathy-related disorders of the gastrointestinal tract

Clinical

In the esophagus, stomach, intestine and gall bladder, neuropathy makes its presence known in particular through motility disturbances. Clinical symptoms have been described particularly for type I diabetics. They appear in advanced

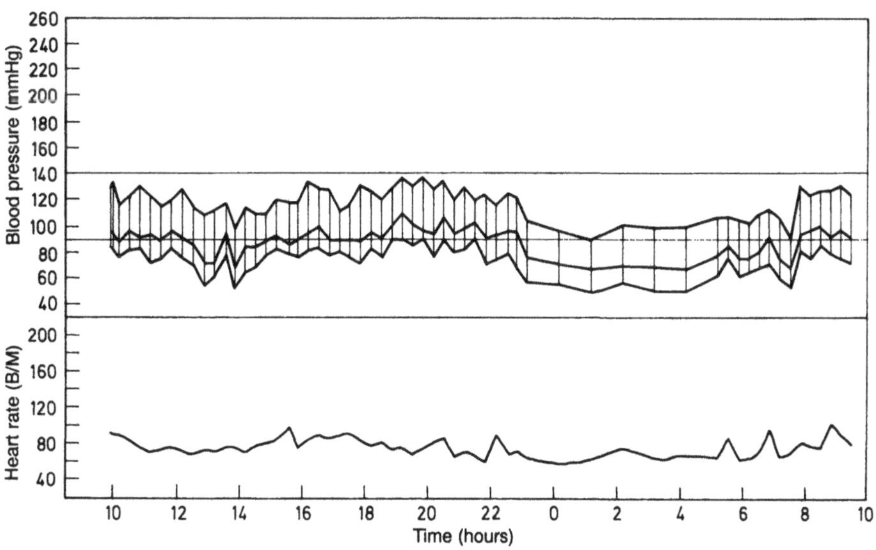

Fig. 3: 24-hour blood pressure profile in a patient without indication of sympathetic nervous system damage, normotension and nocturnal blood pressure drop are physiologically present 52-year old type II female diabetic, HbA_{1C} 7.5% (SpaceLabs, original).

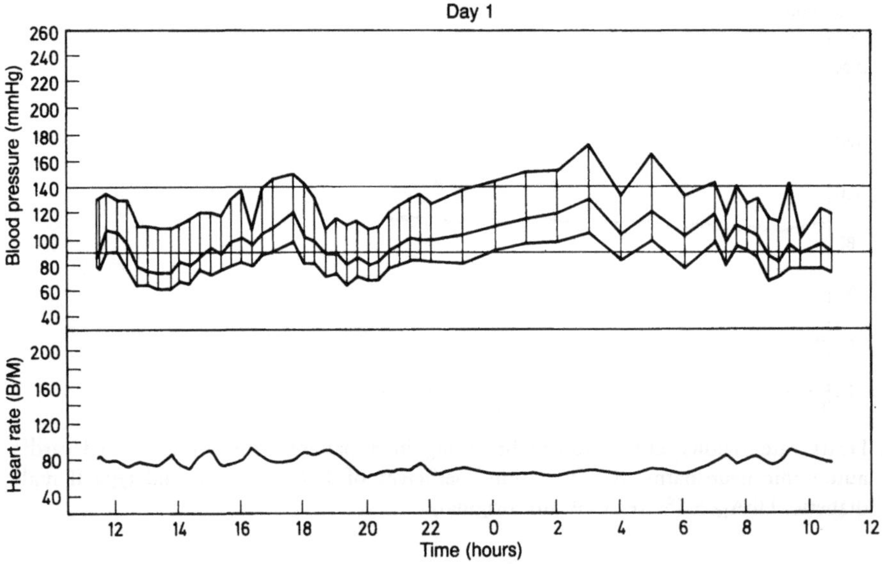

Fig. 4: 24-hour blood pressure profile in a diabetic with pronounced nocturnal hypertension, 57-year old type II male diabetic, HbA_{1C} 9.3% (SpaceLabs, original).

polyneuropathy. Significant delays in the stomach emptying with subsequent absorption disorders can cause significant problems in the dietary and insulin treatment. Particularly torturous for patients are the disorders of intestinal motility. The constipation of the colon seen in up to 20% of all diabetics presents the lesser problem. Watery diarrhea, as a result of an autonomic neuropathy of the small intestine is unfortunately not uncommon. Here, germ ascensions in the intestine and bacterial dysenteries occur, which result in additional therapeutic problems. Innervation disorders of the anal sphincter can lead to incontinence. Disturbances in gall bladder emptying, which can be sonographically detected, are of minor clinical importance according to today's knowledge, but are attributed co-responsibility for the frequent occurrence of gall stones in diabetics.

Special diagnostics

Motility disorders of the esophagus and stomach can be detected through cineradiography. Next to radiological and nuclearmedical methods, the less inconvenient ultrasound-supported observation of stomach emptying after fluid intake has been recently frequently practiced according to the respective experience of the investigators. Here, however, divergent results are not infrequent. Thus there may be examination days where the disorder is more pronounced and others where it is less so. The investigation method with the greatest descriptive power appears to be the stomach intestinal passage with standard porridge marked with 99m technetium.

Polyneuropathy-related disorders of the urogenital system

Clinical

Detrusory weakness must be seen as an important consequence of nerve damage, and contributes to development of atonic bladder with urine volumes of frequently not more than 500 ml. Urinary frequency, stress incontinence and residual urines over 50 ml are importance signs of a diabetic cystopathy and indicate a further complication, the possible development of a chronic urinary tract infection.

Disorders of sexual function are often overlooked in the case history. An important symptom is erectile impotence with unimpaired libido. Orgasm abnormalities have also been described. Here, with a normal orgasm, normal ejaculation may be lacking. This results in retrograde ejaculation into the bladder. Innervation disorders of the suprarenal gland with disorders of cortisol secretion have particular significance for type I diabetes.

Special diagnostics

Retrograde ejaculation can be detected through sperm traces in the catheterized urine. The residual urine volume can be easily evaluated with sonography.

Peripheral disorders of the autonomic nervous system

The syndrome of the diabetic foot is also a consequence of the diabetic autonomic polyneuropathy. The first symptom here is foot instep edema. Due to its prominent clinical importance, the appropriate chapter should be referred to.

Additionally important is a disorder in sweat and sebaceous gland excretion. Next to the typical dry skin, pronounced sweat abnormalities occur on the trunk. Patients thus often find themselves with night sweats. These symptoms are more common in type I diabetes than in type II diabetes.

9.2.5.2 *The distal symmetric, sensorimotor polyneuropathy*

Here we are dealing with a classical form of the disease group. It is the most common form, because it is clinically relatively simple to diagnose. The first symptoms are pruritus, dysthesia and paresthesia in the lower extremities. In the further course of the disease, typical neuropathic pains may occur, making their presence known to the patient especially at night. As soon as the patient rests, these complaints begin at different elevations on the legs. It is often difficult for those affected to keep the legs still, e.g., to leave them under the blankets. They feel a relief with movement, also with nocturnal walking about. Due to this symptomatic, the terms

"burning feet" and *"restless feet"*

have emerged as very apt for clinical description. The complaints described can also lag weeks and months behind rapidly advancing forms of polyneuropathy and overlap by the time of the examination due to the accompanying loss of sensitivity.
The diagnosis is supported by case history information and by clinical findings:

- affects chiefly the lower extremities, arms are very infrequently involved
- primarily loss or decrease in the Achilles tendon reflex, but also in the patellar tendon reflex and in the radial reflex
- sensory deficiencies, ascending up from the feet, in which the deep sensitivity of the leg musculature is also particularly affected
- pathologically reduced sensitivity to vibration
- often severely disturbed warm-cold sensation up to analgesia.

The *tuning fork test* representative for the *sensation of vibration* is a subjective examination method. It is suited to orienting examinations and to observations of disease process. It is simple to conduct and can be recommended as a reliable diagnostic tool. In order to insure that the patient can feel the vibrations of the tuning fork, it is recommended that a reference examination point with high sensitivity, e.g., in the shoulder area, be tested at the beginning of the examination. On the leg, different levels are examined, toes, mid-foot, the inner and outer malleoli, lower leg in side comparisons. It is important to observe strict points of examination, so that the individual examinations are comparable with one another. One must also take the learning curve of the patient into account. The vibrational intensity of the tuning fork ($f = 128/s$) can be read in 8/8. The sensitivity decreases distally and with age. Taking subjectivity into account, the following lower limits can be used for orientation [3]:

Examination of the inner ankle

Lower limit norm up to an age of 40: 6/8
Lower limit norm over the age of 40: 4/8

The results obtained with a tuning fork are dependent on many influencing factors. The cooperation of the patient is of critical importance. The method is clearly not suited to a systematic examination, but is suited to an orienting examination. The methodologically more exact vibratometry is cannot be performed at bedside without a great deal of inconvenience, but is, however, imperative for systematic data gathering.

Simple sensation tests can complement the examination:

- Localization of the point of stimulation
- Sharp/dull differentiation
- Warm/cold differentiation (a temperature difference of 10 degrees should still be recognizable)

- Stimulus discrimination with a pricking circle (the points of stimulation are normally recognized as two stimulations if they are separated by 3 – 5 mm on the fingertips and by 30 – 40 mm on the insteps)
- Examination of the motor and sensory velocity of nerve conduction
- The search for motor pareses
- Walking disorders and frequent falls occur occasionally as symptoms of the loss of deep sensitivity.

The bilateral distal-sensory, sensorimotory polyneuropathy occurs in both type I and type II diabetes. It is rather difficult to characterize in the clinical progression and in the prognosis. Healing is infrequent. In poorly controlled diabetes, the manifestation does not infrequently show a rapid progression. In general, with the optimization of the diabetes therapy, there occur partial remissions with persisting neuropathic complaints, complaints which, however, often improve to a convincing degree for the patient. The total reversal of symptoms is the exception.

9.2.5.3 *Focal neuropathies*

Only in type II diabetics do disorders of the various individual nerves occur, which, in general, are followed by motor paralysis. The duration and severity of the metabolic imbalances seem to be of limited importance to the manifestation. Here, the accumulation of additional diseases is conspicuous. The so-called amyotrophic, asymmetric, proximal polyneuropathic attacks the torso musculature in particular. The results are paralyses of the mm. quadriceps and psoas, with, for example, retained patellar tendon reflex. Other muscles can also be affected, such as the on the shoulder girdle (m. deltoidens). As a rule, atrophies are conspicuous. A 25% portion of all neuropathies is attributed to the focal forms. The changing picture of the paralysis in the course of the disease is characteristic for this nerve damage.

Though cranial nerves (III, IV, VI, VII) are affected as well, it is principally the ocular muscle nerves which are affected. Ophthalmoplegia takes acute effect and shows a one-sided asymmetric attack. The paralysis are cloaked by significant periorbital facial pain. Facialis pareses occur more frequently in diabetics than in persons with normal metabolisms. In addition, carpal tunnel syndrome is more common, as well as peroneus paralysis as a result of pressure damage. Infrequently, the intercostal nerves and the phrenic nerve can also be affected. These nerve lesions have a good prognosis, much better than the sensorimotor form. Rapid remissions do occur, with an only very slight tendency toward defective healing.

9.2.6 *Differential diagnosis of diabetic polyneuropathy*

Diabetes mellitus and toxic alcohol effects cause two thirds of all polyneuropathies. It should be noted that with the presence of both noxae, the course of the disease can take a severe course. Representatively named from the long list of the remaining causes are:

- Uremia
- Folic acid and vitamin B12 deficiency
- Hypothyroidism and other endocrinopathies
- Porphyria
- Heavy metal poisoning
- Vasculitis
- Paraneoplasia
- Parainfectious genesis.

9.2.7 *The therapy of diabetic polyneuropathy*

An optimal metabolic control with normoglycemia is the most important means of influencing diabetic polyneuropathies. It is important to remember that a reversal of the symptoms is only possible as long as the damage has not reached the point where the nerve cells have lost the ability to regenerate ("the point of no return"). The therapy prospects are thus to be viewed as being from without effect to the full reversal of the complaints, but in any event in terms of the prevention of the progression of the changes. This leads to the obligatory conclusion that the therapy of diabetic polyneuropathy should be initiated as early as possible. The measures for optimizing metabolism can be accompanied by drug therapy, and differ with respect to type and staging of diabetic neuropathy.

1. In general, severe forms of neuropathy can only be influenced and their progression halted with sufficient metabolic control, such as, for example, with an intensified insulin treatment. Recently, the use of insulin pumps has been recommended for the optimization of metabolism in complicated cases.
2. As a naturally occurring substance, alpha-liponic acid acts on the energy metabolism of nerve cells through an elimination of the glycolysis blockade and reduction in ketogenesis. Convincing improvements in the symptoms, especially a mellowing of nocturnal pains and a return of sensitivity, have been seen from high-dosage parenteral administration of the substance. The effects on the autonomic vegetative polyneuropathy is currently being intensively investigated. The efficacy of an unaccompanied oral therapy is still disputed.
3. Bentofiamin, as a lipophilic vitamin B1, is reported to be better able to penetrate the lipophilic nerve membrane. It is said to be orally effective. In

order to assure the effectiveness of the substance, further placebo-controlled studies will be required.

4. A general vitamin B deficiency is not uncommon in older patients, so that a vitamin B therapy can show a good clinical result in these cases. A vitamin B deficiency in patients with additional alcohol consumption is common. In contrast, a general vitamin B deficiency among diabetics cannot be assumed [11].
5. If no improvement is attained with intensified insulin therapy (insulin pump) and liponic acid, the use of analgesics and tricyclic antidepressants for the sensorimotor form of neuropathy cannot be avoided. Salicylates are also often effective. Local capsaicine therapy has also proven itself effective.
6. An accompanying physiotherapy is of great benefit.
7. Fludrocortisone has proven beneficial in treating a tendency to orthostasis.
8. The disorders of the gastrointestinal tract are extremely resistant to therapy:
   - Therapy attempts at treating motility disorders with metoclopramide and cisapride.
   - Doxycycline for bacterial dysentery, erythromycin is reported to have additional beneficial effects on motor control.
     Cholestyramine can be tried against diarrhea.
   - Clonidine has not fulfilled the hopes placed in the substance.
   - Occasionally, treatment with opiates and atropine derivatives may be necessary on a symptomatic basis.
9. A consistent infection treatment is to be carried out on the urogenital system. Cave: chronic pyelonephritis through chronic urine retention!
10. For the treatment of disorders of the sexual function, especially of erectile impotence, cavernous body auto injection treatment has to date proven very effective. The therapy should be introduced in centers, because of the fact that an individual dose is necessary in order to prevent an eventual priapism. Mechanical aids have also proven to be successful. The treatment should be conducted in a center.

9.2.8 *Summary*

Through diagnostic and therapeutic efforts, diabetic polyneuropathy has found a central place as an essentially diabetes-associated form of disease. Descriptions of diabetic polyneuropathy are found in every standard work of diabetology. Many investigations are available regarding its pathophysiology, though the final elucidation of the pathogenesis still awaits. Not infrequently, clinically manifest polyneuropathy falls into a subordinate position in the therapeutic efforts, due to its poor symptomatic results. An early diagnosis from the time of the first neuropathic changes is necessary for an improvement of the often still inadequate treatment success. Here, the autonomic diabetic polyneuropathies should be given particular attention. Optimal diabetes control is the most effective prevention as well as the single proven therapeutic principle of improvement in the polyneuropathy and in the prevention of its progression. For the therapy of manifest diabetic polyneuropathies additional medications are available, the effectiveness of which is in part disputed. Successes in the symptomatic therapy give rise to the search for ways to alleviate the complaints. Though often under taboo, erectile impotence can be treated in a therapeutically satisfactoy manner.

The therapy should be conducted from the beginning with the intent of guarding against diabetic polyneuropathies, in order to prevent reaching of the "point of no return".

References

[1] Boulton, A. J. M., J. Drury, B. Clarke et al.: Continuous subcutanous insulin infusion in the management of painful diabetic neuropathy. Diabetes Care 5 (1982) 386–91.

[2] Brown, M. J., J. R. Martin, A. K. Asbury: Painful diabetic neuropathy: a morphometric study. Arch. Neurol. *33* (1976) 164–71.

[3] Claus, D., V. P. Carvalho, B. Neundörfer et al.: Zur Untersuchung des Vibrationsempfindens. Nervenarzt 59 (1988) 138–142.

[4] Ewing, D., J. I. W. Campbell, B. F. Clark: The natural-history of diabetic autonomic neuropathy. Q. J. Med. *49* (1980) 95–108.

[5] Hasslacher, C., G. Bässler: Prognose der kardialen autonomen Neuropathie bei Diabetikern. MMW *125* (1983) 375–377.

[6] Lilja, B., B. Nosslin, B. Bergstrom et al.: Glomerular filtration rate, autonomic nerve function and orthostatic blood pressure in patients with diabetes mellitus. Diabetes Res. *2* (1985) 179–81.

[7] Melton, L. J., P. J. Dyck: Epidemiology. In: P. J. Dyck, P. K. Thomas, A. I. Winegard et al. (eds.): Diabetic Neuropathy, 27–35. WB Saunders, Philadelphia 1987.

[8] Pfeifer, M. A., C. R. Weinberg, D. L. Cook et al.: Autonomic neural dysfunction in recently diagnosed diabetic subjects. Diabetes Care 7 (1984) 447–53.

[9] Pirart, J.: Diabetes mellitus and its degenerative complications: A prospective study of 4,400 patients observed between 1947 and 1973. Diabetes Care *1* (1978) 168–188, 252–263.

[10] Porte, D., R. J. Graf, J. B. Halter et al.:: Diabetic neuropathy and plasma glucose control. Am. J. Med. *70* (1981) 195–200.

[11] Schiffter, R., W. Reuter, K. Borner: Ist Vitamin B1 ein Mittel gegen Neuropathien? Deutsches Ärzteblatt *46* (1979) 3044–3046.

[12] Terkidsen, A. B., N. J. Christensen: Reversible nervous abnormalities in juvenile diabetics with recently diagnosed diabetes. Diabetologia 7 (1971) 113.

9.3 Retinopathy

J. Schulze

Even in the times of modern diabetes therapy, microangiopathic diabetic eye complications remain the leading cause of blindness in the working age population of the industrialized world. The rate of blindness resulting from diabetic retinopathy can be reduced by about 60% with the early use of modern laser photocoagulation. Because high risk retinopathy is not accompanied by visual disturbances in the early stages, where it can be treated, the patients often obtain therapy too late.

9.3.1 *Epidemiology*

At present there are about 3 million symptomatic or known diabetics in Germany. Diabetic retinopathy develops in 50% diabetics after 10 years of disease, and in 80% after 20 years and, if allowed to progress unchecked or insufficiently treated, results in serious eye changes and visual impairment [6], fig. 1 [2].

According to Standl [8] the prevalence of diabetic retinopathy in type II diabetics at the time of diagnosis is 10%. In the DIS, more than 4% of purely diet-controlled NIDDM patients were found to exhibit the early exudative and occlusive stages of so-called "background" retinopathy, at the time of the

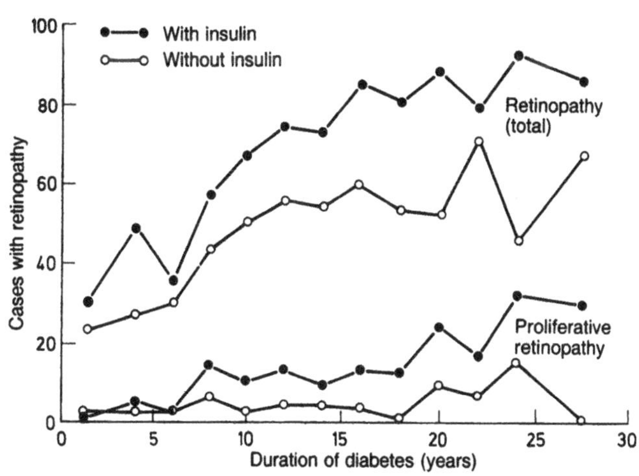

Fig. 1: Frequency of retinopathy, as dependent on the duration of diabetes (diabetes diagnosis as of 30 years of age) [2].

diagnosis [3]. It can not go unmentioned however, that by means of fluorescence angiography initial preretinopathies were observed in over 40%, i. e. 10-fold more often. Hypertensive and atherosclerotic retinal changes, which were found in 33% of the DIS diabetics between the ages of 30 – 55, are further expressions of the "vascular strain". It was possible to show in this intervention study that the long-term treatment of associated risk factors leads to a slowing of the progression of microangiopathic eye background changes. The avoidance, early detection and treatment has therefore moved more and more into the realm of physicians, self-help groups and health officials working in the field of diabetes.

The WHO group set a realistic goal in the St. Vincent Declaration which calls for a 30% (or more) reduction in the rate of blindness by 1995 by means of regular eye examinations [5]. The classification of diabetic retinopathy into stages is a prerequisite for establishing adequate therapeutic measures and follow up evaluation.

9.3.2 Diagnosis, clinical picture and stages of diabetic retinopathy

The phenomenology of diabetic retinopathy is multifaceted, varying and characterized by phases of progression and regression or the persistance of microangiopathy in the background of the eye. From the many proposals for a classification of the stages of diabetic retinopathy, a division into two, based on morphological and therapeutic criteria, has proven itself best suited:

1. The non-proliferative diabetic retinopathy (known as background retinopathy) (fig. 2)
2. The proliferative diabetic vitreoretinopathy (fig. 3)

ad 1.: An eye examination should follow soon after the diagnosis of diabetes mellitus, because typical signs of diabetic background retinopathy such as microaneurysms, discrete hemorrhagic foci, exudates, vascular obliteration or ischaemic retinal edema may have developed in the long period of latency of the diabetic metabolism until clinical manifestation.

It is not uncommon for the ophthalmologist to refer patients with such pathognomonic findings to the internist. On the other hand, there are some discrete early changes on the diabetic fundus that can only be detected with the aid of fluorescence angiography. Following the injection of fluorescein, it is possible to perform retinal angiograms, in which pre-retinopathic changes can be detected, long before this is possible clinically-ophthalmoscopically (figs. 4a, 4b).

In cases of diabetic metabolic disorder, regular eye examinations are required in 6-month to 1-year intervals even in the early stages of fundus changes, so as to not miss the time for photo coagulation therapy. It is often difficult to convince patients of such check ups and treatment, because despite obvious vascular changes there is no disturbance of the vision.

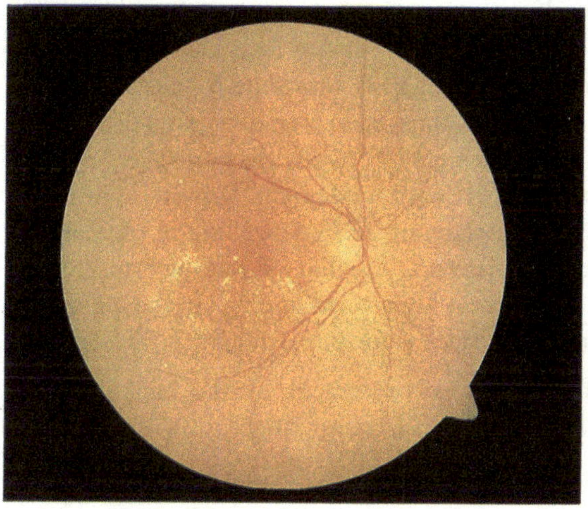

Fig. 2: Diabetic fundus retinopathy (Background)

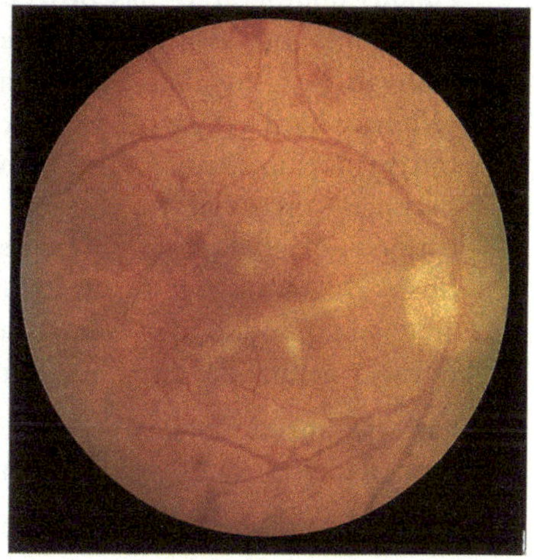

Fig. 3: Proliferative diabetic retinopathy

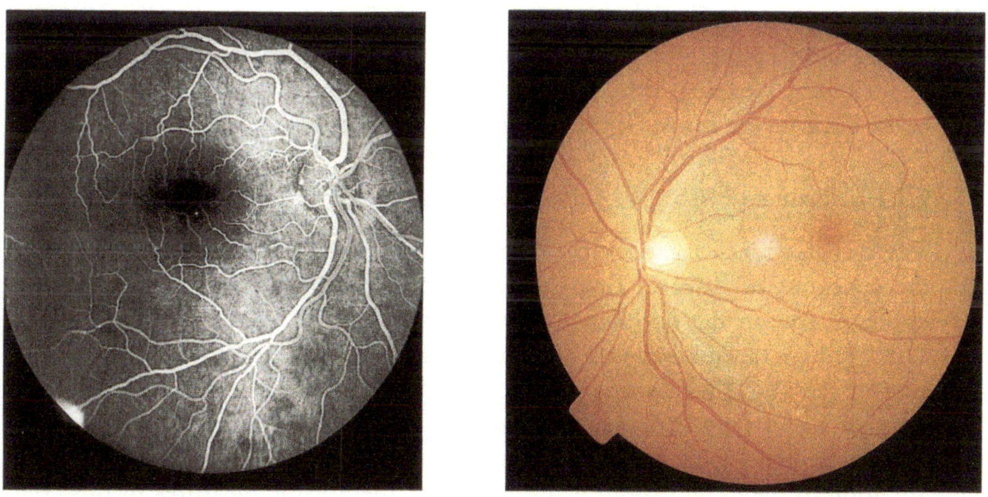

Fig. 4: (a, left) First manifestation of a diabetic angiopathy as determined by fluorescent angiography, which is not detectable ophthalmoscopically (b, right).

Fundus photography has proven itself important in our opinion, for objective documentation, assessment of the course and, last but not least, for the patient motivation. Other important retinal findings such as intraretinal exudate (syn. yellow or hard exudates), as an expression of sometimes reversible lipoid deposits, can be documented. A distinction must be made between these and the more fleeting "soft exudates", which also occur with malignant hypertension, or cottonwool exudates as an expression of ischaemia related swelling of the nerve fibers. Dilatation and tortuosity of the retinal veins, capillary shrinking (avascular area) and in some cases even macular disorders are typical findings in the diabetic retina, whereby the latter are accompanied by obvious impairments in the vision.

The therapeutic objective is to hinder the advancement of the background retinopathy to the dangerous proliferative diabetic retinopathy.

ad 2.: The proliferative diabetic vitreoretinopathy is characterized by the irregular vascular growth from the retinal level into the back vitreous body layer. This neovascularization of pathologically changed retinal vessels can lead to vitreous body hemorrhages on the one hand and tractive retinal detachment on the other as a result of shrinking or scarring processes. The "extracellular modification factors", meaning vascular growth induced chronic retinal ischaemia, which cause an angiogenic or proliferating stimulation, are discussed nowadays. The clinical pictures, which can range from marginally impaired vision to blindness also correspond to the multifaceted pathologic-anatomic processes – with and without traction, bleeding, proliferation and destruction of the retina and vitreous body. Such severe forms of the disease play a secondary role in type II diabetes.

9.3.3 *Course and therapy of the diabetic retinopathy*

The diabetes type, duration, the degree of metabolic compensation (HbA_1) and the concomitant diseases (hypertension, obesity and smoking habits) play an impotant role in the development, course and severity of diabetic retinopathy. With well-controlled diabetes, measured using HbA_{1c}-values $< 7.5\%$, and exclusion of the above-mentioned risk factors, the incidence of diabetic retinopathy for type I and type II diabetics could be significantly reduced [1, 4]. With the increasing life expectancy of diabetics, it becomes necessary to pay careful attention to the early diagnosis and adequate therapeutic measures of this complication.

9.3.3.1 *Basic therapy*

An optimization of the metabolic syndrome in accordance to the Euro-Norms (see Chapter 7) (normalization of blood glucose, lipids, body weight, blood pressure $< 140/90$) and strict avoidance of nicotine, alcohol and sodium chloride abuse are the primary targets of treating micro- and macroangiopathy. It is possible to favorably influence the development of the non-proliferative retinopathy with these basic measures, whereby the influence of these on proliferative retinopathy appears to be considerably less. The textbook explanation still holds for this situation, if the oral therapy does not satisfactorily adjust the diabetic, and vascular changes are present, insulin must be applied. To realize the optimal therapeutic concept requires the close cooperation of the general practitioner, diabetes consultants and ophthalmologists.

9.3.3.2 Drug therapy

The use of medication to influence the non-proliferative retinopathy with vascular permeability-inhibiting drugs like calcium, vitamin C, rutin and hemostatics have not succeeded. No definite therapeutic effect could be proven for either these preparations or for calcium dobesilate, anticoagulants, vasodilatators, dextrans, prostaglandin inhibitors or aldose-reductase inhibitors. The need for an effective drug therapy for diabetic retinopathy is great. The profile of action for the ACE-inhibitor group appears to offer a new, hopeful approach.
Heroic procedures such as adrenal and hypophysectomies have been abandoned due to doubts about the effectiveness and hormonal consequences.

9.3.3.3 Focal and panretinal laser therapy

Therefore an effective therapy is even sought for the finding of widespread non-proliferative retinopathy, which can be accompanied by pathologically changed retinal vessels, hemorrhages, edema or lipid deposits. This can serve as a relative indication for focal laser application, depending on the location and severity of the findings [7].

An absolute indication for photocoagulation in the slightest indication of change from non-proliferative to proliferative fundoscopic changes. By means of fluorescence angiography and photodocumentation, it is now possible to obtain a standstill or regression of proliferative vascular growth by means of panretinal laser coagulation, if this is performed soon enough.

9.3.4 Summary

Advanced retinopathies are still the most frequent cause of blindness in industrialized countries. The avoidance, early detection and complex treatment of the basic disease and local manifestation on the background of the eye have taken the interest of physicians working in the field of diabetes, self-help groups and health authorities. Diabetics should undergo eye examinations every 6 months to 1 year, maintain normal blood pressure and eumetabolization, and the progression from background retinopathy into dangerous proliferative diabetic retinopathy should be avoided.

Because all of the alternative therapeutic procedures and particularly the variety of drug treatments have not shown any definite effect on the progression of the diabetic retinopathy, the exploitation of internistic therapy and the use of light and laser coagulation are of utmost importance for the maintenance of eye sight in diabetics.

References

[1] Chase, H. P., W. E. Jackson, S. L. Hoops et al.: Glucose control and the renal and retinal complications of insulin-dependent diabetes. JAMA *261* (1989) 1155 – 1160.

[2] Klein, R., B. E. K. Klein, S. E. Moss et al.: Wisconsin Epidemiologic, Study of Diabetic Retinopathy when age at diagnosis is 30 or more years. Arch. Ophthalmol. *102* (1984) 527 – 532.

[3] Klein, R., E. M. Beer et al.: Epidemiologie, Klinik und Verlaufskontrolle der diabetischen Retinopathie bei Diabetes mellitus Typ-II. Klin. Mbl. Augenheilk. *189* (1986) 374 – 375.

[4] Klein, R., B. E. Klein, S. E. Moss et al.: Glycosylated haemoglobin predicts the incidence and progression of diabetic retinopathy. JAMA *260* (1988) 2864 – 2871.

[5] Krans, H. M. I., M. Porta, H. Keen: Diabetes care and research in Europe: the St. Vincent Declaration action programme. Giornale Italiano di Diabetologia *12* (suppl. 2) (1992) 2 – 44.

[6] Kroll, P., P. Berg: Diabetische Retinopathie und ihre Behandlung. Dt. Ärztebl. *88* (1991) 1147 – 1154.

[7] Lucke, K., H. Laqua: Die stadiengerechte Behandlung der diabetischen Retinopathie. Internist *31* (1990) 236 – 242.

[8] Standl, E.: Diabetische Retinopathien – internistische Aspekte. Verh. Dtsch. Ges. Inn. Med. *93* (1987) 195 – 201.

9.4 Nephropathy

J. Schulze

Renal complications are common in diabetics, whereby the knowledge about kidney diseases in type II diabetes is considerably less than with type I diabetics.

Definition: In diabetic nephropathy there are various combinations of glomerulosclerosis, athero-/arteriolosclerosis, pyelonephritis with papillary necrosis. An early subtle diagnosis has in recent years brought improved therapeutic and prognostic results.

9.4.1 *Epidemiology*

In comparison to IDDM, the development and prevalence of diabetic nephropathy in NIDDM differs greatly, whereby the improvement of the metabolic regulation and an optimal blood pressure control have led to reduction of the incidence of nephropathy. The prevalence of clinically manifest proteinuria with NIDDM fluctuates in various studies of between 3–16% [2, 4], for microalbuminuria 15–55% have been reported [5, 8]. With NIDDM, the time from clinical diagnosis to the proof of nephropathy is shorter than with IDDM, because there are often several years between manifestation of diabetes and diagnosis.

9.4.2 *Diagnosis*

The leading biochemical symptom of diabetic nephropathy is the persistent albuminuria, which as a rule is accompanied by decreasing glomerular filtration rate and increasing blood pressure (tab. 1), [6].

A urine protein excretion of > 0.5 g per day on at least two consecutive collection days in diabetics without coronary insufficiency or other renal diseases indicates a dangerously persistent proteinuria, which unfortunately indicates the irreversible stage of the renal insufficiency. This stage is preceded by long phases of the beginning diabetic nephropathy, which can be diagnosed by the detection of microalbuminuria (30–300 mg per day or 20–200 μg/min) by means of sensitive analysis (e.g. radioimmunoassay) (fig. 1), [1]. Urine albumin excretion of about 300 mg per day or 200 μg/min can be clearly determined by means of the albumin strip test.

For the prognostic value of a constant proteinuria, the patients may not present with any deranged metabolic conditions, because these cause an increase of the albumin excretion rate per se. Physical stress, hypertension, cardiac decompensation, independent of a diabetes-related glomerular disease, can also lead to

Tab. 1: Stages of diabetic nephropathy [6]

Stage	Renal findings	Duration of diabetes (years)	Therapeutic prospects	Albuminuria
I	Renal hypertrophy, hyperfunction	0–2	Reversible	<20 µg/min <30 mg/24 h
II	Glomerular lesions w/o clinical symptoms	>2	Progression can be halted	Microalbuminuria (<30 mg/24 h) only under physical stress
III	Beginning nephropathy	10–15	Possibility for improvement	20–200 µg/min 30-300 mg/24 h
IV	Clinically manifested nephropathy	10–20 (some years after III)	Slight improvement possible	Macroalbuminuria >200 µg/min >300 mg/24 h
V	Renal insufficiency	20–25	Irreversible	Proteinuria (>500 mg/24 h)

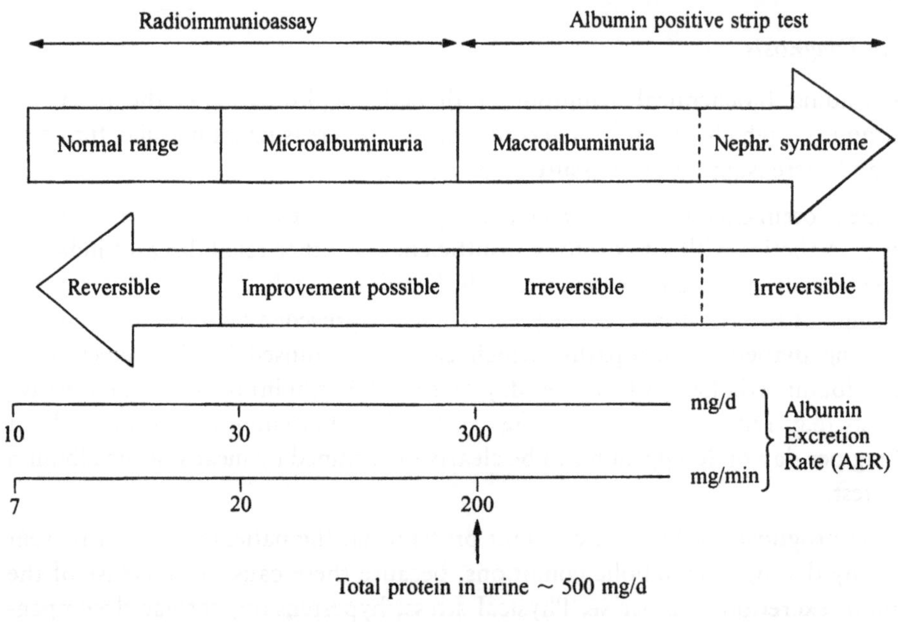

Fig. 1: Threshold values for normo-, micro-, and macroalbuminuria [1].

increased albumin excretion in urine. Other diagnostic measures such as blood pressure monitoring, assessment of the fundus oculi, urine sediments and cultures as well as measurement of the glomerular filtration rates and lipid status are needed for final clarification. A renal sonography offers information about the form and size, infectious consequences, cysts and anomalies. If, as a result of atypical course, a secondary disease, e.g. a glomerulonephritis, is suspected beside the diabetic nephropathy, a kidney biopsy should be considered with a nephrologist. Mogensen [5] lists the following as indications for a renal biopsy:

- nephropathy without retinopathy
- rapid deterioration of the renal function
- decrease in renal function without previous proteinuria.

9.4.3 *Clinical course*

Parallel to the functional renal changes with microalbuminuria and glomerular hyperfiltration, there is increased renal bloodflow and hypertrophy of the kidneys. In the early stage these changes are basically reversible, they can however, be the prestage for the later development of a clinical nephropathy. In such cases, the genetic disposition, male sex, and quality of the diabetes and blood pressure control determine the course. The developing capillaropathy at the glomerula is not only accompanied by an albuminuria, but is also the expression of a generalizing vasopathy on the microvascular system.

Other abnormalities in patients with persistant albuminuria are increasing blood pressure and metabolic disorders with increasing LDL cholesterol, triglycerides and fibrinogen and reduction of HDL cholesterol. This atherogenic constellation leads to a 10-fold increase of cardiovascular mortality in comparison to patients without proteinuria [7]. The incidence of proliferative retinopathy is also increased many fold. The causes of death of type II diabetics with nephropathy are myocardial infarction, cardiac failure and cerebrovascular accident, and renal complications such as renal failure or uremia are only secondary [3].

One of the most frequently occurring infectious renal complications, particularly in diabetic women, is in the form of the ascending urinary tract infections. Cystitis with ascending pyelonephritis is diagnosed much more frequently in diabetics than in non-diabetics. If the diabetes was not diagnosed early enough and inadequate antibiotic treatment was given, there is a tendency to chronicity and complications. Perinephritic abscesses, papillary necrosis and "creeping" renal insufficiency are particularly feared.

9.4.4 *Prevention and therapy*

Because there are still no methods to determine which individuals are at risk for nephropathy before the occurrence of microalbuminuria, early and repeated controls of these parameters and other renal function tests are necessary (see sec.

Tab. 2: Diagnosis and therapeutic proposals in diabetic nephropathy (modified according to [9])

	Follow up controls	Therapy
Stage *micro*albuminuria	– Blood pressure (all 3 months)	– Blood pressure control
	– Glycemic controls (BG, HbA_1, fructosamine)	– Metabolic optimization
	– Proteinuria detection (protein, albumin, ß2-microglobulin)	– Moderate protein restriction
	– Laboratory: creatinine, electrolytes, uric acid, electrophoresis, urine sediment or cultures, coagulation analysis)	– Adequate substitution with disturbed homoiostasis
	– Paraclinic: renal sonography, ECG	
	– Control of cardiovascular risks (lipids, smoking, sodium chloride)	– Correction of risk factors
In addition to the above-mentioned measures		
Stage *macro*albuminuria	– Glomerular filtration rate (GFR) – Creatinine clearance (6 – 12 months)	– Strict protein restriction
	– ECG-blood pressure monitoring (annually) – Cardiac and renal sonography (annually) – Autonomic nerve function tests – Uroflow measurement; residual urine – Ophthalmoscopy with fundus photography	– Differentiated treatment of diabetes and its complications in team!

6.2). The early detection and treatment of pyelonephritis also plays an important role. Euglycemic metabolic control with HbA_{1c} values of 6 – 7% are the goal. Type II diabetics have to receive insulin – if necessary – and be instructed in blood glucose self-monitoring.

The diet should be rich in carbohydrates which do not easily breakdown and take into account a protein limitation to 45 g/d as early as the detection of a microproteinuria and/or compensated retention. Previously propagated sharp sodium chloride restrictions are only relevant for hypertension which is difficult to compensate.

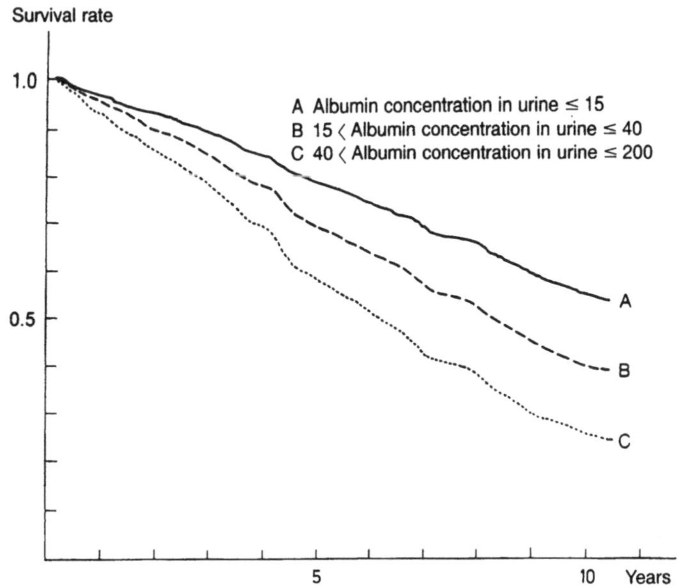

Fig. 2: Mortality in NIDDM patients (n= 503) with different albumin concentrations in morning urine (μg/ml) at the first examination [5].

With increased blood pressure, stricter dietary and drug therapy to obtain normotension are necessary. In principle, in cases of nephropathy, the same limits apply as with type I diabetes. The risk factor albuminuria/proteinuria has to be seen in context with the remaining life expectancy and possible side effects of a rigorous decrease in the blood pressure. Carbohydrate-metabolism neutral and "lipid-friendly" antihypertensives are highly recommended (see sec. 8.1). The treatment of hyper- and dyslipoproteinemias should first be dietary – if necessary drug-assisted – whereby the doses should be reduced with renal function impairment so as to avoid accumulation.

The improvement of diabetic care has led to a reduction in the incidence of diabetic nephropathy of 30%. Only early detection, frequent control and complex intervention can maintain or even improve this prognosis (tab. 2).

9.4.5 *Summary*

A 3–16% prevalence of nephropathy is expected with type II diabetics. The leading symptom of diabetic nephropathy is a constant albuminuria of > 300 mg/d, which is accompanied by a drop in the glomerular filtration rate (GFR) and an increase in the blood pressure. This manifest stage of nephropathy is often preceded by many years of a beginning nephropathy with a microalbuminuria of 30–300 mg/d which can only be diagnosed with sensitive methods, e.g.

radioimmunoassay. If the urine albumin excretion is detectable with albumin-sensitive test strips, there is already a macroalbuminuria with decreasing GFR.

The albuminuria in diabetic nephropathy results from the destruction of glomeruli and is generally accompanied with increased incidence of diabetic retinopathy. Type II diabetics with nephropathy have a manifold increase in cardiovascular mortality. Due to the serious complications, an early evaluation of the indicator proteins and other risk factors is necessary and therefore a proper assessment of the stage and the appropriate treatment possible. It has been shown that microalbuminuria is not only a predecessor of subsequent proteinuria, but a "signum mali ominis" for other complications and early mortality in these patients (fig. 2).

The progression of nephropathy can be stopped or slowed by eumetabolization and aggressive decrease in blood pressure. The cardiovascular mortality decreases in parallel.

References

[1] Deckert, T., A. Grenfell: Epidemiology and natural history of diabetic nephropathy. In: J. C. Pickup, G. Williams (eds.): Textbook of Diabetes, 651–656. Blackwell Scientific Publications, Oxford 1991.

[2] Fabrè, J., L. P. Balant, P. G. Dayer et al.: The Kidney in maturity onset diabetes mellitus: A clinical study of 510 patients. Kidney Int. *21* (1982) 730–738.

[3] Friedmann, E. A.: Diabetes with Kidney failure. Lancet *1* (1986) 1285–1288.

[4] Garancini, P., G. Gallus, G. Calori: Microalbuminuria and its associated risk factors in a representative sample of Italian type II diabetics. J. Diabetic Compl. 2 (1988) 12–15.

[5] Mogensen, C. E.: Microalbuminuria predicts clinical proteinuria and early mortality in maturity onset diabetes. N. Engl. J. Med. *310* (1984) 356–360.

[6] Reinauer, H.: Stadien der diabetischen Nephropathie. Internist *31* (1990) 13 (modified).

[7] Schmitz, A., M. Vaeth: Microalbuminuria: A major risk factor in non-insulin-dependent diabetes. A 10-year follow up study of 503 patients. Diabetic Med. *5* (1988) 126–134.

[8] Standl, E., B. Rebell, H. Stiegler: Prevalence and risk profile of incipient diabetic nephropathy in type 2 (non insulin dependent) diabetes mellitus. Diabetologia *30* (1987) 584 A – 585 A.

[9] Grenfell, A.: Clinical features and management of established diabetic nephropathy. In: J. C. Pickup, G. Williams (eds.): Textbook of Diabetes, 677–697. Blackwell scientific publications, Oxford 1991.

10 Medical-social aspects and legal determinations

Silke Meisel

Diabetes and career choice

Diabetics without complications and who are not being treated with insulin should be able to have the same careers as non-diabetics. Occupations seen to be particularly well-suited to diabetics are those which have a regulated work time and where the possibility of self-monitoring exists at the workplace. These include all business and sales careers, teaching, dental technician work, medical university and trade school careers and precision mechanics.

In contrast to these professions are ones in which, during the performance of duties, the maintenance of the diet is not always possible and the danger of metabolic imbalances seems preprogrammed, such as in the careers of baker, cook and waiter. These careers are therefore not suited to diabetics and cannot be recommended. Work in a shift system is also ill-suited for diabetics.

The greatest limitations to career choice or the continued performance of a job exist for insulin-requiring diabetics, for whom hypoglycemia can result in a danger to themselves or others. For this reason, pilots who evidence a carbohydrate metabolism disorder are denied licences internationally. The fitness of diabetics for the Bundesbahn (German Federal Railway) is evaluated in a more differentiated fashion. For diabetics who can be treated purely dietetically, there are no limitations. All those who are treated with oral hypoglycemics must undergo an industrial medical fitness examination. This is also the case for professional truck drivers and crane operators. Work with a hypoglycemia-related elevated risk of falling (roofers, chimney sweeps) should not be performed by insulin-injecting diabetics, nor should work underground. As insulinized diabetics are, as a rule, not allowed to perform work with weapons – they are released from German military service, they are naturally also not suited to police work, though desk jobs are possible.

Diabetes and drivers' licences

The related regulations have been published in the report "Disease and Driving" by the Joint Council on Transportation Medicine of the Federal Ministry of Transportation and the Federal Ministry for Youth, Family, Women and Health. According to these regulations, diabetics who wish to apply for a driver's licence must provide a medical certificate. This should contain the form of diabetes, including duration and possible frequency of self-monitoring, the therapy and the danger of hypoglycemia.

Differentiations between three risk groups are made on the basis of the risk of hypoglycemia:

Risk group 1: Diabetics with purely dietary treatment
Risk group 2: Diabetics with dietary and oral hypoglycemic treatment – above all sulfonyl ureas
Risk group 3: Diabetics treated with insulin.

Diabetics in risk groups 1 and 2 are allowed to operate all motor vehicles, as long as they have a balanced metabolic state and have been at least three months without hypoglycemia. With the exception of Class 2 vehicles or vehicles used for personnel or public transport, the same applies for risk group 3. In addition, the eye doctor decides on the ability to drive for diabetics with retinopathy.

Diabetic motor vehicle operators are recommended to always bring their diabetes record book with them, above all in order to be able to prove regular medical metabolic monitoring and the frequency of urine and blood glucose self-monitoring.

Diabetics with an unstable metabolic condition and tendency towards hypo- and hyperglycemia are not suited to the operating of motor vehicles. Diabetics, who have been injecting insulin for less than three months, should not drive in this time period.

Diabetes and severe disability

Whether a diabetic is considered legally severely disabled or not depends on the degree of the impairment. The foundation for this is the severe disability law in the version of August 26, 1986 (Federal German Law Statute 1.I pp. 1421 – 1550) with the changes related to the Treaty of German Unification. In the first section of the law, the terms "disability", "severely disabled" and "those of equal status" are defined

Severe Disability Law
First section
Protected category of persons
§ 1 The severely disabled

As used in this law, the severely disabled are those persons with a degree of disability of at least 50, providing they – legally in terms of the range of applicability of this law – have their legal residence, their actual residence or their occupation at a work place in the sense of law 7, paragraph 1.

§ 2 Those of equal status

1) Persons with a degree of disability of less than 50, but at least 30, who meet the additional requirements of § 1, should given a status equal to the severely disabled on the basis of a determination of their application by the Employment Office according to § 4, if, as a result of their disability, they are not able to obtain or retain an appropriate job (as defined in § 7, section 1) without this equal status. The equal status takes effect on the date of the application. It can be limited.
2) For those given equal status, this law is to be applied with the exception of § 47 and the eleventh section.

§ 3 Disability

1) As used in this law, disability is the effect of a non-temporary functional impairment, which is due to an abnormal bodily or psychological condition. An abnormal condition is one which deviates from the typical condition for the respective age group. As non-temporary is considered a time period which lasts more than 6 months. In the case of multiple, mutually-influencing functional impairments, their total combined effect is used for the determination.

2) The effect of the functional impairment is established as a degree of disability (DOD), in increments of ten degrees, from 20 to 100.

3) The appropriate scale established in § 30, section 1 of the Federal German Social Service Law is applied in determining the degree of disability. According to the "Reference points for medical opinions in social compensation law" of November 1983, diabetes mellitus is evaluated as follows:

	Degree of disability
Well-controlled through diet or diet and oral hypoglycemics, without complications	0–10%
Less well-controlled, with large tolerance variations	20%
Controlled with insulin and diet, without complications	30%
Difficult to control with insulin	40%

Organ complications are to additionally evaluated.

The application for recognition as severely disabled is to be filed at the appropriate Social Services Agency. These authorities prepare a certificate with the characteristics of severe disability. The severe disability is retrospectively recognized as beginning at the time of manifestation of the impairment (medical state of affairs). According to § 15 of the Severe Disability law, the severely disabled have a strengthened right of giving notice. In addition, they have a claim to an additional paid vacation of 5 days per calendar year.

Those given equal status enjoy the strengthen right of giving notice, not, however, the additional vacation. Through the determination of the degree of severity, however, it becomes clear that severe disability cannot be recognized for the majority of NIDDM patients.

Diabetes – education and health care

Every physician should always keep in mind how critical a diagnosis of "diabetes mellitus" is for the patient. As a chronic complaint, diabetes influences the future life. Many patients find themselves in a state of denial at the outset, and, following the doubt, in a fight with the diabetes. In the best cases, this results in a conscious living with diabetes. Thus the prognosis for the disease is largely dependent on whether the patient accepts the disease and the lifestyle associated with it or not. The acceptance of the disease is easier the better informed the diabetic is about it. Therefore, the education of diabetics, along with the diet, physical activity and drug therapy, is today seen as an important cornerstone of the treatment. Various training programs have been developed, especially over the past 15 years, where, on the one hand, the emphasis is placed on multi-day hospital training programs (in particular the many universities in the USA, the Diabetes Training Center at the University of Düsseldorf), on the other, a continual training through the general practitioner is favored (e.g., practices in Great Britain and Australia). The truth lies, as it so often does, in the middle, meaning starting training in the hospital and continuing with life-long, effective and well-organized training and motivation by the general practitioner and the specialized out-patient programs. A valuable addition can be made by the self-help groups of the Society of German Diabetics.

The medical training of NIDDM patients in groups was introduced nationwide in Germany for clients of health insurance companies on July 1, 1991, and in part for clients of public health programs. After a preparation seminar, the diabetes training program – NIDDM – is deductible for approved doctors, as long as the permission is requested by the insuree. The main points of the group training (conducted by a team consisting of a doctor, a diabetes nurse and, if possible, a dietician) are the definition of diabetes and symptoms of diabetes mellitus, urine glucose self-monitoring, proper diet and late complications, whereby particular emphasis should be placed on the diabetic foot. The goal is for every non-insulinized type II diabetic to achieve good control through a training program. In these programs, the EBM No. 15 can be billed up to four times for each participant and meeting, the EBM No. 8015 only once.

Diabetes training materials can be obtained from the German Physicians' Press. At present the following training packages are offered:

- Package set for training of 10 patients at DM 9.38 per patient
- Package set for training of 5 patients at DM 11.40 per patient
- Package set for the training of one patient at DM 13.70.

The billing for the training materials takes place through the billing form (insurance form or bank transfer form) with EBM No. 8015 – complete provisions with diabetes training material per patient (DM 12.50) and EBM No. 15 – programmed medical training and supervision of type II diabetics in groups in the practice of the attending physician with a participation of 4 to 10 persons, per participant and meeting (DM 15.00/in the treaty area of eastern Germany for the time being only DM 9.00).

Diabetes and health spas

A visit to a spa is requested by the diabetic through the health insurer or the respective office of Social Security. Here the patient can have some influence on the time and place of the cure. The diabetes cure is considered a rehabilitation measure. Therefore, the necessity of the cure must be medically evaluated by the attending general practitioner or diabetologist.

Diabetics in our society

"Diabetes affects everyone" – under this motto, the first World Diabetes Day was begun on June 27, 1991. The goal was to sensitize the public to the problem of diabetes through an educational program. The sole German event on the day proclaimed by the WHO and IDF was the presentation of the "Diabetes Diagnostic Bus" in Berlin. It was shown that there was a large deficit in public understanding regarding the wide-spread disease diabetes. Therefore, it was decided to declare June 27 as World Diabetes Day on an on-going basis.

Already in 1989 with the St. Vincent Declaration, complaints were made regarding the insufficient care for diabetics and the thereby related health problem with increasing importance in Europe. Demands for the offering of means and solutions in the form of national and international programs were also issued to governments and health authorities. The non-profit German Diabetic Association (GDA) was founded on January 2, 1951. The purpose and goals of the organization lie in the informing and training of diabetics, representing diabetics with regard to officials and authorities, insurance companies etc., teaching the public about the problems faced by diabetics and supporting diabetes research through close cooperative work with diabetologists and dietary consultants under the motto "together we are stronger". In September 1963 doctors working in the field of diabetes joined together to form the German Diabetes Society (GDS), which currently has 1300 members. A close cooperation between the GDA has been a goal from the outset. First with the founding of the German Diabetes Union on September 28, 1990 in Düsseldorf were the GDS, GDA and ADCY (the Association of Diabetic Children and Youth) joined under one umbrella organization.

Authors

Dr. med. habil. Sabine Fischer
Prof. Dr. med. habil. Markolf Hanefeld
Prof. Dr. med. habil. Ulrich Julius
Dr. med. Silke Meisel
Dr. med. Hannes Rietzsch
Prof. Dr. med. habil. Jan Schulze
Dr. med. habil. Matthias Weck
Universitätsklinikum Carl Gustav Carus
der Technischen Universität Dresden
Klinik für Innere Medizin
Abteilung für Stoffwechselkrankheiten und
Endokrinopathien/Fettstoffwechselforschung
Fetscherstraße 74
D-01307 Dresden
Germany

Prof. Dr. med. habil. Hans-Egbert Schröder
Universitätsklinikum Carl Gustav Carus
der Technischen Universität Dresden
Medizinische Klinik III/Medizinische Poliklinik
Fetscherstraße 74
D-01307 Dresden
Germany

Bei Fragen zur Produktsicherheit wenden Sie sich bitte an:
If you have any questions regarding product safety,
please contact:

Walter de Gruyter GmbH
Genthiner Straße 13
10785 Berlin
productsafety@degruyterbrill.com